ASIAN
AMERICAN
HERBALISM

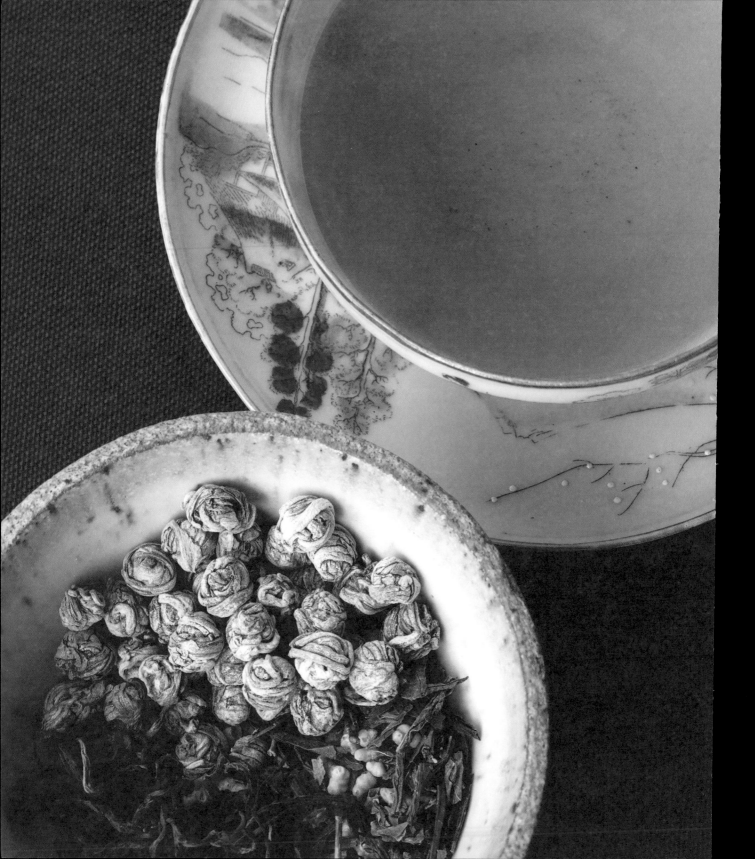

TRADITIONAL AND MODERN
HEALING PRACTICES
FOR EVERYDAY WELLNESS

ASIAN AMERICAN HERBALISM

アジア系アメリカ人ハーバリズム

Erin Masako Wilkins

photography by **Kristen Murakoshi**   *illustrations by* **Ayako Kiener**

PA PRESS

PRINCETON ARCHITECTURAL PRESS · NEW YORK

Dedicated to mama, Gail Yamamoto Seymour

———

For Zoë and Weston

Published by
Princeton Architectural Press
A division of Chronicle Books LLC
70 West 36th Street, New York, NY 10018
www.papress.com

© 2023 Erin Masako Wilkins
All rights reserved.
Printed and bound in China
26 25 24 23 4 3 2 1 First edition

ISBN 978-1-7972-2331-5

Every reasonable attempt has been made to identify
owners of copyright. Errors or omissions will be corrected
in subsequent editions.

Editor: Holly La Due
Designer: Paul Wagner
Stylists: Alysia Andriola, Kristin Bickle

Library of Congress
Cataloging-in-Publication Data
available upon request.

Credits:
p. 12: Photograph by Michelle Westling
p. 15 (bottom): Photograph by Sarah Deragon
p. 18: Photograph by Sarah Deragon

Kombu Shiitake Dashi and Wakame Miso recipes adapted from
Japanese Home Cooking: Simple Meals, Authentic Flavors by
Sonoko Sakai (2019), courtesy of Roost Books

Barley and Greens Congee recipe adapted from *Book of Jook:
Chinese Medicinal Porridges* by Bob Flaws (1995), courtesy of Blue
Poppy Press, Inc.

I don't think that we are original formulators of really anything that has to do with herbs. I think it's something that travels through us; It's part of our ancestors' teaching. If we stand in the right place with our hearts open, our minds ready, oftentimes this information moves through us, in service to be passed out.

So, it's part of that teaching—you just let it flow in, you accept it, you share it, and then you let it flow back out. And it becomes part of that great underground stream that's circling around this world nourishing all of us.

—**Rosemary Gladstar**

CONTENTS

CHAPTER ONE

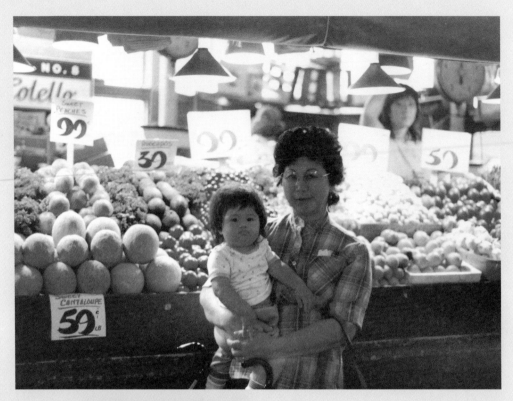

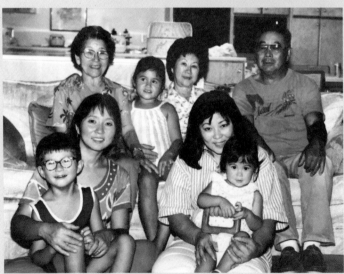

above:
Erin and her grandma Masako,
Sacramento, California, 1983

left:
Four generations of the Kaku-Yamamoto
family, Sacramento, California, 1990

INTRODUCTION

——————

My earliest memories are of my grandma Masako's kitchen. The memory of her hands shaping steaming hot gohan into rice balls. How she would grate gobo and carrots for inari zushi and mix ginger and shoyu in a suribachi. I remember the joy of receiving baskets full of juicy ripe strawberries from her garden. And how she put leftover umeboshi pits into lukewarm chawans of genmaicha green tea.

I know and hold these memories with all my senses. The sounds, scents, rhythms, and feel of these daily moments connect me to my family's traditions. They connect me to myself and reflect the comforting food and wellness traditions that each of us holds across cultures and generations.

Asian American herbalism is rooted in the wellness that we cultivate at home, in the lessons we learn in the kitchen about how to take care of a stuffy nose, ease everyday ailments, and find comfort in difficult times. Herbalism not only offers us remedies to maintain good health but also ways to feel greater ease and balance daily. From the garden and kitchen, Asian American herbalism is rooted in complex, sophisticated healing systems of ancient Asian medicine that predate written history and the scientific method. We know that Asian American herbalism works not because of randomized controlled experiments but because this medicine has been developed and passed down for thousands of years. It is an earth-based medicine that is written in our blood and bones.

Herbalism is one of the ways that our species has learned to thrive from generation to generation—the original form of accessible health care. For those who can't see a doctor for social, economic, and cultural reasons, knowing the remedies in our kitchens, gardens, and community

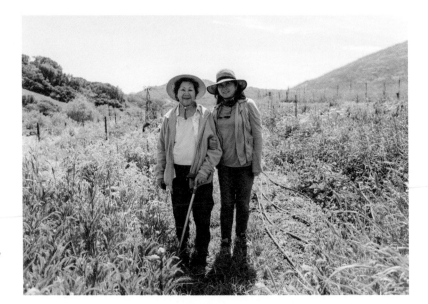

Grandma Masako Yamamoto and mom Gail Yamamoto Seymour at a wellness workshop at Tara Firma Farms, Petaluma, California, 2019

spaces is not only an act of wellness but one of survival and resilience. Unfortunately, the very individuals who need this care most, often don't have access to it.

In my clinical practice, I quickly noticed the disparities in who came in to receive consistent holistic care. The lack of accessibility for Black, Indigenous, and people of color in the community I was serving was alarming and reminded me of my own experience growing up in a working-class family. I know firsthand what it's like not to have the resources or time to seek out private wellness services including herbalism and acupuncture. With this realization and a desire to make Asian American herbalism more accessible, I began developing seasonal wellness workshops in my town. I shared herbalism basics and practical ways to empower others to learn about this medicine. As the classes developed, many folks in the community came together with a genuine interest in learning not only about self-care but also about creating paths for community care. Together, we navigated how our ancestors used herbs and earth-based medicine to heal from illness and create more balance individually and as a community.

From these workshops, I began to teach more in-depth traditional East Asian energetic medicine around themes including Qi, Blood, Yin, Yang, and the energy of illness. My intention was and remains to open up the world of Asian American herbalism and inspire others with the theory, practice, and cultural roots of this work. I found that deepening the cultural content in these workshops drew in a diverse community with people from many cultures, including the Asian diaspora.

At each workshop, someone would ask me which books I recommend for deeper learning and many folks asked specifically for books written by Asian or Asian American authors. I realized that the books I reference are either dense text-books from my time in graduate school or books that speak to Asian herbalism through a Western lens. I found almost no modern books written by practitioners of Asian descent. To fill the need and appetite for books on Asian American herbalism written by an Asian practitioner, I started writing and self-publishing zines, in which I wrote about the seasons, healing practices, locally grown herbs, and home remedies. I found my stride in sharing this information freely on social media and had fun weaving in stories of my family history. As I did so, I was inspired anew by my family's generational connections to the land where we live in Sonoma County, California, the land of the Coast Miwok and Southern Pomo people, past and present. Revisiting my Japanese American family's rich history, I connected my modern-day herbalism practice more fully to the generations of farm laborers, conservationists, educators, and healers that came before me. This led me to believe, with my whole heart, that the time is now to honor our ancestral connections and amplify voices that have not historically had a platform.

My path of learning traditional medicine and Asian American herbalism has been a process of reclaiming Asian American culture with respect and pride. I learned Asian herbalism through a graduate program, but I had to overcome a major roadblock before enrolling. Upon reflection and soul searching, I realized that I am deeply uncomfortable with how Asian medicine has been exoticized and commodified in America. Think ancient secrets, endangered animals, and massage parlors. Growing up Asian in the United States is to experience layers of internalized shame from

how our cultures are dismissed, mocked, and misrepresented in mainstream culture. However, when I entered the Acupuncture and Integrative Medicine College in Berkeley, California, I was taken aback by my feeling of connection to the cultural roots of this medicine. As a yonsei—fourth-generation Japanese American—graduate school was the first time I had the opportunity to learn from Asian teachers. These teachers reminded me of my own family and instilled a sense of pride in my culture's depth, beauty, and significance. They gifted me, by their very presence, a powerful example of how to practice and embody traditional Asian medicine in modern times.

As I shadowed Dr. Hideko Pelzer in the clinic, I came to understand the nuance and feeling of Japanese energetic medicine. As I learned about herbs and classical Chinese formulas with Dr. Xin Zhu (Hualing) Xu, I found that the umeboshi plum, gobo (burdock root), ginger, and green tea from my grandma's kitchen held powerful medicinal properties. Connecting the theory and medicine to my most comforting, sacred childhood memories allowed me to see beyond the textbooks, lectures, and clinical rotations. It allowed me to see the necessity of learning by cultural feeling, instinct, and ancestral connection. It is the kind of learning that comes from teachers who carry decades and generations of cultural integrity in their work. And for this, I am thankful to my teachers Dr. Xin Zhu (Hualing) Xu, Dr. Hideko Pelzer, Zhi-Bin (Benny) Zhang, Dr. Emmie Zhu, and Daju Suzanne Friedman.

I wrote this book because I believe that Asian American herbalism is meant to be shared with people of every culture while honoring the Asian

Symbol Key

| Qi | Blood | Stagnation | Damp | Yin | Yang |

roots of this medicine. This book was written for you to have at home, so you can create remedies using culturally relevant herbs and things that you can find at your local market. The pages are filled with ideas to inspire you to try new recipes and techniques when your energy and spirit need lifting. There are remedies to ease aches and pains, both physical and emotional, and medicine that empowers you to reconnect with the rhythm of the natural world, as well as the rhythms within.

Asian American Herbalism intends to lovingly open up the worlds of traditional Asian medicine and folk herbalism. It aims to make Eastern philosophy accessible and relatable to your everyday life by breaking down concepts including Yin and Yang and the five elements within the context of herbalism and folk traditions. This mix of theory and practical techniques will help you develop a deeper understanding of your health and well-being, so you can feel better now and on your own terms. This work is meant to be one of your guides as you remember the wisdom already within you. For times when you know in your heart that it's up to you to find the answers for your healing. And for times when you are in tune with your authentic self and learning what that feels like, again and again.

How to Use This Book

This book does not intend to cover every aspect of Asian medicine, folk traditions, or the full scope and magic of each herb. This text is drawn from years of study and experience as a working clinical herbalist. Its purpose is to increase understanding and confidence in practicing herbal medicine at home and to empower the reader to move through the world in a softer, more peaceful way.

My perspective on healing is specific to East Asian and North American herbalism. Some of my work is from ancestral knowledge but much is not. I am a Japanese American woman practicing a modern interpretation of traditional Chinese and Japanese medicine. With that in mind, I recognize that my singular voice and perspective do not and cannot encompass all of the Asian American experience. Asian American herbalism is simply how I identify the work that I do and how I embody herbal medicine. I invite you to consider how these words and this work speak to you.

The information presented in this book is for educational purposes and is not intended to diagnose, treat, cure, or prevent any disease. Always consult a qualified healthcare professional before taking new herbal supplements or changing your diet, especially if you are pregnant, nursing, immunocompromised, or on medications. As always, seek outside help if something doesn't feel right for you.

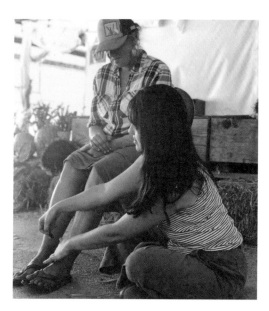

Erin demonstrating how to do moxibustion with Mandy O'Doul, Petaluma, California, 2018

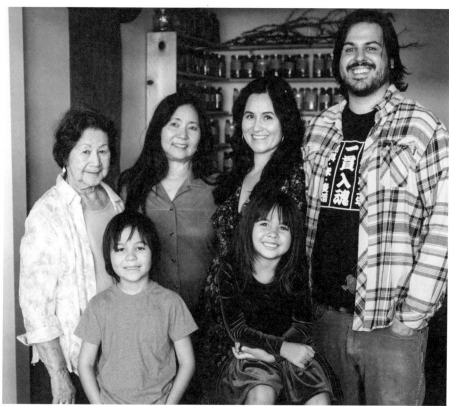

Left to right: Grandma Masako Yamamoto, Weston Wilkins (author's son), Gail Yamamoto Seymour (author's mom), Erin, Zoë Wilkins (author's daughter), and Derek Wilkins (author's husband) at Herb Folk, 2020

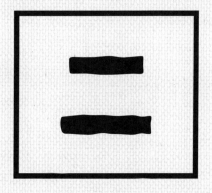

CHAPTER TWO

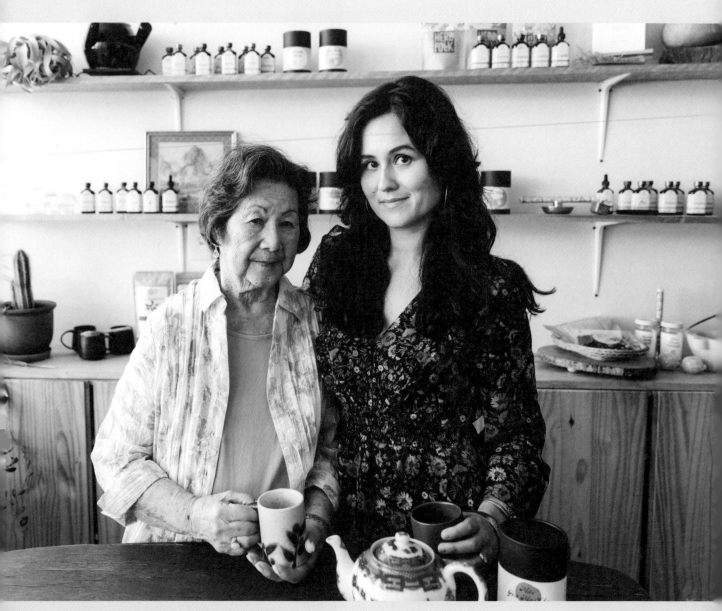
Grandma Masako and Erin at Herb Folk, 2020

THE PRINCIPLES OF ASIAN AMERICAN HERBALISM

———

Beloved community is formed not by the eradication of difference but by its affirmation, by each of us claiming the identities and cultural legacies that shape who we are and how we live in the world.

—bell hooks

Asian American herbalism is folk traditions in modern-day practice. These folk traditions center around knowing how to use plants to heal, uplift, and improve the quality of daily life, knowledge passed down through generations. The herbs and folk traditions that have served humanity since before written history are still relevant to modern life. A cup of herbal tea, a soup, a comforting bath, and a healing massage are examples of folk traditions that are shared across many cultures. Thus, this work is an awakening of the wisdom that is already in us and all around us. These are not mystical secrets that need discovery. On the contrary, this work is about the humble ways that healing takes place in our homes, gardens, and community spaces every day.

Asian American herbalism is meaningful because it is not just about how the herbs can benefit health—it's about empathy, resilience, and understanding the human condition on an energetic level. I believe that it is meant to be shared with people of every culture while honoring the cultural roots of the medicine. While this book is specific to my East Asian heritage, I hope that it will inspire you to look into your family's traditions as well. People of every race, ethnicity, and culture have ancestral connections to herbs and healing practices with wisdom that stands to benefit us all.

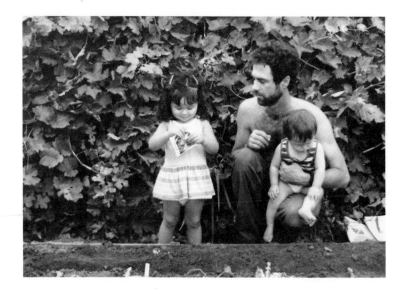

Erin in the garden with dad, John Seymour, and brother, Sean Seymour, Sacramento, California, 1985

Why Asian American Herbalism

In the summer of 2020, I found the words that spoke to my wholeness as a human and herbalist: Asian American herbalism. Until then, I had not expressed how my identity as a mixed-heritage Japanese American woman influenced my work as an Asian herbalist and acupuncturist. I had labeled myself an East-West herbalist without thinking through the problematic implications of that binary paradigm. I certainly do not think that herbalism is either Eastern or Western. However, I realized that the label reflected how I had compartmentalized my professional and personal life, a reflection of how I felt safest presenting one way at home and another way in public. Beyond professionalism, I'm talking about double consciousness and instinctually trying to fit in with the dominant culture.

In *The Souls of Black Folk,* W. E. B. Du Bois defined double consciousness as the internal conflict of experiencing your identity as being divided into different parts. That experience makes it difficult to feel whole, authentic, and understood. Shifting the language of how I identify myself and my work has been a profound source of healing and emergence. With this shift, my confidence grew, and I became more vocal about my work as an Asian American herbalist. I felt empowered to share more of my true self and my family history in classes and in my writing. And my sense of community deepened as others came forward with an interest in learning about the reclamation of Asian healing practices.

You Are Nature

We do not often question the wisdom of the natural world, the growth of the giant redwoods, or the ocean's tides. Nature is not just something we experience; it is what we are. You are nature. However, I've witnessed how often people hold on to self-judgment when experiencing difficult times, change, a healing crisis, or growing older.

At its highest potential, Asian American herbalism offers us ways to understand our real pains, discomforts, and need for healing without judgment. It provides us with a way to trust our own nature.

When considering that we are an integral part of nature, embodied herbalism is a way to learn by feeling and experience. This means learning which herbs work for your body by trying them out. Herbal medicine, by its very nature, is steady and deliberate. So, it is only by taking herbs consistently and over time that one can truly understand a plant's energetics and vibe. It is not a quick fix but an enduring one that can be used safely and healthily throughout a lifetime. With this principle, we can learn about herbalism based on our bodies' imbalances, energetics, and constitutions. Unlike our earliest ancestors who used plants by trial and error, without ways to know if they were poisonous or detrimental, we have many resources to draw from, including this book.

Heal Locally

The best herbal medicine is that which grows in abundance where you live. Herbs that thrive in your local environment share a resonance with you. Locally grown herbs are also the freshest and most delicious. My first taste of locally grown chamomile tea changed my perspective on herbalism. Freshly dried chamomile maintains an apple-like sweetness and depth of flavor that is lost through the months it takes to process and ship imported herbs. I now have a modest garden that is also one of my greatest teachers. The lemon balm, rose, comfrey, and chrysanthemum spilling out of my garden beds are incomparable. Mugwort has taken over a corner of my yard, making me wonder why I once only bought it from

Research your own experience. Absorb what is useful, reject what is useless, and add what is essentially your own.

—Bruce Lee

distant companies. Growing our herbs, reseeding, and seed saving are ways to maintain a steady local source right in our own sacred spaces. It's an opportunity to explore our connection to the earth, the rhythms of the seasons, and the ancient tradition of making do with what you have at home.

Not everyone has the space, desire, or time to grow an herb garden. Unlike our ancestors, who survived by growing their own food, our modern-day experience is shaped by grocery stores, restaurants, and convenient meals. Although I'm a huge proponent of locally grown herbs, I still use many herbs grown and shipped from afar. In my busy life, as in everyone's lives nowadays, we should encourage ourselves to be considerate consumers by frequenting farmers' markets, natural food shops, community gardens, CSA farms, specialty growers, and herb shops. When we purchase food and herbal medicine locally, we are part of a sustainable economy within our communities. And we benefit from the freshest items, while also supporting the livelihoods and survival of our people. I'm not a purist, but my experience with Asian American herbalism has been an exploration of how to cultivate more of this within my own life, and I invite you to do the same.

AT-RISK
MEDICINAL PLANTS

Sandalwood
Kava Kava
American Ginseng
Goldenseal
White Sage
Osha

Echinacea
Yerba Mansa
Black Cohosh
Slippery Elm
Arnica
Gentian
Frankincense
Myrrh

For the Earth

A common misconception is that because herbal medicine is of the earth, it is a more ethical or earth-friendly practice. However, human exploitation, environmental degradation, supply chain issues, and quality and safety problems exist like in other industries. Considerations of carbon footprint and the environmental impacts of importing herbs are another reason to grow and source locally whenever possible. Sourcing herbs from growers and suppliers who sustainably steward the land with a transparent supply chain is essential.

With climate collapse, increasing demand, and overharvesting, we must also be vigilant about threatened and endangered plants. Asian American herbalism asks us to consider not only the plants and remedies of our ancestors, but also the ones that we will pass down to the next generation. We do right by the earth and our people by focusing on the plants that thrive in abundance where we live and the plants that provide essential habitats for native wildlife to sustain the web of life.

For the Culture

Asian American herbalism is for the culture. The culture is about reclaiming healing traditions in deeply personal ways. It's the tenderness of discovering the parts of ourselves that we didn't even

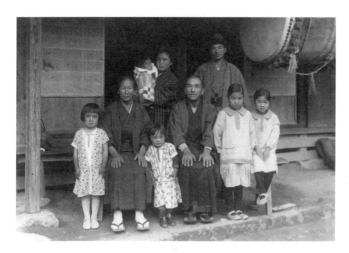

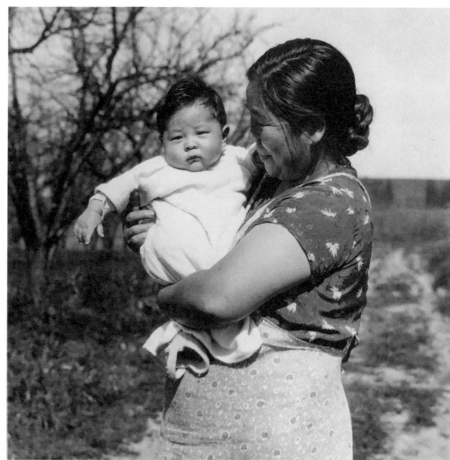

above:
Tanaka-Sonoda
family, Kyushu,
Japan, 1926

right:
Great-grandma
Katsu Yamamoto
and her son, Bob
Yamamoto, Utah,
1940s

realize were missing. And it's the emergence and authenticity that takes place when we stand in our truth.

Reclamation of herbal culture includes identity herbalism, which is the work of learning the healing traditions of one's ethnicity and ancestry. Identity herbalism resonates because it reminds us of our cultural connections to the earth. The earth-based lessons are there for all of us to discover.

With so much access to information through the internet, it's easy to look up cultural practices and recipes. However, it has become increasingly difficult to find in-depth information on healing traditions because so much knowledge has been lost due to colonialism and the genocide of indigenous peoples. I hope this book will inspire us to cultivate a greater awareness of our cultures' herbs and healing traditions. And to honor our living elders by receiving, documenting, and preserving the healing wisdom that can only be passed down by word of mouth. Herbalism will always be an oral history tradition.

Cultural Appropriation

Cultural appropriation is the act of taking, misrepresenting, and misusing elements from another culture. This often includes healing practices, such as yoga, that have been repackaged and sold in ways that purposefully remove the cultural context. And the real sting is when folks from one culture sell an element from another culture as a new or proprietary thing for personal gain.

Appropriation of Asian food is an example in which we often witness people disrespecting cultural foods as needing to be fixed, made healthier, or made cleaner. The exploitation and disrespect of culinary traditions and heritage is always harmful. It harms the people of that culture in multifaceted ways, including but not limited to threatening the livelihoods of artisans and professionals, but it also harms the people with whom it is shared, as it strips and distorts the heritage, history, and cultural feeling from the food.

On the other hand, cultural appreciation and exchange are about seeking to understand another culture through community connection and learning in a cross-cultural way. The key here is reciprocity and understanding the vulnerability of sharing yourself to bring forward a mutual exchange of culture and knowledge. So, while the American part of Asian American herbalism speaks to change and evolution, the foundation of this medicine is based on traditional East Asian knowledge. Coming from this perspective affords us the possibility of approaching this medicine with deep cultural appreciation for the fact that it is passed down to us and through us. This work is fluid and ever evolving, but its roots are always steeped in tradition.

The Asian Diaspora

Asian and Asian American culture means different things to everyone. Identity is shaped by where you were born, the languages you speak, the food traditions you follow, citizenship, access to community, and the histories of violence that led to assimilation. Asian American is a political designation that groups together people from many different cultures and countries—the Asian diaspora. There are hundreds of Asian countries and ethnic groups, and there is no monolithic Asian identity. According to a U.S. census analysis from 2021, Asian Americans are the

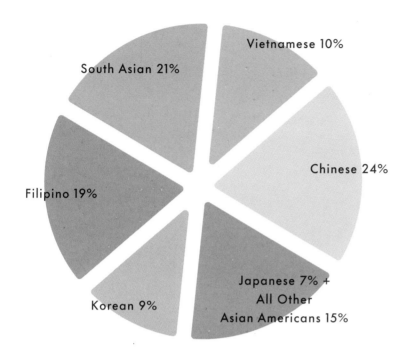

ASIAN AMERICAN POPULATION BY RACE AND ETHNICITY

(18.9 million)

Vietnamese 10%

South Asian 21%

Chinese 24%

Filipino 19%

Korean 9%

Japanese 7% +
All Other
Asian Americans 15%

Note: Because individuals surveyed often identified with more than one Asian nationality, the numbers in this chart do not add up to 100 percent. The "All Others" category includes people who identified as "Other Asian, not specified." Source: Pew Research Center

fastest-growing population of all racial or ethnic groups in the United States. The same study illustrated that the Asian American diaspora is made up primarily of Chinese, Filipino, South Asian, Korean, Japanese, and Vietnamese Americans. The collective category of other ethnicities includes Bangladeshi, Burmese, Cambodian, Hmong, Indonesian, Laotian, Malaysian, Melanesian, Micronesian, Nepalese, Pakistani, Polynesian, Sri Lankan, and Thai.

Asian American herbalism is an evolving, living system of herbalism that should reflect the diversity of people of Asian descent. This herbalism is influenced by traditional and modern medical systems, such as traditional Chinese medicine hospitals in China, Kampo herbs prescribed by medical doctors in Japan, and Ayurvedic medicine in India. As I researched for this book, I was startled by just how little I knew about Asia in many ways—the vast number of countries, geopolitical borders, cultures, and ethnicities. The Asian continent is so expansive that it is humbling to see how the Asian diaspora touches nearly every corner of this earth. And while my work relies heavily on the herbs of East Asia, I am in awe of the diversity of herbs from each region. I recognize that the following list of herbs (see page 26) is incomplete, and I apologize for what I have inevitably left out. I am also still learning.

Herbs and Locations

Herbs of East Asia
Atractylodes, bupleurum, chrysanthemum, cordyceps, dang gui, forsythia, ginger, ginseng, goji berries, isatis root, kombu, licorice, mint, mugwort, white peony root, poria, rehmannia, and tea

Herbs of Southeast Asia
Ampalaya, basil, camphor, cardamom, citronella, coriander, curry leaves, galangal, ginger, guava, lemongrass, makrut lime leaves, moringa, pandan, peppercorn, sambong, tamarind, tiger milk mushroom, tongkat ali, and turmeric

Herbs of the Pacific Islands
Awa, banana, basil, gardenia, ground cherry, hibiscus, kava kava, kukui flowers, maltadati, noni, papaya leaves, and ti

Herbs of Southern Asia
Ashwagandha, bacopa, cardamom, cloves, coriander, cumin, fenugreek (methi), gotu kola, mustard seeds, tulsi, and turmeric

Herbs of Northern Asia
Eleuthero, dodder, knotweed, mugwort, pine, rhaponticum, rhodiola, rhododendron, rippleseed plantain, scutellaria, silky wormwood, and thistle

Herbs of Central and Western Asia
Basil, black pepper, calendula, castor, cilantro, cumin, dang gui, dill, elecampane, fennel, flax, greater celandine, jujube dates, lavender, milk thistle, mint, motherwort, nigella, parsley, parsnip, sage, sesame seed, skullcap, and valerian

Our ultimate objective in learning about anything is to try to create and develop a more just society.

—Yuri Kochiyama

Health Justice

The ability to access and receive healthcare is a fundamental human right. Health justice is a movement that removes economic and social barriers and improves healthcare for all people. This work is done with the purpose of not only healing ourselves but also reclaiming our power in the wellness industry by reviving culturally relevant healing practices that have been dispelled by systemic racism. Empowered healing practices are needed now more than ever as we live and work through many modern-day pressures, including the COVID-19 pandemic, the climate crisis, challenges to civil and human rights, and the reckonings of injustice in our personal lives. Reviving ancestral healing practices and building new, more inclusive ones will create a more equitable and safer world.

My experience in America is that we are conditioned to see Western as the norm and Eastern as the other. Biomedicine, or Western medicine, is the standard, and Chinese medicine is the obscure alternative. And when people are labeled as the "other," they are seen as exotic, unworthy, and dangerous. We see this with the rise of Asian hate crimes, racially motivated violence, and the murder of Black men and women in the United States. Racial discrimination has grown exponentially in recent years, and the implicit biases we all carry have real-life implications. But this is not new.

I grew up witnessing generational trauma from the systemic racism and violence of the forced internment of Japanese Americans in concentration camps during the Second World War.

Systemic racism relies on stigmatizing, dismissing, and invalidating the people and the pride in our cultures. Asian American herbalism is meant to act in opposition to systemic racism as it centers the Asian American experience and creates access to the knowledge of culturally relevant healing practices. In solidarity with the Black, Brown, and Indigenous communities committed to achieving racial equity, we must remain committed to prioritizing our health, both mentally and physically. When we heal ourselves, we honor our ancestors and our children, as we release the generations of grief held in our consciousness from systemic racism and colonialism. The absence of healing will only exacerbate our collective pain, so we must integrate ancestral wisdom into our very being.

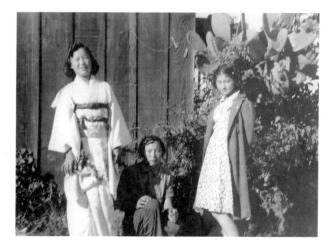

Left to right: Tomiko Inouye, Grace Inouye, and Grandma Masako Yamamoto, Sunnyvale, California, 1930s

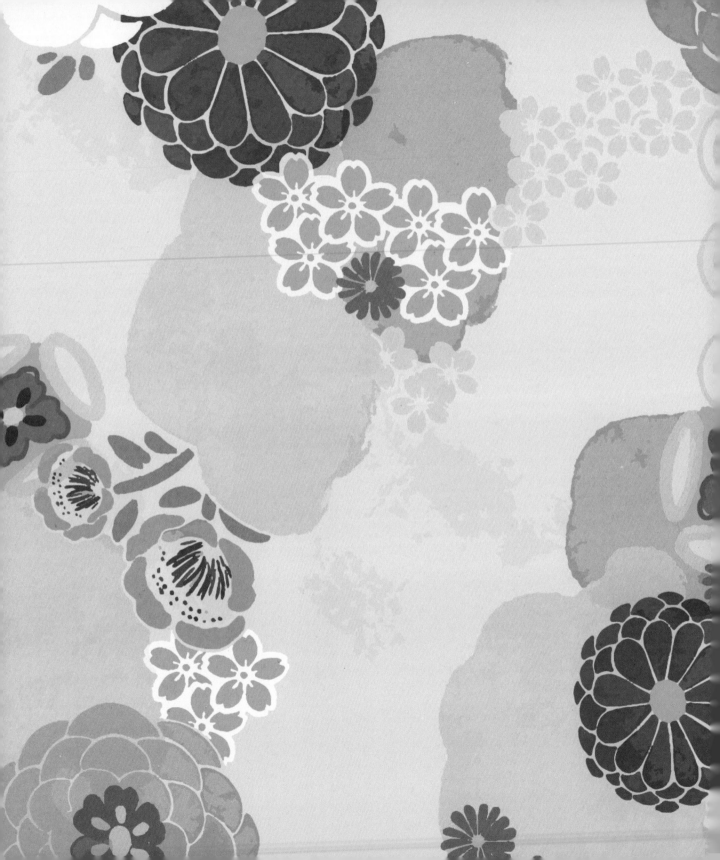

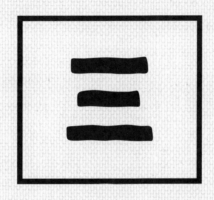

CHAPTER THREE

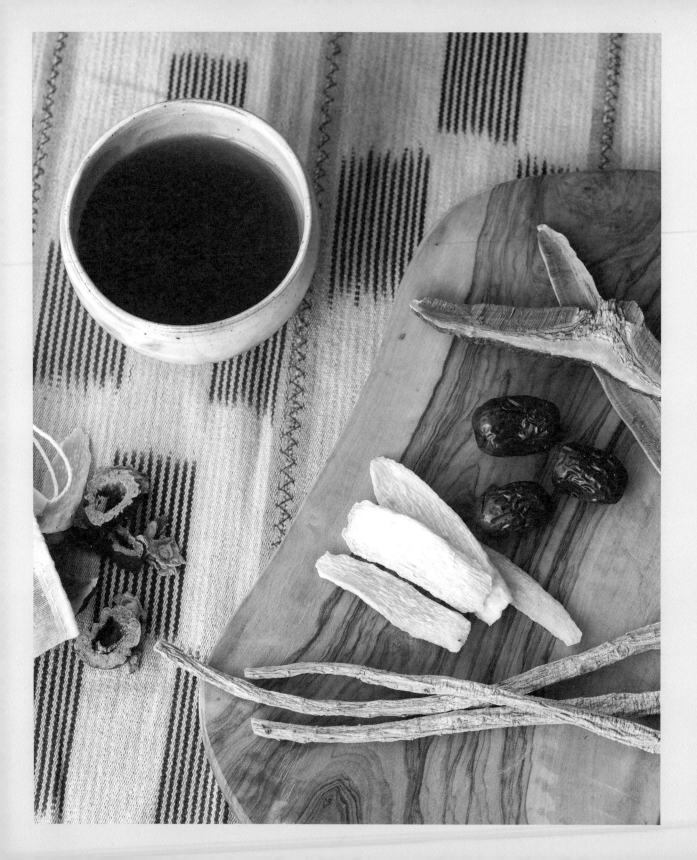

HERBALISM BASICS

W hen preparing herbs, consider the following: Are you treating a specific ailment or solely increasing vitality and wellness? How fresh and robust are the herbs? What is the size, age, and constitution of the person taking the herbs? How sensitive are they to food, herbs, and medicines generally? All these considerations will inform precisely how and why a person takes herbs.

Dose and Course of Treatment

Herbal medicine is, by its very nature, slow medicine. The effects are cumulative, whether herbs are taken over a few days, months, or years. Consistent and proper dosing of herbal medicine is vital for experiencing the full benefits of the herbs. And understanding the reason and intention for taking an herbal remedy is the heart of Asian American herbalism.

The most important aspect of dosing is to give enough to affect a noticeable change but not so much as to cause an adverse effect. When determining the dose, it is best to start small and then increase if there is no noticeable effect. There should be a tangible effect, even if quite subtle, after one to two days. If no results are felt, and it's an herb that is generally safe for consumption and your constitution, increase the herb by fifty percent or to the maximum dose for that specific herb (see single herb profiles for dosing guidelines on page 300).

For acute situations, you want to take many doses of herbal medicine within a few days. When menstrual cramps, a tension headache, or cold is coming on, treat those immediately by taking small doses every few hours over a few days to prevent worsening symptoms. The condition should be resolved within three days.

For acute conditions:

TEA: ½ cup (120 ml) every hour until symptoms are resolved (up to 4 cups [960 ml] per day for one to three days)

TINCTURE: ½ tsp every hour until symptoms are resolved (up to 4 teaspoons per day for one to three days)

For chronic or long-term issues, consistently taking herbal medicine over a long period is often needed to heal the root causes. However, I find that many folks are put off by having to take something multiple times a day. In my clinical practice, I give people some flexibility around how and when they take their herbs. I recommend that people start with a three-day commitment and increase it to one week as they notice a specific, meaningful change. This allows some grace in taking herbs because consistency over time is generally more effective than consistency for a few days. And over time, taking the medicine becomes an embodied practice that leads to an instinct and sense of how the medicine works, so that it can be used when needed and on your own terms.

For long-term conditions:

TEA: 1 to 3 cups (240 to 720 ml) per day for one to three months

TINCTURES: 1 tsp twice per day for one to three months

DECOCTIONS AND HEALING SOUPS: 1 cup (240 ml) twice per day for one to three months

HERBAL DOSING FOR ADULTS

ACUTE AND SUDDEN CONDITIONS

—

Herbs are taken frequently over 2 to 3 days until symptoms resolve.

—

Tea: ½ cup every hour until symptoms are resolved
Tincture: ½ tsp every hour until symptoms are resolved

CHRONIC OR LONG-TERM ISSUES

—

Herbs are taken slowly over 1 to 3 months for cumulative effect.

—

Tea: 1 to 3 cups per day
Tincture: 1 tsp twice per day
Decoctions and healing foods: 1 cup twice per day

Consistency

Consistency is the key to herbal medicine. Like exercise and eating well, it's about the cumulative effect. Herbal formulas are most effective when taken fifteen to thirty minutes before eating so that the body can quickly receive and digest the medicine. However, they should be taken with food for folks prone to an upset stomach. Herbal medicine that is applied to the skin, like salves and liniments, also benefit from consistent application. These topical preparations should be massaged into injured areas for fifteen minutes three times per day until there is relief.

Taste

Taste is one of the most important ways that we experience herbal medicine. The five tastes—pungent (spicy), bitter, sweet, sour, and salty—are key to understanding how herbs heal energetically and therapeutically. For example, spicy herbs are usually warming, while bitter herbs tend to reduce heat in the body. Taste is also a way to accurately identify herbs. Learning herbalism through taste is key to developing a working, embodied knowledge of the plants.

Taste and flavor are often an intentional part of herbal medicine. For example, the taste of a bitter herb like dandelion signals the brain to stimulate digestion and the production of saliva. The taste of something sweet has energetic properties that strengthen Qi energy and increase moisture to benefit body fluids. For more on the five tastes and Qi, see pages 53 and 83.

Preparing an Herbal Workspace at Home

When stocking your herbal workspace, first make use of what you already have. Many of the tools needed are things you will find in your kitchen—bowls, pots, glass jars and bottles, good knives, scissors, a cutting board, chopsticks, and wooden spoons. Many other ingredients and specialty items can be found locally, and I encourage you to support your local markets and herb shops to purchase any unique supplies. Here are my most used and beloved specialty tools for a well-stocked herbal working station.

Amber Glass Bottles

Amber glass bottles are the standard for minimizing exposure to light and protecting herbal preparations from oxidizing and spoiling. I prefer to use 1 to 8 fl oz (30 to 240 ml) bottles with flat lids.

Blender

A blender can take the place of a mortar and pestle in many cases. A high-powered blender is an efficient grinder for breaking down hard plant material. I store locally harvested herbs in larger pieces and break them down to size in a blender right before use.

Clear Glass Jars

Glass jars with good lids are a necessity for herbal preparations. Pint (480 ml), quart (960 ml), and half-gallon (2 L) jars are particularly useful. Glass jars safely store a variety of preparations without leaching chemicals as plastics do. A wide-mouth funnel is handy for pouring herbal preparations and dried herbs into the glass jars.

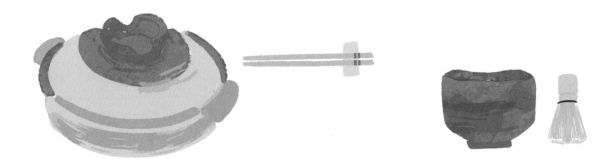

Dehydrator

A quality dehydrator with an adjustable temperature gauge is a vital tool when processing fresh herbs. Dehydrating leaves and flowers preserves and locks in their delicate shapes, color, and Qi. Qi refers to the energy and vitality of the herb. Even when using quainter drying methods, such as hanging bundles of fresh herbs in the kitchen or drying them over racks outdoors, finishing herbs in a dehydrator allows you to ensure that they are completely dry. In the late summer and early fall, the plants in my garden are ready to harvest all at once! A dehydrator helps to quickly preserve large amounts of herbs before mold or bugs can take hold.

Enamel Pot with Lid

A heavy enamel-coated pot serves various purposes and is my preference for decoctions and large herbal preparations. I always keep one reserved solely for making medicine because the white enamel will stain over time. A heavy stainless-steel pot is a good substitute. Never use aluminum or nonstick cooking vessels because the materials can adversely react with some plants and minerals, such as ginseng and he shou wu. I don't recommend traditional glazed clay pots out of concern for heavy metal contamination from the glazes.

Fine-Mesh Sieve

A fine-mesh sieve, also known as a chinois, is used when a clear liquid or uniform texture are desired. The layers of fine mesh strain out the tiniest of particles, which is ideal when working with herbs that have fine hairs, such as mullein and loquat leaf. This tool is a special investment, but it alleviates the need for cheesecloth in many herbal preparations and recipes in this book. Alternatively, a cheesecloth-lined colander is a good substitute.

Kitchen Scale

A kitchen scale is needed for formulating traditional and more complex herbal recipes. Traditional Chinese herbal formulas are written in grams, but this book's recipes are measured in both imperial and metric units. Weight is a more accurate unit of measure than volume, which is why a scale is important.

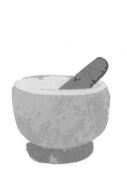
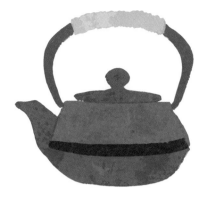
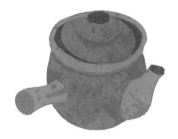

Mortar and Pestle

A mortar and pestle are synonymous with herbal medicine making. I use a heavy marble mortar and a wooden pestle to combine herbal tea blends, break down plant material into uniform sizes, and crush seeds such as cardamom and jujube date seed. I use a Japanese-style suribachi with abrasive ceramic ridges that combine substances such as ginger and miso to make pastes and sauces.

Tea Kettle

A stovetop kettle is a centerpiece in the kitchen and a daily reminder for tea. In my kitchen, I also have an electric tea kettle with a temperature-setting dial that is necessary for making green and black tea. Green tea needs to be steeped in barely simmering water (170 to 180°F [75 to 80°C]) for one to three minutes. If you do not have temperature settings on your kettle, the temperature for green tea is called "fisheye" because the bubbles look like tiny fisheyes. Black tea benefits from a stronger steep in simmering to boiling water (180 to 200°F [80 to 95°C]) for three to five minutes.

Tea Pot and Strainer

Teapots and strainers come in various sizes and styles and speak to the different tea cultures worldwide. I prefer a basket tea strainer so the herbs and tea leaves have plenty of space to expand and release their medicine. When using tea bags, ensure that they do not have plastics, adhesives, or bleached materials.

Building an Herbal Pantry

A well-stocked herbal pantry starts by shopping for your first recipe. From there, it is a joy to build a collection of healing herbs that speak to you and your family's needs. You'll find that many herbs and medicines will keep for many months and come in handy when needed for an ailment. Many of the herbs I recommend in this book can be sourced from a local herb shop or purchased online. Some of the herbs can be found in well-stocked grocery stores, Asian markets, or at local farmers' markets. For fresh herbs and berries, such as mulberries and jujube dates, a post on your local foodie social media groups can connect you with people who have fruiting trees in your area. For my preferred herb companies, please see the list of Where to Buy Herbs and Seeds at the back of the book under Resources on page 312.

Herbs for a well-stocked herbal pantry:

DRIED FLOWERS AND LEAVES
Calendula

Chrysanthemum

Lemon verbena

Marshmallow leaf and root

Mint

Nettle

Rose petals and buds

DRIED SPECIALTY HERBS
Aged tangerine peel (chen pi)

Astragalus

Codonopsis

Dang gui

Longan fruit

POWDER EXTRACTS
Eucommia

He shou wu

Reishi mushroom

FOUND AT THE MARKET
Black and green tea

Black sesame seeds

Burdock root, fresh

Ginger, fresh

Goji berry, dried

Jujube dates, dried or fresh (seasonally)

Mulberries, dried or fresh (seasonally)

Mushrooms, fresh and dried (i.e., shiitake, maitake, lion's mane, etc.)

Seaweed, dried (i.e., kombu, nori)

Tangerine and citrus peel, fresh

Working with Locally Grown Herbs

How you source herbs for making medicine influences the strength, taste, and overall experience. I believe there is also a positive, energetic impact on the medicine when we grow our own herbs or cultivate friendships with local growers and farmers. Our relationships with each other and with the plants are the foundation of Asian American herbalism.

One of the perks of sourcing herbs from well-respected companies is trust in the quality of their products. I implicitly trust the Chinese herbs imported by Andy Ellis of Spring Wind Herbs in San Leandro, California, because he has built personal relationships with the herb growers, and he diligently tests all the herbs for purity and quality before selling them to the public. There are many places to buy herbs, especially online, and it is important to know what to look for when selecting herbs grown locally and from afar.

Good Quality Herbs

We can consider several specific elements to determine the quality of herbs, including their smell, taste, appearance, and potency. It is like shopping for fresh produce at the grocery store. The look and color of a plant immediately indicate its quality and strength. Freshly dried herbs retain their natural colors. Herbs that are gray, dusty, or faded suggest that they have been exposed to sunlight, stored improperly, or expired. Herbs should also have a distinct, unmistakable scent. When herbs lose their scent, it is a sign that they have lost their Qi and medicine as well. And finally, quality herbs should be potent and effective medicine. Plant quality could be the issue if your herbal preparations are not working. Imported herbs are

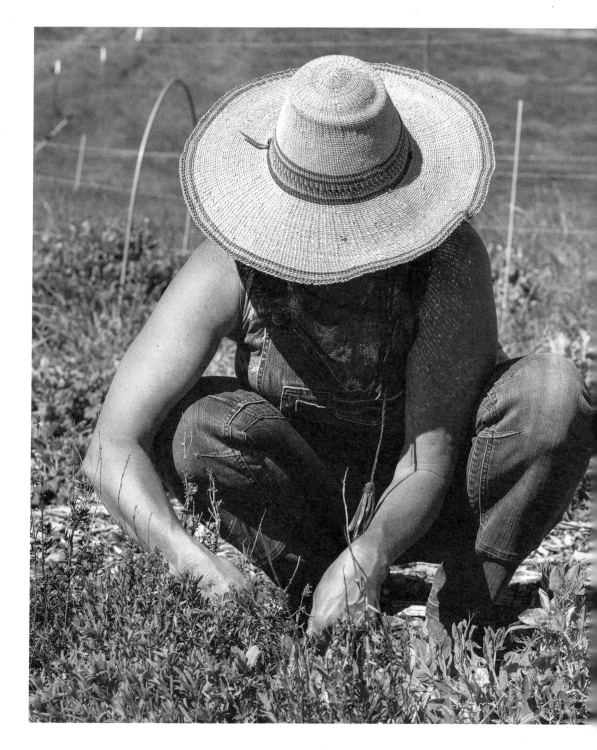

Mandy O'Doul
harvesting herbs
in her flower
fields, Petaluma,
California, 2022

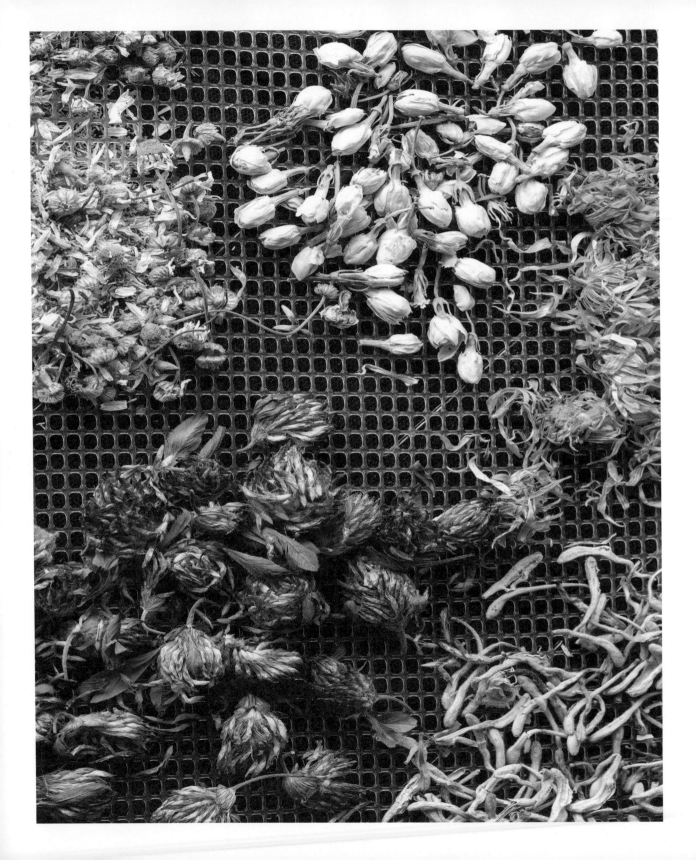

often exposed to high heat and long storage times during FDA inspections. This ages delicate leaves and flowers and dissipates their volatile oils and medicinal constituents. This is not to say that imported herbs are ineffective, but rather they will expire more quickly than freshly dried herbs. I primarily make medicine with imported herbs but I prefer to work with freshly dried herbs when available.

Harvesting and Preserving Fresh Herbs

Harvesting and preserving herbs for later use is a cornerstone of traditional herbalism. This can look like growing your own, finding fresh herbs at a market, gleaning from a local source, or harvesting in the wild. The first consideration is ensuring the plant material is as clean as possible. Do not harvest plants that grow near roads with high traffic because of the chemical pollution from motor vehicles. When foraging and wildcrafting herbs, by gathering them in their natural habitat, make sure that the plant is growing in abundance and is not a sensitive or at-risk species. Take only what you need, and never more than half of a given plant, so it can regenerate. Consider that the plants you are taking provide food, shelter, and nesting materials for a variety of wildlife. Remember to ask for permission and give thanks to the plants, earth, and people who are providing for your wellness.

Harvesting Leaves, Flowers, and Fruits

The best time of day for harvesting is in the morning, after the dew has evaporated and before the heat of the day, when harvesting is stressful to the parts of the plants that you leave behind. Handle fresh plant material gently, so that it doesn't bruise. Choose strong stems with healthy looking plant material and cut close to the base of the stem so that the main plant can produce new stems. Shake and tap off any dust or rogue bugs from the garden. If necessary, you can quickly rinse any dirt off with water.

Leaves and flowers can be harvested year-round but are particularly abundant from late spring to early autumn. When harvesting flowers, I like to break them off right under the flower head. They can also be harvested on the stem for airdrying in bundles (as described in this chapter). For roses, cut the stem just above the first leafy offshoot with five leaves. After harvest, remove any plant materials that are damaged, wilted, crispy, or munched on by insects. Keep the herbs in the shade, in thin layers with good airflow. It is important that you process the herbs for drying as soon as possible.

Fruit and berries tend to have a short window for harvest during the late summer and autumn months. Harvest ripened fruit and berries directly from their branches. Each fruit will require specific preparations before drying. For example, longan fruit needs the husk and seed removed. Jujube dates can be dried whole, pitted before drying, or eaten fresh like a tiny apple. Berries, like mulberries, can be stored in the refrigerator immediately after harvest, but they will spoil and mold after a few days if not dried. There is a lot of great information and videos online about how to harvest various Asian herbs and fruits.

Harvesting and Cleaning Roots

Roots are harvested in the late fall or early spring when there is just enough plant material to identify the herb but before the new growth of early spring begins. Many plants go dormant in autumn and store Qi and medicine in their roots over the winter months. You'll need a clean digging tool or shovel to carefully loosen the soil around the plant to get down to the roots. As always, take only what you need and do not harvest the entire root system, so the plant can regenerate.

Clean the harvested roots as well as possible because any remaining dirt will end up in your herbal preparations! Cut any twisted roots to get the dirt out of the folds and crevices. Fill a basin with cool water and meticulously clean away the dirt using a scrub brush—a vegetable brush or new toothbrush works well. When the roots are very clean, slice them into smaller pieces. I prefer root slices to be as thin and long as possible. As the roots dry, they will be more difficult to cut up. Roots are more challenging because some, such as codonopsis and mai men dong (ophiopogon root), need to grow for many years before harvesting. For more in-depth information on harvesting, see Resources on page 313.

Drying

When drying herbs, time is of the essence. The faster herbs are dried, the less chance of mold, oxidation, and discoloration. When drying large batches of herbs, I complete the drying in a food dehydrator at the lowest setting to eliminate any residual moisture. However, traditional drying methods that don't require a dehydrator can work well if the environment is conducive. For instance, it is nearly impossible to air-dry herbs in humid or damp environments. On the other hand, places with dry heat during the summer and autumn months are ideal for air-drying herbs.

Bundling Herbs for Air-Drying

This method is best for light plant material such as leaves, stems, and flowers. Keep leaves and flowers on the stem and tie them into small ½ in (12 mm) bundles with twine or a rubber band. Removing thick stems or woody branches is important, as they will slow the drying time. With the herbs in bundles, hang them, with the stems pointing up, in a space that is out of direct sunlight and has good air circulation. Drying can take up to a week. When properly dried, leaves and flowers crumble when rubbed, and the stems snap when bent.

Air-Drying with Baskets and Drying Racks

Airflow is key to quickly drying plant material. Large shallow baskets work well for drying smaller quantities of herbs, but there are many affordable drying rack options online. Spread the plant material in a single layer, without any overlapping, on a rack or in a basket. Set it in a place with good airflow but out of direct sunlight. Large roots and stems should be cut down with a sharp knife to improve and expedite their drying. Gently shuffle the herbs every day to ensure that any damp or heavy parts are fully exposed and able to dry. When preserving flowers, remove the buds from the stems. It's easier to dry flowers with the petals separated, but I prefer to leave the flower heads intact to capture as much plant material as possible. Whole flowers take extra time and care to ensure no moisture remains in the flower heads. Drying berries and fruits can be tricky because of the moisture content and sweetness, so I always use a dehydrator.

Storing

It is best to store herbs as soon as possible after drying. They lose Qi when left out for too long after drying or when exposed to light, moisture, heat, or air. Each herb should be kept in a dry, clean glass jar and labeled with its name, the date it was prepared or purchased, and its location of origin. Leaves, flowers, berries, and chopped roots can go into a jar as is. They will stay fresher longer if you leave them in larger pieces to prevent oxidation. Strip the leaves, flowers, and berries if they are still on their stems before storing. Remove any discolored plant material. You don't need to be as gentle here as you were when the herbs were fresh. The general rule is that flowers and leaves can be kept for one to two years. Denser plant materials, like roots, can last for two to three years.

Medicine Making

Making medicine with locally grown herbs is different from using store-bought herbs that have been processed by machines. Store-bought herbs are processed by being cut into small uniform pieces and this makes them heavier when measured using teaspoon, tablespoon, and cup measurements. Locally grown herbs will be much lighter and airier because they're left in larger pieces with small stems. The recipes in this book use both volume and weight measurements, and the weight measurements are more accurate for both local and store-bought herbs.

When making medicine with locally grown herbs, after thoroughly drying, I recommend pulsing them in a blender until the large leaves break down to a more uniform size, similar to the texture of store-bought dried herbs, such as oregano or sage. Breaking down the herbs increases their surface area, which helps extract all their medicinal components. However, it also speeds oxidation, so it's best to use ground herbs within twelve months. For more on herbal preparations, see Maintaining Health – Herbal Preparations on page 288.

When to Ask for Help

Always ask for help! As you experiment with herbs, please seek out an experienced herbalist to discuss questions as they come up. This can be a highly trained practitioner or a trusted friend with some herbal knowledge and perspective. Working with seasoned practitioners and herbalists in your community is a vital part of learning herbalism. If any remedies cause a headache, nausea, upset digestion, dizziness, or allergic reaction, stop immediately and consult your health care provider as soon as possible. We are all susceptible to adverse reactions when taking new herbs, foods, or supplements. As always, trust your intuition.

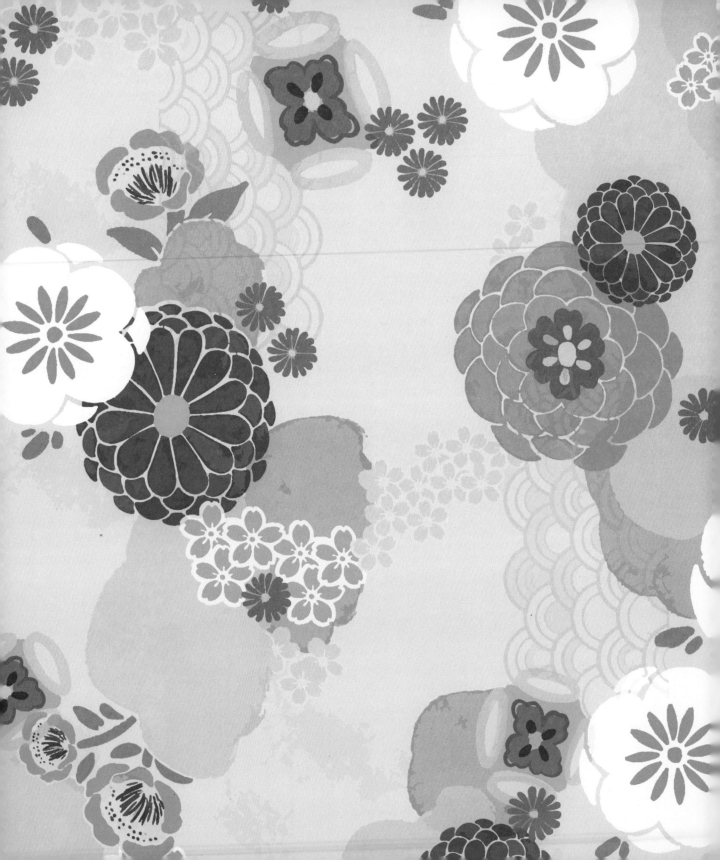

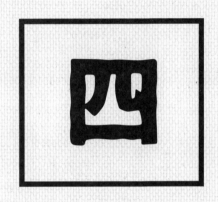

CHAPTER FOUR

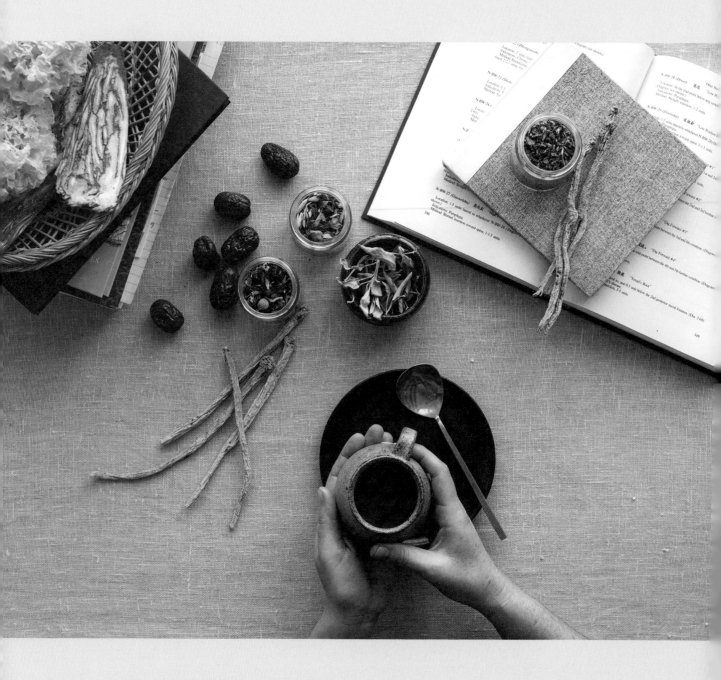

TRADITIONAL CHINESE MEDICINE THEORY

———

Traditional Chinese medicine theory is a framework and language for Asian American herbalism. Traditional East Asian philosophies include Yin-Yang, the five elements, the Zangfu organ system, and the vital substances. Understanding these theories is essential for learning about Asian herbalism as it is practiced traditionally and in modern times. Yin-Yang and the five elements are theories based on the wisdom of the natural world that view disease as interconnected to lifestyle, circumstance, and the rhythms of nature. These theories departed from old beliefs that illness was caused by demons and evil spirits. The Zangfu organ system and the vital substances are theories that view the human body and mind as a complex, integrated system. They are akin to anatomy and physiology in biomedicine.

Zangfu Organs

The Zangfu organs are the 12 energetic organs. They are parallel yet different from the anatomical organs in the body. The Zangfu organs are capitalized (i.e., Liver, Spleen) when used in reference to Asian medicine theory.

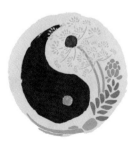

All symptoms and signs
[of illness] are ultimately due
to an imbalance between
Yin and Yang.

—Giovanni Maciocia, from The
Foundations of Chinese Medicine

Yin-Yang Theory

Yin and Yang symbolize duality in the natural world—hot and cold, activity and rest, internal and external, day and night. It is a conceptual framework for observing and understanding the natural world from ancient China's Yin and Zhou dynasties (1050–256 BC). Yin and Yang symbolize how all natural phenomena are interconnected, including the workings of the human body and mind.

Yin is the dark side of the Yin-Yang symbol. Yin is associated with coldness, tranquility, slowing down, completion, darkness, fluids, the earth, nighttime, and the cold winter months. When Yin is depleted in the human body, symptoms are insomnia, night sweats, dryness, anxiety, and a restless mind.

Yang is the light side of the Yin-Yang symbol. Yang is associated with heat, excitement, activity, expansion, light, Qi energy, the heavens, daytime, and the warm summer months. When Yang is weak in the body, the symptoms are feeling cold, fatigue, water retention, digestive upset, and a waning libido. For more on Yin and Yang, see page 105.

The Vital Substances

The five vital substances are Qi, Blood, Jing, body fluids, and Shen. The theory is that the vital substances make up the body and mind, and each plays a role in maintaining health. Qi is the building block for all the other vital substances as well.

Qi

Qi, pronounced "chi," is often translated as "energy" or "life force." It is the basis of how all things exist in the universe—both the form and the function. When Qi condenses, it becomes a physical form such as plants, water, and the human body. When Qi is dispersed, it creates movement including the pulse of the heartbeat and the rhythm of the breath.

Although Qi is not something that can be seen or held, all the activities of the human body can be explained by changes in the movement of Qi. When Qi is weak, symptoms are spontaneous sweating, fatigue after eating, weak muscles, weak voice, loose stools, poor digestion, and foggy, unclear thinking. Qi is a physical manifestation of Yang, so a long-term imbalance of Qi can lead to Yang deficiency, and a Yang deficiency always indicates Qi deficiency. For more information on Qi and Qi herbs, see page 83.

Blood

The understanding of Blood in Asian medicine is not the same as blood in biomedicine. In Asian medicine, Blood with a capital "B" includes all the healthy fluids and substances that nourish and moisten the body. It consists of the red blood we see when we get a cut, but also hydration, moisture in the body, spinal fluid, hair, menstrual blood, and breast milk. Therefore, issues with dryness, thinning hair, the menstrual cycle, and milk supply signal depletion of Blood. Blood also supports mental functioning by providing nourishment to the mind. Issues with mental clarity, anxiety, depression, restlessness, insomnia, memory, and mental health often indicate a Blood imbalance. For more information on Blood and Blood herbs, see page 96.

Jing

Jing, often translated as "essence," is unique to Asian medicine theory. I consider it parallel to hormones and the endocrine system. Jing is a precious, energetic substance that is inherited from parents at the time of conception and becomes the essence of a person. Jing is stored in the Kidney, and so it is also called Kidney Jing. The strength of your Jing determines critical factors and stages of growth over a lifetime, including physical and mental development, puberty, fertility, menopause, and aging. It is used gradually over the course of one's lifetime, so Jing tonics and Kidney herbs are used to enhance graceful aging, vitality, and longevity. Herbs that benefit Jing include he shou wu, black sesame seed, gotu kola, ashwagandha, cordyceps, eucommia, walnut, schisandra, and lotus seed.

Body Fluids

Body fluids are the healthy fluids of the body, including lymph, tears, sweat, saliva, gastric and intestinal juices, urine, and synovial fluid. The distribution of body fluids nourishes and provides moisture to the body and organs. Circulation of body fluids is dependent upon the healthy flow of Qi. Qi stagnation and deficiency will cause fluids to dry up. Body fluids and Blood share many similarities in how they operate, and when there is Blood loss, there will also be a loss of body fluids. When making medicine for someone with depleted body fluids, astringent and tonic herbs are called for, such as yam, he shou wu, white peony root, gotu kola, nettle, sage, and burdock root.

Shen

Shen, which translates as "the mind and spirit," is the most obscure and intangible of the vital substances. The Shen resides in the Heart and is what makes us conscious beings. The Shen and the Heart work together to ensure healthy emotional processing and mental activities, including consciousness, sleep, feelings, thinking, memory, insight, cognition, intelligence, wisdom, ideas, and the senses. Herbs that benefit the Shen are often Yin tonics and Blood herbs, such as motherwort, longan fruit, mai men dong (ophiopogon root), lily root, California poppy, jujube date seed, lotus seed, mimosa tree bark, reishi mushroom, and schisandra.

Five Element Theory

From the seasons to the life cycles, the five element theory is an ancient philosophy that poetically describes the flow and balance of

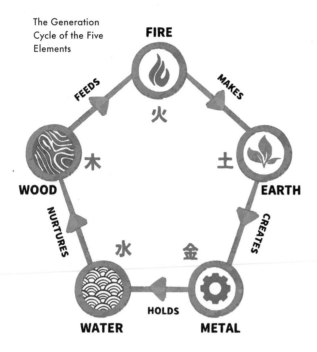

The Generation Cycle of the Five Elements

FIRE
火

FEEDS

MAKES

WOOD
木

NURTURES

水

EARTH
土

CREATES

金

HOLDS

WATER

METAL

nature. The five elements are wood, fire, earth, metal, and water. This theory significantly influences East Asian culture, including medicine, astrology, design (feng shui), music, and martial arts. The Mandarin Chinese translation of five elements is "wu xing"—wu means "five" and xing means "movement, process, or behavior." Thus, some consider the term "five phases" to be a more accurate translation and description of this philosophy.

Each element is associated with a Zang (Yin) organ and various aspects of nature, such as the seasons, emotions, senses, colors, and sounds. Notably, the elemental associations are tidy categories that can also be used for diagnosis. For example, when a person has brittle nails and eye issues (i.e., redness, dryness, blurred vision, floaters), I immediately consider if there is an underlying wood imbalance connected to the

nails, eyes, and Liver. When someone comes to me with cravings for sweets, I consider an earth imbalance which might also be connected to weak muscles and excess weight (damp).

Just as in nature, the elements follow cycles of generation and destruction or life and death. The generation cycle (Sheng cycle) signals how the elements feed into one another. The clockwise movement around the five-element chart represents how wood feeds fire, fire regenerates the earth, earth bears metal, metal collects water, and water grows wood. The destruction cycle (Ko cycle) is more nuanced and follows the path of a five-pointed star. It illustrates how imbalances in one organ affect the other organs. For example, if there is an issue with the wood element (Liver Qi stagnation), it will attack and weaken the earth element across from it (Spleen Qi deficiency). Five element theory is a stand-alone philosophy that is distinct from yet overlaps with the Zangfu organ theory.

Zangfu Organ Theory

The energetic organs in Zangfu organ theory are separate from our everyday understudying of the organs in biomedicine. They support the production, maintenance, transformation, and movement of Qi, Blood, and the vital substances and are capitalized in writing to distinguish them from anatomical organs. While Zangfu energetic organs are loosely related to the anatomical organs, they are more importantly associated with specific functional relationships,

opposite:
The Five Element Association Chart

Asian American Herbalism

Element	wood	fire	earth	metal	water
Zang (Yin) Organ	liver	heart	spleen	lung	kidney
Fu (Yang) Organ	gallbladder	small intestine	stomach	large intestine	bladder
Season	spring	summer	late summer	autumn	winter
Climate	wind	heat	damp	dry	cold
Tissue	tendons nails	blood vessels complexion	muscles lips	skin body hair	bones hair
Sense Organ	eyes	tongue	mouth	nose	ears
Emotion in Balance	discernment patience	insight optimism	integrity empathy	inspired spiritual	wise aware
Emotional Disharmony	anger unfocused	mania apathy	worry needy	grief emptiness	fear recklessness
Taste	sour	bitter	sweet	pungent spicy	salty
Sound	shouting	laughing	singing	weeping	groaning
Color	green	red	yellow	white	indigo

as seen in the element association chart on page 49. One of the most common things I tell patients is that issues with the energetic Liver (i.e., Liver Qi stagnation) don't mean that something is wrong with the physical liver! On the contrary, issues with the Zangfu organs are rooted in energetic imbalances rather than physical disease.

The Zangfu organ system is the primary theory used in traditional Chinese medicine because it is an efficient, systematized way to diagnose and treat illness. For those same reasons, it is the primary diagnostic tool for Chinese medicine and acupuncture schools in America, as it lends itself well to standardized testing for medical licensing.

Each Zangfu organ has various associations that reflect one's health. For example, the Lung physically manifests in the skin and is emotionally connected to grief. So, when someone has skin issues, I always consider if there is an issue with the Lung. The Lung's connection to grief can be felt as a heaviness in the chest or as cough, shortness of breath, asthma, and sighing. For more on the Zangfu organs, see the Energetics of Illness on page 63.

ZANGFU ORGANS (YIN + YANG ORGANS)

Lung	Large Intestine
Spleen	Stomach
Heart	Small Intestine
Kidney	Urinary Bladder
Liver	Gallbladder
Pericardium	San Jiao

THE ENERGETICS OF HERBS

Herbal medicine affects changes in the body based on energetic properties. The energetic properties of each herb are like its personality based on its inherent tastes, temperatures, movements, and therapeutic properties. The energetics of the herbs are also a way to categorize herbs, so we know what to expect and how to determine if the herbal medicine is working. For example, the five tastes describe the flavors of the herbs as healing properties. The temperature, or thermal nature, of each herb speaks to how it cools or warms the body. And the herbal actions describe the energetic movement and therapeutic properties. For Asian American herbalism, I've drawn from Asian and North American herbal theories to cultivate a holistic understanding of the energetics of the plants. For the energetics of individual herbs, see the single herb profiles on page 300.

Herbal Actions

Tonic Herbs

Tonics strengthen the body and mind and improve overall health. The energy buzz of a ginseng shot you would find at an Asian market is a perfect example of a Qi tonic. Many of the most famous herbs in traditional East Asian medicine are tonic herbs because they address the profound exhaustion that is so common to the human condition. Tonics including cordyceps, yam, and he shou wu increase life force by tonifying Yin and Yang. Qi and Blood tonics including ginseng and dang gui strengthen the vital substances for everyday energy and vitality. Tonics can also benefit specific organ systems. For example, hawthorn (Western) is a heart tonic, raspberry leaf is a uterine tonic, and oats are nerve tonics. Many tonics have consolidating action that draws energy inward to maintain and protect Qi, Blood, Yin, and Yang. They are also helpful for people with weak constitutions that lead to leaking symptoms, including spontaneous sweating or the tendency to give too much energy away to others.

> ## Considerations When Taking Tonic Herbs
>
> *Tonic herbs are becoming more well-known and accessible as supplement pills and powders. It's often necessary to take tonic herbs over a long period for the full, cumulative effect. However, tonics are not a panacea. Tonic herbs should not be taken during acute cold, flu, infection, or illness, because just as these herbs strengthen healthy energetics within the body, they can also strengthen pathogens. When sick, replace tonics with herbs that are right for treating the ailment at hand, such as those included in the Everyday Ailments— Cold, Flu, and Allergies section on page 156.*

Harmonizing and Invigorating Herbs

Harmonizing and invigorating herbs increase circulation and the movement of Qi, Blood, and fluids in the body. Harmonizers are some of my favorite herbs because they help bring balance and create greater ease in the body and mind. The way a cup of ginger or mint tea settles an upset stomach is the experience of harmonizing energy. Licorice, jujube date, and fresh ginger are often added to tea blends and herbal medicine to harmonize the recipe and make it easier to digest. Invigorators, such as safflower and motherwort, tend to be more aggressive in creating movement and breaking through stubborn holding patterns including Qi and Blood stagnation. Some have ascending energy that draws energy and medicine toward the head, face, and mind. Both harmonizing and invigorating herbs have a variety of uses for the health of the Zangfu organs, body systems, and mental health.

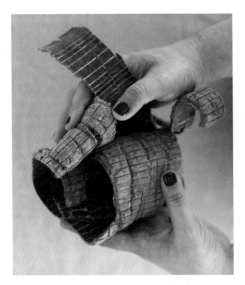

Eucommia

Reducing and Clearing Herbs

Reducing and clearing herbs remove excesses from the body, such as stagnation, dampness, food, Qi, Blood, heat, and cold. Reducing herbs also decrease *severity* of excess in the body, for example, burdock root reduces heat, honeysuckle reduces toxins, and Chinese hawthorn reduces indigestion due to stagnant food. Clearing herbs often have descending energy that strongly resolves and moves things down and out. The clearing action often takes place in the form of elimination via bowel movements and urination. For example, astragalus and green tea clear out dampness from the body via urination.

Dispersing and Release-the-Exterior Herbs

Dispersing energy is expansive and dispersing herbs draw energy and pathogens from deep in the body out to the surface. My favorite use for dispersing herbs, including chrysanthemum and lemon balm, is to draw out stagnant Qi and holding patterns in the body to ease pain and reduce stress. For healing the skin, dispersing herbs also vent or expedite the expression of rashes, itchiness, and discomfort below the skin's surface.

Dispersing energy is also known as releasing-the-exterior, which opens the pores and vents pathogenic factors (i.e., wind, heat, cold) out through the skin, our exterior boundary. When used correctly, release-the-exterior herbs, such as elder and yarrow, prevent illness from progressing and worsening. For more on dispersing and release-the-exterior energetics, see page 157.

The Five Tastes

The five tastes are sweet, bitter, pungent (spicy), salty, and sour, and they are often the initial way we experience herbal medicine. Think of tasting the spice of fresh ginger and how it warms the tongue and causes the skin to flush. Energetically, taste speaks to the healing properties and therapeutic actions of each herb. Not only does bitter taste stimulate digestion by encouraging saliva production, it also stimulates movement in the intestines.

Each taste also has healing properties that are associated with the Zangfu organs. The taste associated with each Zangfu organ has the power to strengthen that organ or, when taken in excess, cause an imbalance. Sweetness corresponds to the Spleen and when taken in moderation, in the form of sweet potato or jujube dates for instance, it benefits a healthy digestive system and overall energy. However, when taken in excess or highly concentrated forms, sweet can damage the Spleen and cause issues with digestion, dampness, and weight gain. Cravings for specific tastes can even be used to diagnose organ imbalances, such as craving sweets as a sign of Spleen Qi deficiency. Understanding the five tastes helps us recognize the vibe of an herb and develop our understanding of how to make medicine intentionally.

Sweet

The sweet taste is a gift that brings joy to the senses. Sweet cravings are often deemed unhealthy because sweet is associated with processed sugars, condensed fruit sugars, corn syrup, and the like. However, more subtle, natural forms of sweetness are energizing,

> **The Five Tastes associated with the Zangfu Organs**
>
> **Bitter** – *Heart*
> **Pungent** – *Lung*
> **Salty** – *Kidney*
> **Sour** – *Liver*
> **Sweet** – *Spleen*

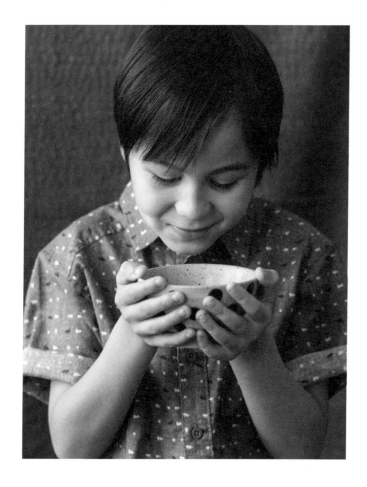

nourishing, and uplifting. Sweet also protects precious fluids, including Blood and Yin, such as when adding honey to tea for soothing a dry, scratchy throat. An excess of sweetness leads to internal dampness that slows metabolism, inhibits digestion, and has a negative effect on daily energy.

—

HERBS: Astragalus, boat seed, cinnamon, ginkgo, ginseng, honey, honeysuckle, jujube date, lemon balm, licorice, lotus seed, mimosa, mullein, passionflower, red clover, reishi mushroom, rice, and tulsi.

RECIPE: Yin Oatmeal (page 113)

Bitter

In modern-day society, the bitter taste gets a bad rap and is limited to coffee and tea in modern diets. However, many traditional food cultures use herbal bitters to stoke the digestive fire after a meal. Bitter is stimulating, as it draws energy downward to promote healthy bowel movements and cool the mind-body by draining heat.

Dry and cooling in nature, bitter also heals dampness and heat issues, such as cold sores and herpes. However, when taken in excess, it is too drying and depletes Blood and body fluids. Bitter directly affects the Blood and is associated with the Heart. Combining bitter herbs with nourishing Blood tonics is a strategy to buffer any harsh effects.

—

HERBS: Artichoke, burdock root, cacao, chamomile, coffee, dandelion, gentian, and tea.

RECIPE: Burdock Root Bitters (page 202)

Pungent

The pungent taste awakens the senses and increases the circulation of Qi. Also known as spicy or acrid, it is characterized by a sharp, stinging, and strong taste or smell. Many common kitchen herbs, such as black pepper, cinnamon, garlic, and thyme, are pungent. So, it is no surprise that they stimulate the appetite and benefit digestion. These herbs are warm and dispersing in nature and are beneficial for people who run cold, damp, and stagnant. However, dispersing pungent herbs can deplete Qi and should be used in moderation for people who are deeply exhausted, constitutionally very weak, or recovering from illness. Pungent taste is associated with the Lungs.

—

HERBS: Black pepper, cinnamon, garlic, ginger, peppermint, rosemary, sage, and thyme.

RECIPE: Kkaenip Kimchi (page 281)

Salty

The taste of salt connects us to our humanity and the earth, and its vitamins and minerals are essential for life and proper nervous system function. The energy of salt is cold in nature, regulates fluids, and has a very stabilizing effect. People who crave salt may have or be on the brink of burnout, exhaustion, or adrenal fatigue. The salty taste corresponds to the Kidney. When the Kidney energy is weak, natural salt in the diet or in a bath is wonderfully therapeutic. However, when taken in excess or in highly processed forms (i.e., monosodium glutamate, nitrates in processed meat), there is a negative effect on the Kidney that leads to fluid retention (edema), puffiness, inflammation, and pain. Salty medicinals, such as seaweed and nettle, have a softening effect, soothe tight muscles, and soften cysts. Sea salts that are high in naturally occurring minerals should be used for seasoning daily meals.

—

HERBS: Chickweed, cleavers, nettle, oat straw, pearl, seaweeds, and violet.
RECIPE: Creamy Nettle Soup (page 259)

Sour

Sour is a fun, provocative, and exciting taste. The sour of an umeboshi plum stimulates digestion, benefits metabolism, and aids in assimilating nutrients from food and drink. A squeeze of lemon in drinking water makes it easier for the body to absorb the water due to the fruit's sour, astringent nature. Sour directly affects the Liver and is beneficial for people prone to irritation, edginess, and Liver Qi stagnation. However, in excess, the sour taste can hurt the digestive system by slowing digestion and absorption.

The sour taste is energetically cool, dry, and astringent. Astringency speaks to not only the taste but also the function of preventing fluid loss. Astringent herbs, including schisandra and lotus seed, prevent and address issues that are marked by leaky body fluids, such as spontaneous sweating, watery diarrhea, incontinence (lack of bladder control), and vaginal discharge.

—

HERBS: White peony root, elder, hawthorn, jujube date seed, lemon balm, passionflower, schisandra, and umeboshi.
RECIPE: Genmaicha Green Tea with Umeboshi (page 201)

Temperature: The Thermal Nature of Herbs

Every herb has a thermal nature—hot, warm, cold, or neutral—that tells us about its energy and healing properties. Some herbs are even defined by their thermal nature. We intuitively know that chiles are hot, and peppermint is cold. However, the temperature of many herbs is quite subtle, such as the warmth of chamomile or the cooling nature of chrysanthemum.

Understanding the temperature of herbs is useful when making herbal medicine, because the function of herbal medicine is primarily based on whether the formula is warm or cool. For example, cool or cold herbs have a slow, calming effect, while herbs that are warm to hot in nature are invigorating and increase circulation. Neutral herbs, such as licorice, are neither warm nor cold and often have a balancing effect on the body. The more nuanced herbal formulas include both warming and cooling herbs to create balance within a given formula.

Warm and Hot Herbs

Herbs that are warm or hot in nature are stimulating and energizing. Generally, the feeling of being too cold is treated by taking herbs that are warm and hot in nature.

Warm herbs also have a comforting and invigorating energy, and when taken internally, they benefit circulation, metabolism, and proper functioning of the body and mind. Fresh ginger, for example, improves digestion, reduces inflammation, and eases pain. Warm herbs are gentle, supportive, and recommended for cold symptoms caused by weakness, including Yang deficiency, which can be treated with warming tonic herbs, such as ginseng.

—

HERBS: Astragalus, cordyceps, damiana, dang gui, elecampane, eucommia, fresh ginger, he shou wu, jujube date, licorice, longan fruit, mugwort, safflower, and tangerine peel.
RECIPE: Fresh Ginger Compress (page 190)

Hot herbs are stimulating and powerful. These herbs strongly affect changes in the body. For instance, chiles are hot and contain the medicinal constituent capsaicin, which is famously used in topical pain relief formulas. Taken internally as food or medicine, hot herbs reduce pain, especially in cases involving arthritis aggravated by cold, damp weather. Hot herbs are used with caution, as they can irritate digestion and be uncomfortable to take.

—

HERBS: Cinnamon, dried ginger, and chile peppers.
RECIPE: Cinnamon Decoction for Cold Pains (page 188)

Cool and Cold Herbs

Herbs that are cool or cold in nature tend to disperse, detoxify, and reduce. People who run hot or feel hot-blooded benefit from taking herbs that are cool and cold in nature.

Cool herbs have dispersing energy and are effective for resolving Qi stagnation stemming from mental and physical stress. Herbs such as mint and chrysanthemum cool heat and disperse Qi stagnation from stress that can show up as physical pain, mood swings, and irritability.

This imbalance of heat with Qi stagnation is so common that most tea blends at my herb shop contain cooling, dispersing herbs! Heat symptoms rooted in Yin deficiency, rather than Qi stagnation, are treated with cooling herbal tonics, such as American ginseng and mulberry.

—

HERBS: Chrysanthemum, elder, field mint, gotu kola, lily, mulberry leaf, sage, thyme, and yarrow.
RECIPE: Elder and Mint Tea for General Wind Invasion (page 159)

Cold herbs sedate and detoxify. Honeysuckle and gentian are cold herbs that address extreme heat and fire affecting the body and mind. Heat symptoms in the body include fever, infection, hot arthritic conditions, and pain. The heat that affects the mind can present as insomnia, headaches, anger, depression, and mania. Cold herbs are often paired with warm herbs to balance and offset a strong cooling effect.

—

HERBS: American ginseng, barley, cleavers, marshmallow, motherwort, mulberry, and plantain.
RECIPE: Fresh Mulberry Sweet Tea (page 111)

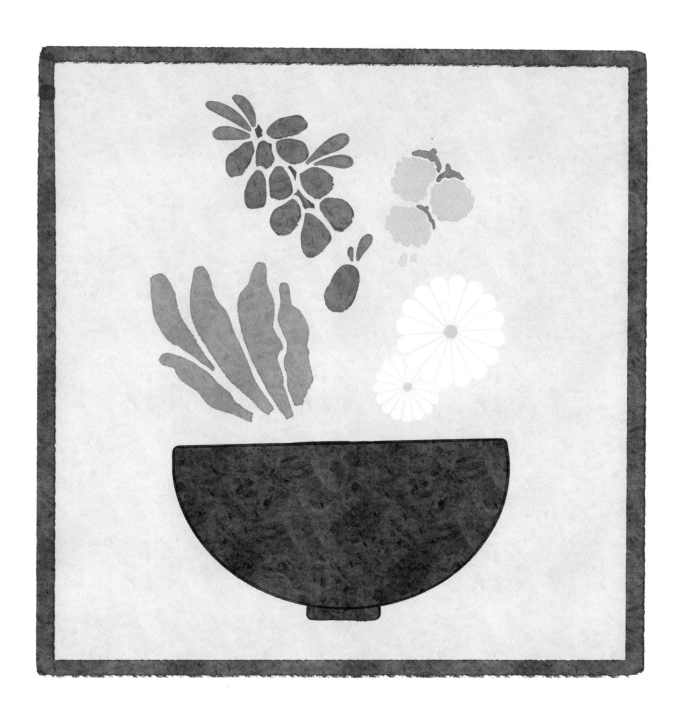

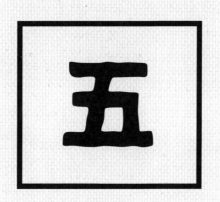

CHAPTER FIVE

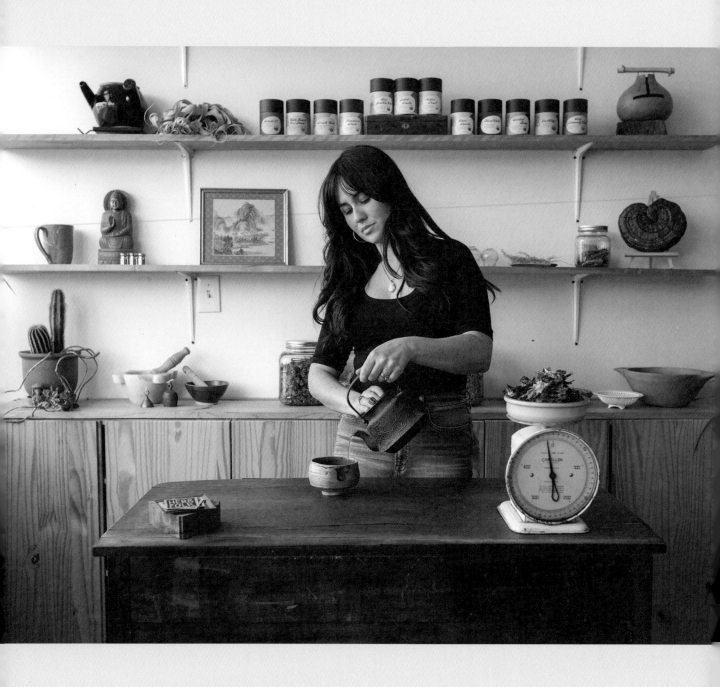

ENERGETICS OF ILLNESS

———

In modern-day culture, we are conditioned to ignore, push through, and become numb to the things that make us uncomfortable or unproductive. And this can make diagnosis, especially self-diagnosis, quite difficult. However, I find that people tend to have a sense of what makes them feel unwell. For example, some people know that they respond to stress with physical symptoms (i.e., low back pain, headaches), while others experience emotional issues (i.e., anxiety, worry, insomnia). Learning how to diagnose energetic imbalances is the key for a deeper understanding of how to apply Asian American herbalism to everyday life.

In Asian American herbalism, diagnosis is mainly done through questioning and observation. The eight principles and the Zangfu organ system are frameworks that help us ask the right questions to diagnose energetic imbalance. Tongue diagnosis, on the other hand, is a diagnostic system based on observation (i.e., observing changes and irregularities on the tongue). All three systems can be used together or separately to offer in-depth knowledge of what makes us feel unwell. And from that understanding, we can take healing into our own hands with herbalism and natural remedies.

THE EIGHT PRINCIPLES

The eight principles are a diagnostic system that brings clarity and focus to an herbal treatment. They apply to nearly every case and are based on the following eight categories: Yin, Yang, excess, deficiency, interior, exterior, hot, and cold. Viewing illness through the lens of these categories provides information on the location and nature of an illness, and why the imbalance is developing. These layers of information give the herbalist information to make treatments more precise, effective, and safe. In Asian American herbalism, the eight principles are the language and system to understand the energetics of illness.

Yin and Yang

Yin and Yang are significant because they are the foundation of East Asian medicine philosophy. Within the scope of the eight principles, they describe two energetic imbalances, Yin deficiency and Yang deficiency. As we explored in the Traditional Chinese Medicine Theory chapter (page 45), the nature of Yin is cold, fluid, and of the nighttime. Therefore, when Yin is depleted (known as Yin deficiency), the associated symptoms are related to heat, dryness, and flare ups in the afternoon and evening. The nature of Yang is associated with heat, activity, and energy. When Yang energy is weak (known as Yang deficiency), the related symptoms are coldness, stagnation, and low energy.

Due to the interdependence of Yin and Yang, they are naturally in a state of balance. However, when Yin is very weak, Yang will overcompensate and cause heat to rise. This condition is called Liver Yang rising and it causes red face and eyes, headaches, migraines, and high blood pressure. We don't typically see excess Yin in the clinic because it is usually in a state of depletion. However, when Yang is very weak, Yin-type conditions, including cold limbs, pain, pale urine, water retention, congestion, depression, and cloudy thinking, show up. For more on Yin and Yang, see page 105.

Excess and Deficiency

When identifying an illness, excess and deficiency are two of the most important principles that I seek clarity on. The distinction between excess and deficiency, also known as full and empty, is a way to understand the nature of an illness.

An excess illness (i.e., Qi stagnation, phlegm in the Lung) signifies the presence of a pathogen or stagnation, such as damp, heat, cold, phlegm, food, and wind. Excess conditions are often related to Zangfu organs, such as Liver Qi stagnation or damp heat in the Urinary Bladder. People with excess constitutions are generally strong, robust, and prone to taking things to excess

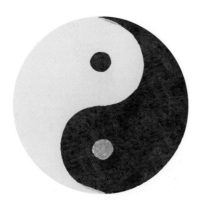

(i.e., overworking, partying, eating, intense hobbies). Excess conditions do well with harmonizing, reducing, clearing, and cooling herbs.

Deficient illnesses (i.e., Qi deficiency, Heart Blood deficiency) are caused by a state of poor health, in which the Qi and vital substances are depleted, and the constitution is weak. Deficient conditions are related to depleted Qi and Blood (i.e., Qi deficiency) and the Zangfu organs (i.e., Liver Blood deficiency). People with deficiency are generally weak, tired, depleted, and respond well to warming and tonic herbs.

Interior and Exterior

Interior and exterior conditions, or internal and external, speak to the depth and location of disease. Exterior conditions indicate that a pathogen (i.e., wind, damp, heat, cold) is trapped just below the skin's surface, such as head colds caused by wind. The body's exterior includes the space between the skin, muscles, and energy meridians. Exterior conditions are acute, superficial illnesses that affect the surface of the body at the nose, mouth, throat, lungs, and skin. If left untreated, exterior conditions have the potential to travel into the body and develop into more complex, interior conditions.

Interior conditions are located deep in the body and deeper than the muscle layer. They are most often caused by emotional strain, such as long-term anxiety leading to Heart Qi deficiency. In fact, any illness that affects the Zangfu organs is considered an interior condition (i.e., Kidney Jing deficiency or Liver cold). Interior conditions can also be caused by exterior conditions, such as when a wind-cold invasion turns into interior wind, leading to muscle cramps, tics, and tremors.

Hot and Cold

Hot and cold describe the temperature or thermal nature of an illness. The simplest way to determine the temperature of an illness is to look at the tongue. In cases of heat, the tongue will either be red and have a thick yellow coat or it will look raw and tender and have no coat. In cases of cold, the tongue will be enlarged, swollen, wet, or have a thick white coat. Hot and cold are also used to describe a Zangfu organ imbalance (i.e., Liver heat) and specific illnesses (i.e., cold in the abdomen causing menstrual cramps).

THE ZANGFU ORGANS

Every herb has a special energetic connection to the Zangfu organs. The term Zangfu is translated in Mandarin Chinese as *Yin* (Zang) and *Yang* (Fu) organs. The Zang, or Yin, organs are the Lung, Spleen, Heart, Kidney, Liver, and Pericardium. The Zang organs are of special importance because they store the vital substances, like Qi and Blood. You will notice that the Zang organs get much more attention in describing the herbs and diagnosing illness. The Fu, or Yang, organs are the Large Intestine, Stomach, Small Intestine, Urinary Bladder, Gallbladder, and San Jiao. The Fu organs are secondary to the Zang organs and are generally in charge of eliminating wastes from the body. The Zangfu organs are all interconnected but each

Zang organ shares a close relationship with a Fu organ, such as Spleen and Stomach.

The Zangfu organs are distinct from the physical organs as we understand them in biomedicine. There are some overlaps in function, such as the Heart being responsible for coursing blood through the body in both Eastern and Western medicine. However, there are also radical differences. For example, in biomedicine, the spleen filters blood, but in East Asian medicine, the Spleen oversees digestion and Qi production. The energetic organs are capitalized in Chinese medicine to distinguish them from the anatomical organs and note their importance in East Asian medical theory.

Key Symptoms of Zangfu Organ Imbalance

Lung – *Breathing issues*
Spleen – *Exhaustion*
Heart – *Heart palpitations*
Kidney – *Low back pain or weak knees*
Liver – *Rib cage pain*

The Zangfu organs are also related to the twelve primary energy meridians, also known as the acupuncture channels, that traverse the entire body. Each meridian is named after the Zangfu organ with which they share common yet distinct energetic properties and functions. While the Zangfu organs store, process, and eliminate energy in the body, the energy meridians are energic pathways that move Qi throughout the body.

Understanding the basics of these twelve energetic organs is needed for in-depth learning of the causes of disease, diagnosis, and healing principles in Asian American herbalism.

Lung – Large Intestine

Lung

When the Lung is healthy, there is confidence in the world and direction in life. The Lung oversees breathing, just like its physiological function in biomedicine. Energetically, the Lung is responsible for taking in energy from the outside (air), assimilating that which is healthy (oxygen), and letting go of that which is not needed (carbon dioxide). In the clinic, I often see Lung imbalances reflected in an inability to process various forms of information from the outside world and an impaired ability to let go of drama, unhealthy behavior, and circular thought patterns. Healing practices focus on self-forgiveness, forgiving others, and finding ways to let go of the past.

The Lung influences:
- Breathing
- The health of the physical lungs
- The health of the skin
- The flow of Qi and body fluids
- Sadness and grief

Physically, the Lung diffuses Qi and body fluids in the body, which manifests as healthy skin and a robust immune system. Lung issues lead to stagnant Qi and fluids, which can cause water retention, edema, and the puffy accumulation of lymphatic fluid below the skin. When the Lung Qi is healthy, there is a good sense of smell. The nose is healthy, well moistened, without congestion or mucous, and the breath is easy. However, when the Lung Qi is out of balance, there are recurrent allergies, colds, flu, sinus infections, nose bleeds, and nasal congestion. For more on Lung conditions, see page 168.

Large Intestine

The imbalance of the Large Intestine is more obscure and not often considered a root cause of digestive issues. Digestion is energetically connected to the Spleen and Liver. However, the health of the Large Intestine is necessary for regular, healthy bowel movements. When bowel movements are too slow or too dry, there can be dryness in the Large Intestine, which will respond well to hydrating herbs, including marshmallow, chamomile, and goji berry. These issues will often also show up via the connection to the Lung—the domain of the skin—in the form of skin irritations, acne, and rashes, including urticaria. Issues affecting the Large Intestine impact our ability to let go of drama or process issues from the past.

Spleen – Stomach

Spleen

In the clinic, when someone reports exhaustion and weakness, I immediately consider the health of the Spleen Qi. The Spleen is responsible for digestion and the production of fresh Qi. It extracts usable energy from food and drink (including herbs!) and sends it to the Lung to make Qi and to the Heart to make Blood. Thus, it is readily benefited by a good diet and healthy lifestyle choices.

The Spleen influences:

- Digestion
- Energy
- The muscles and physical stamina
- The production of Qi
- Dampness
- Worry and pensiveness

When the Spleen is healthy, there is good energy, physical strength, and mental capacity. Weakness of the body is generally a sign of Spleen Qi deficiency (page 86). This commonly manifests as low energy, frequent bruising, and sensations of heaviness or sinking. The Spleen has a strong upward or ascending action such that sinking issues, including hemorrhoids, organ prolapse, and depression, are all hallmarks of a Spleen imbalance.

Water retention and weight gain in the form of dampness also show up with Spleen issues. This looks like holding weight and dampness in the lower parts of the body, such as heaviness and swelling of the legs, weight gain in the lower abdomen, and urinary difficulty. Dampness can also affect the mind, leading to mental fogginess, unclear thought, short-term memory issues, and feeling oppressed or overwhelmed. For more on dampness, see page 270.

When the Spleen Qi is healthy and free of worry, clarity of thought, study, and focus come more readily. There will be an impressive ability to concentrate, think, and memorize material. On the other hand, the Spleen is damaged by constant overthinking and compulsive or circular thoughts about situations, people, and the past. Mindfulness, meditation, and quiet time alone are healing for worrisome folks. Focusing on self-compassion and giving to others from a place of fullness is key.

Stomach

The Stomach is the most important of all the Fu Yang organs because of its close relationship to the Spleen. They are often grouped as the Spleen-Stomach to describe their influence on digestion and the production of Qi. When the Stomach is healthy, the appetite is balanced, and there is an absence of nausea, burping, and acid reflux.

Heart – Small Intestine

Heart

The Heart is considered the most important of the Zang organs. It provides the foundation for overall vitality, balanced emotions, restorative sleep, and consciousness. Like its function in biomedicine, the Heart is responsible for good circulation of Blood in the body. The energetic Heart is so interconnected to the state of Blood in the body that a weakness in one usually indicates a weakness in the other. The state of the Heart Blood is seen in the complexion, meaning a strong Heart will reflect a rosy and dewy face, while a dull or pale face relays a Heart weakness. Holistic beauty treatments with Heart-healing herbs, including rose, hawthorn, and pearl, benefit the Heart and circulation of Blood.

The Heart influences:
- The generation of Blood
- Mental health
- Sleep and consciousness
- Facial complexion
- Joy and emotional processing

The Heart is also said to house the spirit or Shen. Shen translates to both the mind and the spirit, but I think of it more in terms of spirit (page 47). When the Heart is healthy, the spirit has a place to reside, which brings stability to emotions and mental health. The Heart and spirit also have a profound influence on consciousness, sleep, and dreams. Insomnia is often rooted in a Heart Blood deficiency. When there is also heat present (and there usually is), sleep will become more turbulent with frequent waking, disturbed sleep, night sweats, and general restlessness. For more on sleep, see page 228.

When the Heart is healthy, the emotional experience reflects courage, self-worth, and a peaceful mindset. At its best, the Heart maintains a balanced state of joy that is reflected in a friendly, relaxed, and grounded state. When out of balance, the joyful emotion becomes a rollercoaster of excessive desire, compulsiveness, excitement, and mania. Healing takes place through compassion and being more forgiving of yourself. Releasing toxic states of frustration, resentment, jealousy, and guilt are also key. Time in nature, mindfulness, meditation, and gratitude are balms for the Heart.

Small Intestine

The Small Intestine's function is to separate pure from turbid (dirty) and to determine what is useful. It does this in the body by sending unused fluids to the Urinary Bladder to make urine and solids to the Large Intestine to make stools. Energetically, the Small Intestine is about discernment. Discernment ensures that we make decisions in our best interest and have the clarity of thought to know what is not serving us.

Kidney – Urinary Bladder

Kidney

The Kidney holds an elevated position in East Asian philosophy because it stores the Yin and Yang energies of the body. Known as the root of life, the Kidney contains the inherited constitutional makeup that determines our baseline health and development over the course of a lifetime. Thus, issues related to growth and development, especially with the bones, are connected to the Kidney. It's also the central organ for good health and is connected to many vital functions of the body and mind.

The Kidney influences:

- Yin and Yang energy
- The constitution and inherited health
- Sleep and long-term memory
- The ears and hair
- Fear, sleep, and mental health

The Kidney has an important connection with the Heart. Energetically, there is a natural balance between the Kidney's water element and the Heart's fire element. When the Kidney is weak, the Heart fire acts up with symptoms including anxiety, insomnia, and night sweats. On the flip side, when the Heart is weak, the Kidney water overflows, leading to frequent urination, water retention, and swelling in the legs and ankles. In good health, the Kidney and Heart work together to ensure good sleep and mental health. The Kidney has a further connection to the brain by ensuring healthy concentration, long-term memory, and clarity of thought.

The health of the Kidney manifests in the hair and ears. Strong Kidney energy looks like healthy, bountiful, shiny hair, but as we age, Kidney energy naturally declines, and the hair becomes thin, brittle, dull, and gray. The connection between the ears and Kidney energy is a factor in impaired hearing and low-pitch ringing of the ears (tinnitus)—both are indicators of Kidney deficiency. Ear issues are exceedingly difficult to improve in both biomedicine and East Asian medicine. Kidney imbalances run deep, and herbs alone are not a quick fix. For more on the Kidney, see the Yin and Yang section on page 105.

When the Kidney is healthy, there is strong presence, wisdom, willpower, creative spark, and drive. Healing can include time alone, meditation, mindfulness, restorative sleep, and time in nature. On a deeper level, healing will consist of ways to reignite your inner spark or light, such as moxibustion—the burning of mugwort leaves— on the low back and at acupressure point Kidney 3 (See page 287, for more on moxibustion and page 283, for more on acupressure points). And because of the depth of Kidney energy, therapy can help address inherited, generational traumas that are passed down through Kidney energy.

Urinary Bladder

The Urinary Bladder is generally seen as an extension of the Kidney and the function of urination. In the body, it is responsible for receiving, transforming, storing, and eliminating urine. The energetic and emotional component is related to jealousy, suspicion, and holding grudges, so chronic urinary problems can arise or present alongside these mental components.

Liver – Gallbladder

Liver

A healthy Liver keeps us strong, courageous, and resilient. For health of the Liver, harmony and consistency are the names of the game. The Liver oversees the smooth flow of Qi in the body. Thus, any irregularity in the body and mind, from pain to mood swings, suggests issues with the Liver's energy. This dynamic is the most common I see in the clinic and creates problems in nearly all body systems, including digestion, joints, eyes, menstruation, and mental health. Invigorating and harmonizing herbs, such as chrysanthemum, ginger, and mint, are essential for long-term balance. For more on Liver Qi stagnation, see Energetic Healing – Qi on page 83.

The Liver influences:
- The flow of Qi
- The storage of Blood
- Joints, tendons, and ligaments
- The nails and eyes
- Anger

The Liver stores the Blood and regulates blood flow. This impacts the overall vitality and juiciness of the body and tissues. The integrity of the joints is mainly affected by the Liver, and imbalances lead to instability, cramping, pain, inflammation, and arthritis. The Liver Blood also has a special influence on the menstrual cycle. When the Liver Qi and Blood are deficient, there can be delayed, light, or skipped periods. Liver deficiency causes cramps that begin when the period starts in response to the draining effect that the period has on a deficient body.

With Liver Qi stagnation, more severe pain, mood swings, emotional strain, and spotting will be associated with the cycle. A combination of Blood tonic and harmonizing herbs, including dang gui and white peony root, is key for healing.

We can see the state of the Liver in the health of the nails and eyes. In Liver Blood deficiency, the nails become weak, brittle, ridged, and spotted. Eye issues can be related to several things (i.e., allergies and dry weather). However, I always consider the health of the Liver with dry eyes, blurred vision, visual floaters, and chronic irritation.

When the Liver is healthy, there is a benevolent state of generosity, harmony, and creativity. The emotion associated with Liver imbalance is anger, including irritability, frustration, and resentment. Repressed emotions contribute to the stuck energy that causes volatility, anger, and simmering rage over time. When that anger is directed inward, it results in depression, feeling down, or being too hard on yourself. Bring the Liver into balance and healing through acts of service, generosity of spirit, community building, and creative projects that make you feel alive.

Gallbladder

The Gallbladder is an influential Fu Yang organ and shares a special connection with the Liver. Alongside the Liver, the Gallbladder influences joints, tendons, and ligaments. This is key for healthy movement and range of motion— if the Iliotibial (IT) band, which runs along the outside of the thigh from the hip to the knee, is tight, that is a common sign of Gallbladder issues. Energetically, the Gallbladder affects courage, decisiveness, and the ability to make good decisions. As the saying goes, "they have a lot of gall," which tells you that someone has the strength or courage to take something on.

Pericardium – San Jiao

Pericardium

The Pericardium is an outlier of the Zangfu organs. It is technically a membrane that covers and protects the Heart, so its function and influences are connected to the Heart. Pericardium issues typically include the things we see in Heart imbalances (i.e., anxiety and emotional strain), as well as problems affecting the chest and upper body, including nausea and tightness in the chest.

San Jiao

The San Jiao, which translates as the *triple warmer* or *three burners*, is unique to traditional Chinese medicine. There is no anatomically equivalent organ, and the San Jiao is more of a region than a structure. The main function is controlling Qi's movement in the torso—the upper jiao is the chest cavity; the middle jiao is the abdominal cavity; and the lower jiao is the pelvic cavity. In traditional Chinese medicine, the upper jiao refers to the Heart and Lung organs in the chest, the middle jiao is shorthand for the digestive functions of the Spleen and Stomach, and the lower jiao is a non-specific way to encompass all the organs in the pelvis.

TONGUE DIAGNOSIS

Tongue diagnosis is my most trusted and favorite diagnostic tool. It is said that the best herbalists can formulate and diagnose based on tongue and pulse alone. I often joke with patients that no matter what they share with me during the health intake, their tongue will tell me all their secrets!

The tongue gives us clear, objective, and visible markers of a person's current state of health. When looking at the tongue, we consider four main aspects: body color, body shape, tongue coating, and moisture. A healthy tongue is pale red in color and moist, with a thin white coat and a consistent thickness to the tongue body. The tongue is a microcosm of the internal organs, meaning that each area on the tongue's body reflects a different internal organ's health. When changes are isolated to a specific tongue part, it indicates an imbalance in the associated internal organ. The most common areas to see changes in color are the tongue tip (Heart), the sides of the tongue (Liver and Gallbladder), and the center (Spleen and Stomach).

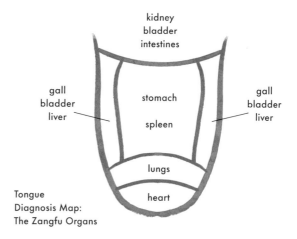

Tongue Diagnosis Map: The Zangfu Organs

kidney
bladder
intestines

gall bladder liver

stomach

spleen

gall bladder liver

lungs

heart

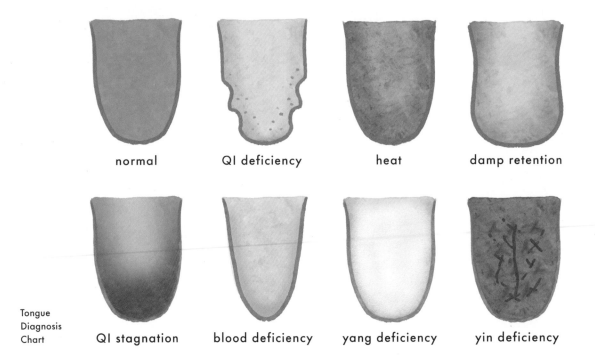

normal   QI deficiency   heat   damp retention

Tongue
Diagnosis
Chart

QI stagnation   blood deficiency   yang deficiency   yin deficiency

When I read the tongue, I expect to confirm what the patient has told me during the question portion of the health intake. For example, I expect a person who has reported debilitating anxiety to have a red tongue tip indicating Heart heat. Next, I consider anything that is surprising or unexpected on the tongue. For example, I assume that a person with insomnia will have a red tongue without a coat, indicating Yin deficiency. However, a thick white tongue coat would indicate a surprising abundance of dampness and relay a more complicated situation. And finally, I look to the tongue to clarify complex patterns and make clear the predominant imbalance at hand. For example, Liver Qi stagnation patterns can be primarily a result of excess (stagnation, heat, pain) or deficiency (Qi, Blood, dampness). The tongue will illuminate if the excess or deficiency is the predominant factor.

It is best to observe the tongue in bright, natural light an hour before or after food and drink. The tongue is a reliable diagnostic tool because it is slow to change, unlike the pulse, which changes at a moment's notice. However, food, drink, and tongue scraping can affect all aspects of the tongue. Black tea and coffee will leave a yellow hue. Heavy foods will increase a thick coat. Tongue scraping will remove coating and moisture. It's best to wait an hour after eating or a full day after scraping the tongue. The following is a guide to what each aspect of the tongue means and how to use the tongue as a diagnostic tool.

Tongue Body Color

In tongue diagnosis, body color is particularly important because it shows the general state of health. The color of the tongue body gives us information on the state of Qi, Blood, and body temperature. A healthy tongue has a pale red body that is uniform in color.

Three colors indicate disharmony: pale pink, red, and purple. Pale pink indicates deficiency, red indicates heat, and purple indicates stagnation. A pale pink tongue reflects Qi deficiency, a pale tongue that is too wet reflects Yang deficiency, and a pale tongue that is slightly dry reflects Blood deficiency. Redness with a normal or thick tongue coat represents an excess internal heat, while redness with a patchy or peeling tongue coat that is dried up is due to Yin deficient heat. The intensity of the color reflects the severity of the condition, for example, a crimson red color indicates severe heat. Purple signals stagnation, with light purple indicating Qi stagnation, and dark purple indicating Blood stagnation.

Tongue Body Shape

The shape of the tongue indicates the state of Blood and Qi, as well as excess and deficiency symptoms. A healthy tongue body is medium in thickness, with a smooth, intact surface, and sits comfortably in the mouth without pressing into the teeth. It's filled with good Blood and Yin fluids. Thus, a thin tongue body indicates a deficiency of Blood or Yin. A thin body with pale color indicates Blood deficiency, while a thin body with red color and a scanty or peeled coat indicates Yin deficiency with heat.

A swollen tongue indicates a deficient condition (Qi or Yang deficiency) that has given way to an excess condition (damp, phlegm, heat). Tooth-marked tongues are very common and indicate a Spleen Qi deficiency with dampness. When the tongue is swollen in a particular area of the tongue, it represents heat or dampness in that specific internal organ. Irritable, edgy, exhausted patients often present with swollen sides of the tongue body (Liver Qi stagnation with heat). Anxious, restless, insomnia patients tend to have a red, swollen tongue tip (Heart heat).

Cracks in the tongue body indicate heat and dryness—the presence of heat dries up and cracks the surface of the tongue. The most common are Stomach and Heart cracks. Stomach cracks are short, superficial cracks in the center of the tongue that indicate digestion issues. A deep and wide Stomach crack indicates severe or long-term problems with digestion. A Heart crack that runs deeply along the midline of the tongue and reaches to the tip of the tongue indicates long-term emotional stress or a tendency to insomnia and mental instability.

Tongue Coat

The tongue coat is the layer of moisture that sits atop the tongue body. A healthy tongue coat has a smooth intact surface with a thin clear or white appearance. Changes in a healthy tongue coat indicate heat, cold, excess, or deficiency conditions. This is an essential tool for diagnosing the presence of dampness or Yin deficiency. The absence of a coat is a sign of Yin deficiency, and the tongue will appear tender, raw, peeled, and cracked. A thick coat indicates dampness and is a visual representation of the thick, dirty nature of dampness. A thick coat can be white, yellow, gray, or black. The most common are thick white coats, which indicate cold and dampness, and thick yellow coats, which indicate damp heat. Black coats are commonly due to medication and signal extreme heat or cold— the thicker the tongue coating, the more severe the pathogenic factor.

Tongue Moisture

Tongue moisture tells us about the state of the body fluids. A regular tongue should be slightly moist, indicating good hydration and the proper transformation and movement of Qi. A tongue that is too wet relays a buildup of dampness due to a weak Yang energy. If the tongue becomes slippery wet or sticky, then retention of damp or phlegm is at play. A dry tongue always indicates heat and is also usually red in color. Just as a kettle will scorch if left on a hot stove for too long, body fluids dry up when there is too much heat.

What is an illness?

An illness is a period of sickness or feeling unwell. In Asian American herbalism, illness is used broadly to cover ailments in biomedicine terms (i.e., anxiety and headache) and energetic imbalances (i.e., Qi deficiency). The term disease is specific to contagious, infectious diseases, such as the flu.

---

100 diseases originate from wind, cold, summer-heat, dampness, dryness, and fire.

—From the Huang Di Nei Jing Su Wen, an ancient Chinese medicine text

CAUSES OF ILLNESS

The causes of illness in ancient times were thought to be related to one's constitution, pathogens in the environment, or the emotions. And these are still relevant causes of illness in modern day life! The constitution is a baseline state of health that each person is born with—for example, someone with a strong constitution is less likely to get sick. Pathogens are things in the environment that cause illness. And the emotions can cause illnesses internally within the body and mind.

There are, of course, other factors that affect health, such as chronic illness, trauma, and pharmaceutical medications. However, the three main causes of illness account for so many everyday ailments and common conditions that they are the focus for Asian American herbalism. Understanding these causes of illness will empower you with the knowledge to both remedy and prevent sickness.

The Constitution

Everyone is born with a constitution that determines baseline health over the course of their life. Our parents' health influences us at the time of conception and the mother's health during

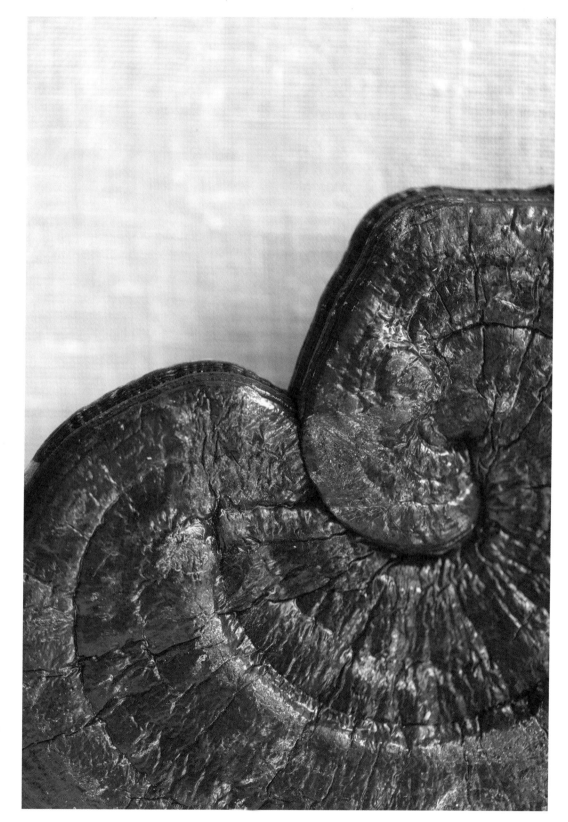

Reishi is a
polypore fungus
(mushroom)
native to East Asia

pregnancy. A strong constitution is the gift of robust health with physical features, such as a well-proportioned face, a strong jaw, full cheeks, firm muscles, and strong bones. Folks with a weak or deficient constitution often struggle with early developmental delays, bone and skeletal issues, chronic disease, and inherited illness.

Constitutions are inherited and based on chance; however, healthy lifestyles can positively affect the constitution we were born with. We can cultivate health with good food, herbs, breath work, and healing practices. So, while a strong constitution is the ultimate gift from our ancestors, true health and longevity are secured by finding healing ways that nourish and replenish us.

The Pathogens

Just as in ancient times, our health is directly impacted by the weather and the natural flow of the seasons. The ancients saw illness as a response to pathogens in the environment, which still holds true today, albeit in slightly different ways. In East Asian medicine, the pathogens include wind, heat, cold, dampness, and dryness. In biomedicine, they consist of bacteria and viruses. Pathogens, pathogenic factors, climates, and climatic factors are common traditional Chinese medicine terms used to describe environmental causes of illness that invade our body's defenses.

The pathogens are naturally occurring climates that we expect to experience seasonally. They only become pathogens that cause illness when the immune system and healthy Qi are weak. And even healthy folks can be affected by pathogens in harsh or unseasonable climates, such as catching a cold after being caught outside on a cold, windy day.

Understanding the pathogens is important to our work in Asian American herbalism, because they are the language we use to describe illnesses—the pathogens both name and describe illnesses. For example, water retention is a damp condition caused by a buildup of dampness. Pathogens can appear individually or in pairs, such as the damp-heat of an infection.

In modern times, we are just as susceptible to pathogens in artificial climates as in natural ones. For example, working under air conditioning or in refrigerated environments can lead to cold issues. Long-term exposure to high temperatures and humidity can be a source of heat and dryness.

Wind

Just as it does in nature, when wind enters the body, it stirs up movement within. Wind tends to disperse outward across skin, muscles, and up to the face and head. Irregularity is the hallmark of Wind conditions, which means symptoms that come and go, and issues that move to different parts of the body (i.e., pain or rashes). Wind invasions occur when the wind from the environment invades the body and takes advantage of a weak immune system. It is akin to an early-stage head cold and is treated with herbs from the release-the-exterior category, such as mint, ginger, chrysanthemum, and honeysuckle. If wind is unchecked, it can travel deep into the body and be marked by arthritic joint pain, muscle cramping, dizziness, and vertigo. For more on wind, see page 156.

Heat

Illnesses due to heat are the most common that I see in the clinic. Everything from inflammation, pain, digestive issues, and minor infections to anxiety and insomnia is related to heat.

Heat symptoms include feeling hot, irritability, red skin, red face, red eyes, thirst for cold drinks, strong appetite, burning sensations, constipation, dryness, bleeding conditions, and a red tongue body with a yellow coat. Hallmarks of heat with a deficient constitution (Yin deficiency heat) are insomnia, feeling hot at night, night sweats, low back pain, memory issues, anxiety, depression, dry mouth, dry throat, and a red tongue body with a peeled tongue coat or no coat. Heat is warming and stimulating, which can create a lot of dryness in the body. Therefore, herbs that are hydrating (i.e., Blood and Yin tonics) are important for healing stubborn heat issues. For more on Yin deficiency heat, see page 107.

Cold

The nature of cold is cooling, slow, and contracted. It is a common cause of pain affecting the muscles, joints, uterus, and abdomen. Cold pain is also experienced as chronic arthritis or menstrual cramps that become more painful in cold weather and wet conditions. Cold illnesses often come from poor diet, overexposure to air conditioning, and working in cold, damp environments.

Classic cold symptoms include feeling cold to the core, poor circulation, exhaustion, dull aches, pain relief with heat, no thirst, frequent pale urination, pale face, and a pale tongue body with a white tongue coat. Common cold symptoms with a deficient constitution (Yang deficiency cold) are feeling cold, a desire to be bundled up, low back pain, knee pain, exhaustion, loose stools, poor digestion, and a pale and wet tongue. For more on Yang deficiency cold, see page 115.

Dampness

The nature of dampness is heavy, fluid, and downward moving. It is one of the most common factors in modern day illnesses, yet we don't have an equivalent word for it in biomedicine.

Damp can come from the environment, such as when living in a humid climate or near a large body of water. In these cases, folks often notice arthritic joint pain that flares up when the climate is cold and damp. But most often, illness due to dampness is rooted in Qi deficiency. Damp conditions are marked by feeling puffy, swollen, waterlogged, sluggish, foggy-minded, and heavy, as well as experiencing swollen joints, nausea, loose stools, congestion, urinary discomfort, water retention affecting the legs and lower half of the body, stubborn weight gain, oozing skin rashes, and a swollen tongue body with a thick coat. For more on dampness, see page 270.

Dryness

The nature of dryness is a lack of moisture and quick evaporation. Symptoms of dryness include dehydration, rough skin, dry sinuses, thirst, dry mouth and lips, constipation with dry stools, chronic cough with little phlegm, and a dry tongue with a thin tongue coat or no coat. Dryness in the air and environment can quickly dry out the body, such as with dry sinuses when spending time in the snow. However, the real damage is done when dryness results in long-term depletion of body fluids, Blood, and Yin.

The Emotions

As humans, we experience a broad range of emotions that are natural and healthy expressions of the human condition. In Asian American herbalism, they are consolidated into five core emotions: anger, joy, sadness, worry, and fear. All illness has an emotional aspect, and emotions cause illness when they carry on for a long time, are very intense, or occur with trauma. Emotions that are repressed, excessive, or extreme, disrupt the mind-body balance and negatively affect health.

There is a reciprocal relationship between the emotions and the Zang (Yin) organs and each organ has a special connection to an emotion. When a person is stuck on a specific emotion, there is often an energetic imbalance with the corresponding Zangfu organ. For example, anger will show up as a Liver imbalance with symptoms including headache, pain in the ribcage, issues with digestion, and eye issues. On the flip side, chronic issues affecting an organ will also cause an increase in related emotion.

The Emotions and the Zang Organs:

Liver – *Anger*
Heart – *Joy*
Lung – *Sadness*
Spleen – *Worry*
Kidney – *Fear*

Anger

The Liver is associated with anger, which can also look like irritability, resentment, frustration, bitterness, and depression. Anger is often a substitute for more vulnerable states such as fear, guilt, and shame. Anger leads to Liver Qi stagnation which shows up as digestive issues, including indigestion, gas, bloating, alternating constipation and diarrhea, and irritable bowel syndrome (IBS). Liver Qi stagnation affecting the Heart leads to anxiety, insomnia, menstrual disorders, and infertility. Healing herbs in these cases will harmonize the flow of Qi and address the Spleen or Heart energy. Intense moments of anger can lead to Liver Yang rising, which happens when the pressure of stagnant energy causes the Qi to shoot upward. Liver Yang rising looks like migraines, dizziness, high-pitched ringing in the ears, high blood pressure, red face, and red eyes. Herbal remedies are always just one part of the healing in these cases. I recommend fully expressing and releasing pent-up anger with the support of a therapist for meaningful deep holistic healing.

Joy

Joy is associated with the Heart and is often seen as a universally positive state. However, Joy is a cause of illness in states of overexcitement, obsessive desire, mania, and compulsive thoughts. Unhealthy behaviors that cause joy-related illness include constant partying with alcohol, drugs, and extreme indulgences. Joy affecting the Heart slows Qi and leads to Blood deficiency with memory issues, feeling ungrounded, and overexcitability. If heat also affects the Heart, then there will be anxiety and insomnia with difficulty staying asleep. A red, sore tongue tip is a sure way to diagnose Heart heat. In these cases, Blood and Yin tonic herbs are deeply healing. Herbs with a special affinity for the Heart, including hawthorn and rose, are also indicated.

Sadness

Sadness is associated with the Lung and affects the Heart as well. Sorrow and regret keep the mind stuck in the past with difficulty letting things go. Sadness related to the Lung can be experienced as a heaviness or discomfort in the chest, breathlessness, crying, depression, and numbness. Sadness as grief carries a heaviness, a heavy heart, that can be detrimental to the body and mind. Grief slows the Lung and Heart Qi so much that phlegm can accumulate and cause a disoriented and foggy mind, exhaustion, shortness of breath, anxiety, and a weak immune system. Having chronic Lung conditions, such as asthma or pneumonia, can also leave a person more susceptible to the depths of grief. In these cases, healing herbs, including astragalus and reishi mushroom, help keep the Lung Qi moving, strong, and uplifted.

Worry

Worry, in the form of compulsive thoughts and actions, is one of the most common causes of emotion-related illness that I see in the clinic. Worry is the emotion associated with the Spleen, and it has a way of knotting the Qi. This dynamic disturbs the Mind and leads to overthinking, nervous energy, and the constant replaying of past situations and memories. Long-term worry weakens the immune system, as seen in people who work to exhaustion and then get sick when they stop to rest. Healing herbs, such as mugwort, poria, and tangerine peel, will tonify Qi and reduce dampness.

Fear

Fear is associated with the Kidney. Fear coexists with anxiety because the brain processes everyday anxieties the same way it registers life-threatening situations. This dynamic causes burnout, exhaustion, insomnia, night sweating, and dry mouth. People who inherit a weak constitution are more prone to being fearful, paranoid, and insecure, and they may easily startle. Long-term fear, such as when living in an unsafe situation, makes Qi descend and causes chronic bladder infections, frequent urination, digestion issues, low back pain, premature aging, and accidentally urinating when startled. Healing herbs include tonics, such as oats and schisandra, that nourish and protect Kidney energy.

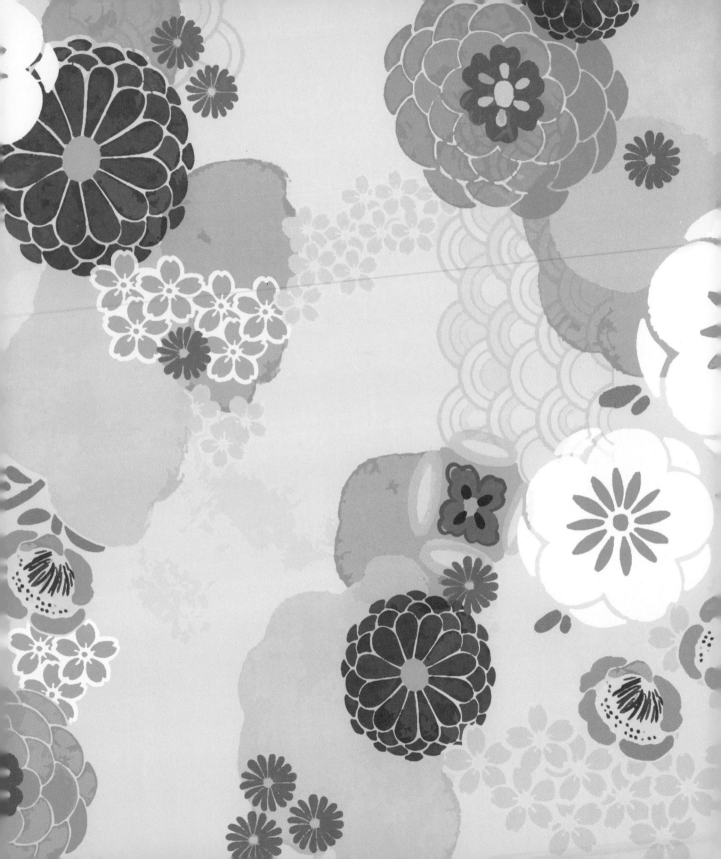

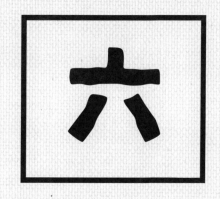

CHAPTER SIX

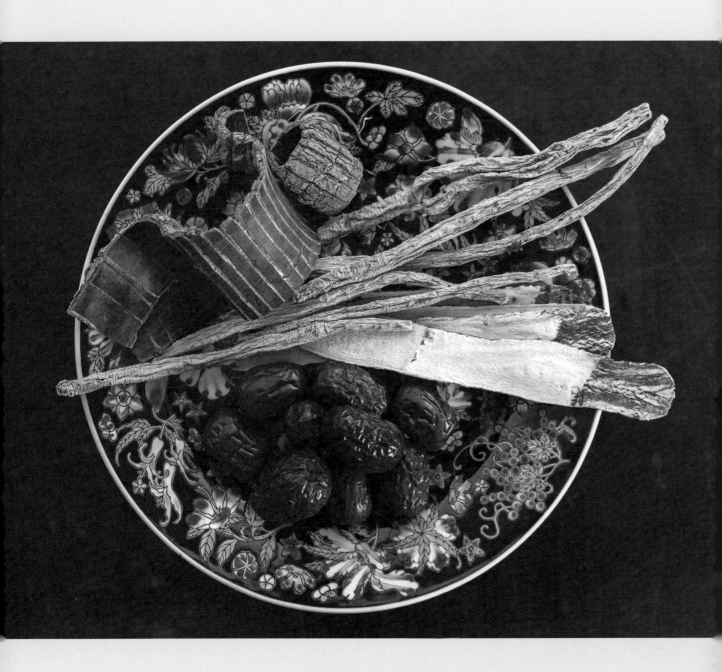

ENERGETIC HEALING

Energetic healing is about improving quality of life by balancing the energy of the body and mind—Qi, Blood, Yin, and Yang. When energy is balanced, there is an ease and authenticity in how we move through the world. Energetic imbalances are not a character flaw; they are a natural part of the human condition. Just as we are all susceptible to common colds, energetic imbalances are not always preventable. A perfect energetic state only happens in theory.

I find that most folks know how they would like their health to improve but are unsure how to create lasting change to increase energy, sleep better, balance emotions, lose excess weight, improve circulation, and alleviate pain. Looking at health concerns through the lens of energetic healing allows us to evaluate not only the symptoms but also their root causes. It also provides us with tools to address issues outside the scope of help we may receive from medical doctors.

Once you sense the energetic imbalance that you are prone to, you can start to work with herbs, nutrition, and healing practices specific to your energetic healing. This chapter is built to be an in-depth guide to energetic healing—how to identify energetic imbalances and healing recipes for you to try at home.

How Do I Do It?

Energetic healing is quite simple to practice. With a basic understanding of how energy shows up in the body, you will find the herbs, remedies, and traditional ways to bring your specific energy into balance.

Learn about your energy

The first step in energetic healing is understanding how energy looks in the body when in balance and when out of balance. Start by reviewing the following Qi, Blood, Yin, and Yang sections. As you read the lists of symptoms for each imbalance, make a note of which ones most closely apply to your current state of health. Do not expect to fit into any box perfectly. Instead, focus on the energy and symptoms you experience most, those that are negatively affecting your daily life. There are usually a few symptoms that will make it very obvious. For example, people with insomnia will focus on Blood or Yin deficiency. Once you are clear on which energy you would like to address, start by considering one to three herbs or remedies to try out.

The rhythm of healing with herbs

There is a rhythm to taking herbal medicine for energetic healing. In the beginning, I recommend committing to three days of herbs at the recommended medicinal dose. This can be tea, powder extract, soup, porridge, tincture, or any combination. By day three, you should feel a difference—even if it's subtle, there should be a noticeable shift in the direction you are looking to go. Someone with Yin deficiency may start waking less frequently at night. With Qi stagnation, there is often an immediate reduction in irritability and tension. Continue taking herbs as directed until you feel a resolution or plateau in your healing. I find that this timeframe is one to three weeks and up to three months for folks with long-term health concerns. When taking herbs to balance the menstrual cycle, a monthly rhythm of herbal medicine can be helpful, as presented in the chapter on Everyday Ailments—Menstruation on page 213.

Incorporate herbs into daily life

The best way to be consistent with herbal medicine is to incorporate it into everyday life. To get a sense of how this might look, I ask clients if they drink tea or coffee and if they cook at home. For tea drinkers, herbal teas are incredibly versatile, and adding herbs to black or green tea is my favorite traditional Asian folk remedy (Hana Bancha Green Tea [page 127] and Mandarin Black Tea [page 90] are good examples). For coffee drinkers, herbal powder extracts blend well with strong flavors and do especially well in drinks with steamed milk (see Blood Tonic Powder [page 102]). I encourage dedicated home cooks to make medicinal stocks with tonic herbs, which are delicious on their own or as a base for many other recipes (see The Qi Herbs [page 88]). And the best options for very busy people are ready-made pills and tinctures found at local herb shops and markets.

Once you find what works best for you, stay curious and try various herbal preparations to keep it interesting and fresh. Just like with our food, it's important to mix it up to get the most benefit from herbal medicine. Overconsumption of any one thing can often do more harm than good.

Be open to change

Learning about yourself on an energetic level is exciting and often life changing. As you learn and experiment with herbs and recipes, you will find that you are . . . healing. And with healing comes change. These changes can be easy to dismiss because they are simply removing the symptoms and ailments that were getting in the way of feeling well. Taking notes in a journal is helpful to track your progress and growth. Healing will also happen because of changes in life circumstances and when undergoing other healing practices including therapy. Our energetic balance and needs change with each season, so it's best to stay flexible and avoid rigidity in paths to healing.

How to go deeper

Energetic healing is deep work. Really, it is *the* work. As you read through the following sections, the energetic theories are broken down in a way that is relatable and accessible to modern life. But even though this information is easy to access, that does not mean that this work is simple or clear-cut. Healing in any tradition is full of nuance and requires a lifetime of learning. When you are ready to take your healing deeper, there is no substitute for working with a professional practitioner. Finding the right herbalist for you can take time, because it is essential to work with practitioners who make you feel safe and heard. See resources for more on finding an herbalist and Asian medicine practitioner.

Building an herbal pantry

As with life, the best way to be ready is to stay ready. As you comb through this book, you will notice an array of items needed to create an herbal pantry. Some herbs can be found at your local grocery store or Asian market. However, many will need to be specially ordered. I recommend starting with the ingredients needed for a few recipes that grab your attention and seem reasonable for your current lifestyle. See page 35 for stocking your herbal kitchen and page 312 for resources on sourcing ingredients.

ENERGETIC HEALING OF QI

Qi is the energy and life force that propels all movement within you and all around you in the natural world. Think of the phases of the moon and the tides of the ocean, the beat of your heart, and the depth of your exhalation. The Chinese character for Qi depicts steam rising from rice, indicating that Qi is both material and immaterial. It is both the ethereal vapors and the material rice. The imagery of rice, the staple grain of the Asian diet, speaks to the fact that the concept of Qi is foundational not only to East Asian medicine but to the culture at large.

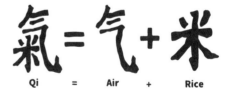

氣 = 气 + 米

Qi = Air + Rice

Qi In Action

Qi is one of the five vital substances that play an essential role in maintaining health. Health depends on the smooth, rhythmic, cyclical flow of Qi coursing through the meridians in the body. When Qi flow becomes deficient (weak) or excessive (stagnation), or takes on the wrong movement (rebellious, rising, or sinking), illnesses may result. We will look at two forms of Qi, how Qi functions, and common Qi imbalances. For more on the vital substances, see page 46.

Ying Qi and Wei Qi

There are various forms of Qi, most notably the Ying Qi and Wei Qi:

YING QI (nutritive Qi) is an internal energy source derived from the food and water we consume. Ying Qi flows deep into the body's interior and internal organs with the Blood.

WEI QI (defensive Qi) is more external, as it extends from just below the skin's surface and radiates out to form an energetic boundary all around the body. The energetic boundary of Wei Qi prevents disease by warding off pathogenic factors that become illnesses, including Wind, Cold, bacteria, and viruses.

Six Functions of Qi

Qi has six functions in the body: It is responsible for transforming, transporting, holding, lifting, warming, and protecting. Here are some common, real-life examples of how Qi functions when in balance:

1. Transforming: The food we eat and the air we breathe are transformed into Qi. This transformation occurs in and by the Spleen.

2. Transporting: Qi transports blood, body fluids, and energy in and around the body. It is a motive force.

3. Holding: Qi is responsible for the integrity of the pores and the holding in of sweat in the sweat glands. When people have spontaneous daytime sweating without exertion, it is a classic sign that the Qi is deficient and weak.

4. Lifting: Qi is responsible for ensuring that body structures are held up in the proper place. Thus, a common symptom of Qi imbalance is sinking symptoms in the body (i.e., heaviness, organ prolapse, down-bearing pressure) and sinking symptoms of the mind (i.e., sadness, depression, feeling down on oneself).

5. Warming: Qi is a source of heat and regulates warmth in the body. Feeling cold all over can be a sign of general Qi deficiency. It's also common for people to have cold hands and feet due to Qi stagnation, which signifies that Qi is not flowing smoothly.

6. Protecting: Wei Qi, often translated as "defensive Qi," is an example of protective Qi. It forms an energetic boundary around the body that wards off pathogens.

Two Patterns of Qi Imbalance

Having covered some of the basics of what Qi is and how it works when it's in balance, let's look at two patterns of Qi imbalance and common symptoms that I see every day in the clinic. Understanding Qi imbalance and how it looks in the body/mind is key to understanding herbs and strategies to improve the quality of daily life by healing imbalance and restoring healthy Qi function.

QI DEFICIENCY: Qi that is weak and depleted. When Qi is deficient, common symptoms are exhaustion, never feeling well rested, issues with digestion and appetite, fatigue after eating, loose stools, spontaneous daytime sweating, weak voice, slight shortness of breath, and foggy and unclear thinking.

QI STAGNATION: Qi that is stuck, tight, slow, or painful. This dynamic often leads to an increase of heat and inflammation in the body. When Qi is stagnant, common symptoms are irritability, mood swings, pressure or pain in the rib cage or mid-back, pain that moves, pain that is dull (rather than sharp), depression, frequent sighing, and generally feeling stuck.

When learning the basics of Asian energetic medicine, I find it most helpful to relate it to your own body. With that in mind, the following allows you to explore the balance of Qi for yourself. Note that these patterns of Qi deficiency and stagnation are very common, and it's expected that you've experienced symptoms from each of the patterns in the course of your life. The key is identifying symptoms that have occurred regularly over the last three to six months. If you have more than two to three symptoms from any one pattern, you're likely experiencing this imbalance. Note that all these Qi patterns are interconnected, so it is common to identify with more than one category.

COMMON QI IMBALANCES

QI STAGNATION
—
tension in ribs,
chest, and shoulders
mood swings
depression
irritability
frequent sighing

QI DEFICIENCY
—
fatigue
weak breath
poor appetite
daytime sweats
loose stools
pale tongue

WITH DAMP
—
foggy mind
heaviness
abdominal fullness
nausea
sticky tongue coat

Qi Deficiency

Qi deficiency often occurs after long periods of exertion under stressful conditions, such as when working long hours, a period of intense study, or when pushing through difficult times. It can also come on suddenly after a high-intensity event. A good example is temporarily losing one's voice after giving a lecture presentation or talking for hours at a party. In such cases there is also a physiological component (i.e., strained vocal cords), but the Qi deficiency is the energetic principle that leads to injury and illness. Qi deficiency is something that you have likely experienced at some point in your life with symptoms such as the following:

- Tiredness and never feeling well rested
- Issues with digestion and appetite
- Loose stools
- Feeling tired after eating
- A tendency toward weight gain and water retention
- Foggy and unclear thinking
- Overthinking and worry
- Spontaneous daytime sweating
- Weak voice or shortness of breath

Although Qi deficiency can affect any of the Zangfu internal organs, it most frequently affects the Spleen, because that is the main organ that produces Qi. When the Spleen Qi becomes very weak and depressed, it is called Spleen Qi sinking, which feels like sinking both physically and mentally—think sinking spirits, depression, hemorrhoids, urgent urination, and bladder or uterine prolapse. If Qi deficiency is not resolved, over time it can lead to dampness. Symptoms of Qi deficiency with dampness include foggy and unclear thinking, difficulty concentrating, a tendency toward weight gain and water retention, a feeling of heaviness or fullness, spitting up phlegm, and urinary problems.

These imbalances are aggravated by stress and overstimulation, poor diet, irregular eating habits, not eating enough, excessive consumption of cold and raw foods, chronic disease, and debility (weakness).

Qi Stagnation

Qi stagnation is one of the most common patterns of illness in our modern culture. The wide range of symptoms is marked by irregularity, meaning that there are periods of increasing symptoms and then times of improvement with little rhyme or reason. The causes of this imbalance are deeply tied to stress, emotional strain, repressed anger, resentment, lack of exercise and time in nature, poor diet, and excess processed foods, processed meat, or alcohol. The most common symptoms are:

- Generally feeling stressed and overstimulated
- Irritability, edginess, and mood swings
- Depression and melancholy
- Dull pain in the ribcage or mid-back
- Pain that moves
- Frequent sighing and yawning
- Irregular and painful menstruation
- PMS
- Breast tenderness

HERBS FOR HEALTHY QI

MOVE AND HARMONIZE QI

—

Tangerine Peel
Chrysanthemum
Mint
Ginger
Vitex
Bupleurum

QI TONICS

—

Codonopsis
Ginseng
American Ginseng
Eleuthero
Astragalus
Chinese Yam
Jujube Date
Licorice
Oat Straw
Milky Oat Tops
Hawthorn

Qi stagnation most frequently affects the Liver because it is the main organ that moves Qi in the body. When the Liver Qi becomes stuck and hot, it is called Liver Qi stagnation with heat. It causes symptoms including red face, irritated eyes, outbursts of anger, headaches, insomnia with dream-disturbed sleep, constipation, dark urine, and a thirst for cold drinks. When there is a concurrent depletion of Blood and Yin in the body, the Liver Qi will rise up as Liver Yang rising and bring on symptoms including migraine headaches, high blood pressure, ringing in the ears, dizziness, a bitter taste in the mouth, and sudden deafness. With Liver Yang rising and Liver Qi stagnation with heat, it is as if there is a fire in the body but not enough water (Blood and Yin) to put it out. This can quickly become a vicious cycle, so Blood-nourishing herbs and heat-clearing herbs must be taken simultaneously.

THE QI HERBS

Makes 1 herbal kit
(enough for 6 cups / 1.4 L of tea
or broth)

INGREDIENTS

10 astragalus slices, each about
2 in (5 cm)

2 dang gui slices, each about 4 in
(10 cm)

⅓ oz (9 g) mugwort

⅓ oz (9 g) white peony root

The Qi Herbs are a blend of herbs that addresses all things Qi, from deficiency to stagnation. Codonopsis and astragalus are Qi tonics that increase energy, aid hydration, and help buffer everyday stress. Dang gui and white peony root regulate the flow of Qi and Blood for regular digestion, a peaceful mindset, and physical ease.

This blend, or kit, is called the Qi Broth Herbs at my shop, because they were originally formulated to make a medicinal chicken stock. However, they are subtle and versatile enough to be infused in fresh water to make a tonic tea and in the various recipes suggested below. Each batch of herbs can be infused into large batches of soup like the Medicinal Herb Stock (on page 274).

In an airtight container, combine the astragalus, dang gui, mugwort, and white peony root to make one batch of The Qi Herbs. Store away from heat, light, and moisture for up to 24 months. Each batch of The Qi Herbs makes 6 cups (1.4 L) of tea or stock (recipe follows).

When preparing multiple batches at once, prefill 3 × 4 in (7.5 × 10 cm) unbleached muslin bags to use as tea bags. Tea bags can also be made by bundling the herbs in a square of cheesecloth and tying the cheesecloth closed with cotton twine. This herb kit can be infused into home-cooked meals and in various recipes in this book.

Buying in Bulk

Tonic herbs like these have a cumulative effect when taken over time, making them ideal for incorporating into daily food and drinks. I purchase these herbs by the pound and make ready-to-use herb kits because it can be challenging to find these ingredients in the U.S. (for sourcing East Asian herbs, see page 312).

TONIC TEA WITH THE QI HERBS

Makes 6 cups (1.4 L)

INGREDIENTS

The Qi Herbs (page 88)

Fresh ginger (optional)

Honey or maple syrup (optional)

Fresh mint or lemon balm
  (optional)

Sauerkraut juice (optional)

Sea salt (optional)

Tonic teas are a modern spin on traditional decoctions, simmered over time to extract the medicinal properties of roots and fibrous plant material. The light, earthy flavors make it easy to enjoy on its own or mixed with stronger flavors, including ginger, mint, or sauerkraut juice. This blend strengthens Qi, Blood, and mental clarity, and benefits digestion. However, Blood-Nourishing Herbs (page 100) or Yama Herbs for Yin and Yang (page 117) can be substituted.

In a large pot, combine The Qi Herbs and 8 cups (2 L) of water. Bring to a boil then turn the heat to low, cover with a cracked lid, and simmer for about 30 minutes, or until the liquid has reduced to approximately 6 cups (1.4 L). Strain the herbs with a slotted spoon and discard. Reserve the tea and add fresh water if there are less than 6 cups (1.4 L) of tea remaining. Store in glass jars in the refrigerator for up to 4 days.

The medicinal dose is 1 cup (240 ml) of tea twice per day for 3 days. It should be taken slowly over the course of each day. Warm each serving of tea before drinking.

For a warming tea, add a 1 in (2.5 cm) slice of fresh ginger. For a sweet tea, add 1 tsp honey or maple syrup. Add a sprig of fresh mint or lemon balm for a cooling tea. For a savory tea, add 1 tsp of sauerkraut juice and a pinch of salt.

MANDARIN BLACK TEA

Makes 4 oz (115 g) loose-leaf tea

INGREDIENTS

2 oz (55 g) loose black tea leaves

2 oz (55 g) loose Earl Grey tea leaves

1 Tbsp aged tangerine peel (chen pi) or the dried peels of 1 small tangerine

1 Tbsp dried calendula petals

Citrus is a symbol of good luck and prosperity. As a medicine, citrus peel from tangerines and mandarin oranges is used to move stuck Qi and reduce water retention. Here, black and Earl Grey teas are blended with aged tangerine peel (chen pi), and calendula petals. Black tea gently warms and moves Qi in the body, while Earl Grey adds a touch of bergamot citrus oil to the mix. The calendula petals play on the color of citrus fruit and soothe the digestive tract, especially when digestion is slow. Aged tangerine peel (chen pi) is dried for two years and is prized in traditional Chinese medicine for its strong ability to address dampness. You may substitute freshly dried tangerine peels in this recipe, but the damp-clearing properties will be less intense. Since learning the benefits of these dried peels, my mom, Gail, and grandma, Masako, diligently dry the tangerine peels from their tree, so that by the end of the citrus season, our family has a bounty of dried peels.

In an airtight container, combine the black tea, Earl Grey tea, tangerine peel, and calendula. Store away from heat, light, and moisture for up to 12 months.

To make a cup of tea, place 1 tsp of the tea in a teapot and pour 1 cup (240 ml) of simmering water (180° F [80°C]) over the tea. Cover and steep for 1 to 3 minutes before straining. Drink immediately.

Note: This tea is not recommended during pregnancy due to the calendula's Blood moving properties.

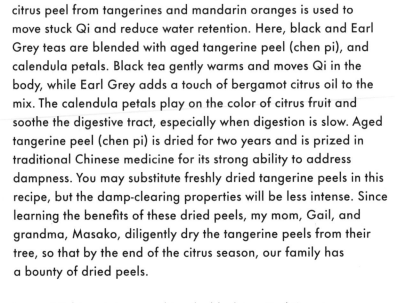

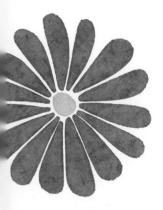

NO SWEAT TEA

Makes 6 cups (1.4 L)

INGREDIENTS

15 astragalus slices, each about
  2 in (5 cm)
5 dried jujube dates
1 Tbsp dried sage or 10 fresh
  sage leaves

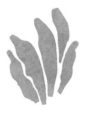

Daytime spontaneous sweating is a unique and pesky symptom of Qi deficiency. This is sweating that comes on without exertion and is sometimes associated with anxiety and nervousness. This is a two-step recipe that combines a decoction and a simple infusion. A decoction is a tea of dense plant material, such as berries, roots, or bark, that needs to be boiled for some time to release its medicine. The decoction of astragalus and jujube dates in this recipe can be taken on its own with good effect, but adding a sage infusion stops spontaneous sweating more effectively. An interesting secondary effect of this tea is that it strengthens energetic boundaries by tonifying the Wei Qi.

In a large pot, combine the astragalus, jujube dates, and 8 cups (2 L) of water. Bring to a boil then turn the heat to low, cover with a cracked lid, and simmer for about 30 minutes, or until the liquid has reduced to approximately 6 cups (1.4 L). Turn off the heat, add the dried or fresh sage, cover, and steep for 8 minutes. Strain the herbs with a slotted spoon and discard. Reserve the tea and add fresh water if there are less than 6 cups (1.4 L) of tea remaining. Store in glass jars in the refrigerator for up to 4 days.

The medicinal dose is 1 cup (240 ml) of tea twice per day for 3 days. It should be taken slowly over the course of each day.

Note: Sage should not be taken when lactating because it will dry up the milk supply.

ON GINSENG

Ginseng is the quintessential Qi tonic and a prized herb in many Asian countries. There are different varieties of ginseng with a range of healing properties, including improved physical strength, circulation, immunity, and mental clarity. Ginseng is a stimulating herb, which means it is best taken during the day so as not to disturb sleep.

As outlined below, choosing the right type of ginseng for your constitution is essential. Taking the wrong kind of ginseng can make you feel ill. Improper use or mild overdose of ginseng can cause dry mouth, diarrhea, headache, insomnia, dizziness, itching, and changes in body temperature or blood pressure. In such cases, discontinue the herb and eat turnip soup (boil turnips in stock until soft, then purée in a blender and season), which neutralizes the effects of ginseng. Seek symptomatic treatment from an herbalist as needed. Tannin-rich foods, including tea, red wine, grapes, and radishes, will also reduce the effectiveness of ginseng medicine. As with all tonic herbs, ginseng should not be taken when you have a cold, flu, or infection as it will worsen the condition.

Red Ginseng (Ren Shen)

Red ginseng is the quintessential Qi tonic herb to increase energy, calm the mind, benefit the nervous system, and give the body and mind healthy vitality. Ready-made ginseng herbal supplements and drinks are usually made with red ginseng. It also increases Blood and body fluids and treats infertility or impotence.

Dried red ginseng can be found at most Asian herb shops or online. It is taken as a tea (1/3 oz or 9 g in decoction) and the dose is 1 to 2 cups (240 to 480 ml) per day for up to two weeks. Red ginseng powder extract can be found online; it is blended into food and drink at a dose of 1/4 to 1/2 tsp per day for up to two weeks.

How to know if it's right for you: A warming and hot herb, red ginseng is for folks who run cold and Yang deficient (i.e., pale tongue with a thick white coat or wet coat). If taken incorrectly, it can cause dry mouth, headache, itching, insomnia, a general feeling of heat, and increased blood pressure.

American Ginseng (Xi Yang Shen)

American ginseng is a common Qi tonic for cases of Qi deficiency and Yin deficiency. It restores vitality and energy, increases strength, calms the mind, and helps with insomnia and anxiety. Its Yin-nourishing properties protect precious body fluids and balance moisture in the body.

Dried American ginseng can be found at most Asian herb shops or online. It is taken as a tea (1/4 oz or 7 g in decoction) and the dose is 1 to 2 cups (240 to 480 ml) per day for up to two weeks. American ginseng powder extract can be found online; it is blended into food and drink at a dose of 1/8 to 1/2 tsp per day for up to two weeks.

How to know if it's right for you: American ginseng is a cooling herb that is suited for folks who are Yin deficient with feelings of heat, insomnia, restlessness, fatigue, and stress (i.e., red tongue body and scanty or patchy tongue coat or no tongue coat). If taken incorrectly, it can cause diarrhea, dizziness, weakness, a general feeling of coldness, and a drop in blood pressure.

Eleuthero (Siberian Ginseng, Ci Wu Jia)

Not a true ginseng, Eleuthero is a Qi tonic that increases strength and endurance. Its ability to strengthen Qi and Yin helps with insomnia, mental clarity, and restorative sleep. In modern times, it is taken to support white blood cell regeneration after chemotherapy and radiation.

Dried eleuthero can be found online or at well-stocked herb shops. It is taken as a tea (½ oz or 15 g in decoction) and the dose is 1 to 2 cups (240 to 480 ml) per day for up to two weeks. Eleuthero powder extract can be found online; it is blended into food and drink at a dose of ¼ to ½ tsp per day for up to two weeks.

Codonopsis as a Substitute for Ginseng

A highly sought-after plant, ginseng is expensive and at risk due to over-harvesting. I, therefore, substitute mugwort in many recipes in which ginseng would typically be used, including The Qi Herbs (page 88). Codonopsis is milder and should be used at two to three times the amount of ginseng in a given recipe. However, the importance of ginseng cannot be underrated in cases of healing from long-term or profound debility.

How to know if it's right for you: Eleuthero is similar in nature to red ginseng (ren shen). See the description of Red Ginseng for more information.

How to Prepare Ginseng

Ginseng is a precious herb, so it is decocted slowly to ensure the complete extraction of the active constituents. When preparing ginseng tea at home, it must be prepared in an earthenware, enamel, or porcelain pot. Do not use metal cookware; it causes an adverse reaction and will not extract properly. Do not use traditional clay pots due to the heavy metal content in the glaze. Ginseng can also be purchased as a ready-made powder extract or liquid extract and should be taken according to the instructions on the package.

Decoction of Ginseng

When preparing ginseng tea at home, it needs to be boiled for some time, which is called a decoction. To prepare, add ⅓ oz (9 g) of ginseng and 8 cups (2 L) of water to an earthenware, enamel, or ceramic pot. Bring to a boil then turn the heat to low, cover with a cracked lid, and simmer for about 60 minutes, or until liquid has reduced to approximately 6 cups (1.4 L). Add an additional 2 cups (480 ml) of fresh water and simmer for 30 minutes more. Strain the herbs with a slotted spoon and discard. Reserve the tea. Store in glass jars in the refrigerator for up to 4 days. Warm each serving of tea before drinking.

NOTE: The medicinal dose is ½ to 1 cup (120 to 240 ml) of tea twice per day for 4 days. Repeat as needed for up to 6 months. For longevity, take a round of ginseng once a month during the autumn and winter.

HAPPY GINSENG TEA

Makes 6 cups (1.4 L)

INGREDIENTS

½ oz (15 g) ginseng, any variety
    described in this chapter
10 licorice slices, each about
    2 in (5 cm)
1 in (2.5 cm) slice of fresh ginger

This recipe is an excellent example of how to prepare ginseng tea. Ginseng on its own doesn't offer much in the way of taste, so when making tea, consider herbs that balance ginseng and add good flavor. Licorice is added to many traditional Chinese teas because it "harmonizes" formulas, meaning it makes the energies work well together and buffers the effects of strong herbs such as ginseng. It also adds a nice sweetness. Ginger is a moving and dispersing herb and works as a counterbalance to the tonic properties of ginseng. It also prevents ginseng from causing indigestion and lends spicy notes.

In an earthenware, enamel, or ceramic pot, combine the ginseng and 10 cups (2.4 L) of water. Bring to a boil then turn the heat to low and simmer uncovered for about 60 minutes or until the liquid has reduced by half. Add the licorice, ginger, and an additional 1 cup (240 ml) of fresh water and simmer covered for 20 minutes more. Strain the herbs with a slotted spoon and discard. Serve warm or store in a glass jar in the refrigerator for up to 4 days. The medicinal dose is ½ to 1 cup (120 to 240 ml) of tea twice per day for 4 days.

Note: This tea is not recommended in cases of kidney disorders, hypertension, and congestive heart failure due to the licorice.

GINSENG QI AND YIN TEA

Makes 6 cups (1.4 L)

INGREDIENTS

⅓ oz (9 g) dried ginseng, any
variety as described in this
chapter

½ oz (15 g) dried mai men dong
(mugwort root)

¼ oz (6 g) dried schisandra

Honey or sweetener, for serving
(optional)

This tea is for someone so depleted that they have generalized weakness, spontaneous sweating, low blood pressure, and a very faint pulse that is hard to find. It is a play on a traditional Chinese formula, Sheng Mai San, used for Qi and Yin deficiency. The ginseng in this recipe strengthens the Qi energy, the mai men dong balances the ginseng by nourishing body fluids and Yin, and the schisandra is an astringent herb that helps the body hold onto the healthy Qi and fluids being generated. This formula is taken until the pulse regains strength and has more force behind it.

In an earthenware, enamel, or ceramic pot, combine the ginseng and 10 cups (2.4 L) of water. Bring to a boil then turn the heat to low and simmer uncovered for 60 minutes. Add the mai men dong (mugwort root), schisandra, and an additional 1 cup (240 ml) of fresh water, cover, and simmer for 20 minutes more. Strain the herbs with a slotted spoon and discard. Reserve the tea and serve warm, adding honey or sweetener, if desired. Store in glass jars in the refrigerator for up to 4 days.

The medicinal dose is 1 to 2 cups (240 to 480 ml) per day for 1 week. It should be taken slowly over the course of each day.

Contraindication: Schisandra can increase the effect of pharmaceutical medications, so consult your doctor before taking schisandra, if you are taking a prescription medication.

ENERGETIC HEALING OF BLOOD

The concept of Blood in East Asian medicine is an interesting topic because it both overlaps and is different from the notion of blood in biomedicine.

Blood is capitalized when referring to it in terms of East Asian medicine and this understanding of Blood with a capital "B" includes not only the blood in our veins but also lymphatic fluids, spinal fluid, hair, and breast milk. The health of our Blood is affected by the amount of blood we have coursing through our veins. When blood is not capitalized, we are speaking strictly about the blood in our veins.

A healthy supply of Blood is essential for good physical and mental health. Let's look at how Blood functions, common Blood imbalances, and how to heal with herbs and foods.

The Functions of Blood

Blood supports mental health, hydrates the body, promotes hair growth, and benefits healthy menstruation. Here are everyday examples to illustrate these functions:

MENTAL HEALTH SUPPORT: Blood is one of the most important factors in mental health and the quality of one's sleep. When Blood is deficient, the mind will be ungrounded, restless, anxious, depressed, foggy, and forgetful. Insomnia is another key sign of Blood imbalance, because a healthy Blood supply allows the mind to rest and dip into restorative sleep.

PROFOUND HYDRATION: Blood is responsible for keeping the body tissues hydrated and healthy. When Blood becomes imbalanced, there are issues with dryness, including dry skin, dry eyes, and dry hair. Breast milk is also an extension of Blood, so any issues with milk supply and lactation go back to the Blood as well.

HAIR HEALTH: Hair loss, thinning, and premature graying are signs of Blood deficiency. Hair is a manifestation of Blood, so the hair is affected when there is a loss of blood. This is commonly seen in folks recovering from surgery, postpartum, and conditions including anemia. Stress is often a culprit for depleting Blood, so it is common for folks to lose their hair during stressful times.

HEALTHY MENSTRUATION: Blood has a direct effect on the quality of the menstrual cycle and menstrual blood. For example, Blood deficiency leads to light, missed, or short periods. Blood stagnation is a cause of cramps and menstrual pain.

Energetics of Blood Imbalance

There are two main ways that Blood imbalances show up in the body and mind. These energetic patterns are quite common, and most of us have experienced some of these symptoms:

BLOOD DEFICIENCY: Blood that is depleted; a state of not having enough Blood to support everyday physical and mental functions. When Blood is deficient common symptoms include dryness, memory issues, anxiety, depression, difficulty falling asleep, blurred vision, dizziness, numbness, missed periods, or low breast milk supply.

BLOOD STAGNATION: Blood that is stuck, slow, and painful. Blood stagnation can result from a trauma or injury like a bruise. Blood stagnation can also occur over time due to Qi or Blood deficiency. Blood stagnation leads to feelings of

BLOOD IMBALANCES

LIVER BLOOD DEFICIENCY
—
dryness
eye issues
achy joints
numbness
dizziness

HEART BLOOD DEFICIENCY
—
insomnia
memory issues
depression
slight anxiety
palpitations

SEVERE DEPLETION
—
thinning hair
dry, itchy skin
withered nails
tics
vertigo

heat, inflammation, and sharp pains. Common symptoms include bruising, fixed stabbing pain, abdominal masses, purple lips, and painful menstruation.

Now let's go deeper and consider Blood deficiency and Blood stagnation related to your own experience. As you read on, focus on symptoms affecting your health now or that are regularly occurring. If you have more than two to three symptoms from any one pattern, you're likely experiencing that imbalance.

Blood Deficiency

Blood deficiency is very common in modern times and reflects what happens to us when living with day-to-day stress and burnout. Blood is all about moisture and hydration, and I find it helpful for people to look at Blood deficiency as an issue of deep hydration. For example, people who drink plenty of water can still experience a surprising level of dry skin and general dryness due to Blood deficiency.

Common Blood deficiency symptoms include:

- Insomnia with difficulty falling asleep
- Poor memory
- Dry skin, itchiness, rashes
- Thinning hair
- Withered nails
- Aching, weak joints
- Depression
- Slight anxiety
- Scanty periods or amenorrhea
- Dizziness, blurred vision
- Numbness and tingling
- Pale or orange tongue, slightly dry coat and tongue body

Blood deficiency primarily affects the Heart and Liver because they are the organs that produce and move the Blood, respectively. When the Heart Blood becomes very depleted, it is called Heart Blood deficiency. It is one of my first considerations in cases of insomnia, anxiety, depression, poor memory, and slow recall. Heart Blood deficiency has a particular influence on mental health because the mind resides in the Heart, rather than the brain, in Asian medicine.

When the Liver Blood is depleted, it is called Liver Blood deficiency and manifests symptoms including vision issues, headache, dizziness, withered nails, aching joints, and various menstrual disorders. Blood is very connected to the menstrual cycle, and people who menstruate benefit significantly from adding Blood-nourishing herbs and foods into their regular diet.

HERBS + FOOD FOR HEALTHY BLOOD

BLOOD TONICS
—
Dang Gui
White Peony Root
Longan Fruit
Blueberry
He Shou Wu
Rehmannia

INVIGORATE AND MOVE BLOOD
—
Calendula
Safflower
Mugwort
Motherwort
Myrrh
Frankincense

HEALING FOODS
—
leafy greens
shiitake
kelp
beets
molasses
dates
rice
egg
black beans
kidney beans
red meat
bone marrow

Asian American Herbalism

Blood Stagnation

Blood stasis is usually at play when the body has fixed stabbing pains. It can stem from acute injuries, such as from a car accident, or chronic issues, such as pain in the hands due to computer work and scrolling on a cellphone. Blood stagnation can also result from depletion because Qi and Blood deficiency cause the Blood to slow and coagulate. Blood stasis can also come from exposure to pathogenic factors including cold. I was a swimmer growing up and spent many years in and out of cold pools. When I started my period, I was plagued with debilitating menstrual cramps that were only alleviated with heat packs. This is an example of Blood stagnation due to cold and could have been remedied by the regular application of moxibustion heat therapy on my lower belly.

Common Blood stagnation symptoms include:
- Pain fixed in one location
- Stabbing or prickling pain
- Abdominal pain or masses
- Deep bruises and bumps
- Dark complexion
- Painful periods with dark blood and clots
- Amenorrhea or irregular periods
- Purple lips, purple nails
- Purple tongue on sides and front

Blood stagnation most frequently affects the Liver because it is the organ responsible for storing and releasing Blood. The classic symptom of Liver Blood stagnation is pain fixed in one location with a stabbing or prickling quality. Blood stasis affecting the uterus is common with painful periods, premenstrual pain, dark blood, and clots. For more on menstruation, see page 213.

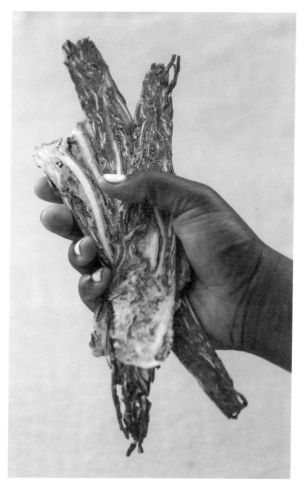

Dang gui

BLOOD-NOURISHING HERBS

Makes 1 ounce (30 g)

INGREDIENTS

3 dried jujube dates

3 dried Chinese yam slices, each
about 2 in (5 cm)

12 dried longan fruits

4 in (10 cm) slice dried dang gui

6 in (15 cm) slice dried reishi
mushroom

This blend of Blood-nourishing herbs addresses the flow and health of Blood. The herbs in this kit are some of the most renowned for their ability to promote longevity and vitality. Reishi mushroom is called the "mushroom of immortality," because it supports youthful energy, restorative sleep, and a healthy immune system. Jujube dates are tonic herbs that benefit both Qi and Blood to increase vitality and glowing skin. Chinese yam nourishes Blood and calms the mind to ease mental chatter. Dang gui is important in this mix because of its Blood invigorating properties; it also balances the tonic effects of the other herbs and prevents them from becoming too cloying.

In an airtight container, combine the jujube dates, Chinese yam, longan fruits, dang gui, and reishi mushroom to make one batch of Blood-Nourishing Herbs. Store away from heat, light, and moisture for up to 24 months. When preparing multiple batches at once, prefill 3 × 4 in (7.5 × 10 cm) unbleached muslin bags to use as tea bags. Tea bags can also be made by bundling the herbs in a square of cheesecloth and tying the cheesecloth closed with cotton twine. This kit can be infused into home-cooked meals and many of the recipes in this book.

FLORAL BLACK TEA LATTE

Serves 1

INGREDIENTS

3 oz (85 g) loose black tea leaves

1 Tbsp dried rosebuds or petals, plus a petal for serving

1 Tbsp dried lemon balm

1 Tbsp safflower petals

½ cup (120 ml) milk or nondairy milk alternative

½ tsp Blood Tonic Powder (recipe follows)

1 tsp honey, or more as needed

Ground cinnamon, for serving

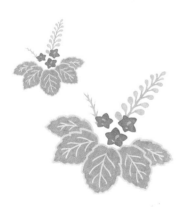

Here is a tea blend to ease stress, tension, and everyday pains. Black tea is a warming and hearty base for carrying a variety of herbs and flowers. The rose in this recipe is a harmonizer, as it gently moves Blood and benefits the flow of energy in the body. It also balances the overall energy of the recipe. Safflower petals are so powerful at moving Blood that they can ease physical pains when taken in small amounts, slowly, and over time. Finally, the milk adds a layer of rich Yin moisture and is a vehicle for the tonic powders. You may substitute a single powdered herbal extract (i.e., chaga or reishi mushroom) in place of the Blood Tonic powder in this recipe for similar effects.

In an airtight container, combine the black tea, rose, lemon balm, and safflower petals. Store away from heat, light, and moisture for up to 12 months.

To make a cup of tea, place 1 tsp of the tea in a teapot and pour 1 cup (240 ml) of simmering water (180° F [80°C]) over the tea. Cover and steep for 3 minutes before straining. In a blender or using a frother, blend the milk, Blood Tonic Powder, and honey for about 10 seconds, or until frothy and just incorporated. Pour the tea into a mug and top with the frothed milk, a sprinkle of cinnamon, and a rose petal.

Contraindication: This tea is not recommended during pregnancy due to the safflower.

BLOOD TONIC POWDER

Makes 5 oz (140 g)

INGREDIENTS

2 oz (55 g) he shou wu powder
    extract

2 oz (55 g) chaga mushroom
    powder extract

1 oz (30 g) reishi mushroom
    powder extract

In an airtight container, combine the he shou wu, chaga mushroom, and reishi mushroom and mix well. Store away from heat, light, and moisture for up to 12 months. Use this powder in tea lattes, coffee drinks, and everyday meals like soups.

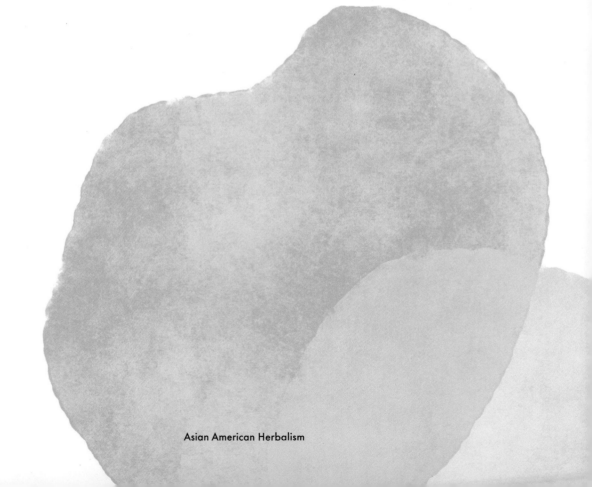

Asian American Herbalism

KINPIRA GOBO / STIR-FRIED BURDOCK ROOT

Serves 4

INGREDIENTS

9 oz (255 g) burdock root

1 small carrot, peeled

1 ½ Tbsp toasted sesame oil

1 ½ Tbsp soy sauce

1 Tbsp mirin

1 Tbsp sake

1 Tbsp cane sugar

1 dried red chile, chopped
    (optional)

2 tsp black sesame seeds

A humble dish often served in a bento box lunch, Kinpira is a quick stir-fry simmered in soy sauce. The star of this recipe is the shredded burdock root, "gobo" in Japanese, which purifies the Blood by clearing heat and toxins. It is a versatile side dish that can be made ahead and stored in the refrigerator for up to 1 week. My grandma Masako often used shredded burdock root and carrots as a base for kinpira gobo, inari sushi, and veggie fritters.

Using the back of a large knife, peel the burdock root then slice on the diagonal into thin rounds. Cut the burdock root slices and carrot into 2 in (5 cm) long matchsticks (julienne). Soak the burdock root matchsticks in water for 10 minutes, changing the water halfway through, to remove the strong astringent flavor. Drain in a colander and remove as much water as possible by pressing with the back of a wooden spoon.

In a wok or large skillet, heat the sesame oil over medium-high heat. Add the burdock root and carrot and stir-fry for 5 minutes, or until tender yet firm. Add the soy sauce, mirin, sake, and sugar and simmer, stirring, until the liquid is absorbed. Serve warm or at room temperature, sprinkled with the sesame seeds and chopped red chiles, if using. Kinpira can be cooled and refrigerated in an airtight container for up to 3 days.

GINGER JUJUBE TEA

Makes 5 cups (1.2 L)

INGREDIENTS

10 dried jujube dates
1 knob of fresh ginger, thinly
    sliced
1 cinnamon stick
Honey, for serving

Ginger Jujube Tea is warming, nourishing, and comforting. The herb combination lifts the spirit, calms the mind, and protects healthy Blood and Qi. Jujube helps to generate healthy body fluids, which benefits circulation. Because of its warming effect on the belly, this tea is also helpful for reducing nausea and indigestion.

In a medium sized pot, combine the jujube dates, ginger, cinnamon and 5 cups (1.2 L) of water. Bring to a boil then turn the heat to low and simmer covered for 30 minutes. Pour the tea through a large fine-mesh sieve into a large bowl. Use the back of a wooden spoon to mash the jujube pulp through the sieve then discard the herbs. Drink warm, adding honey if desired. Store in glass jars in the refrigerator for up to 3 days.

The medicinal dose is 1 cup (240 ml) twice per day for 3 days. It should be taken slowly over the course of each day.

Note: This tea is not recommended during pregnancy due to the cinnamon.

ENERGETIC HEALING OF YIN AND YANG

Yin and Yang are natural phenomena that represent the fundamental dualities of life—life and death, activity and rest, darkness and light. As we see in the iconic Yin Yang symbol, the Yang aspect (the light side of the symbol) contains a seed of the Yin aspect (the dark side of the symbol) and vice versa. Yin and Yang are complementary states of matter, constantly transforming into one another. A great example of this transformation is the seasons, which effortlessly flow from one to the next. Yin and Yang also cycle with purpose over the course of one's life, allowing growth and change to happen rhythmically and according to the laws of nature. And when the laws of nature and the balance of Yin and Yang are violated illness results.

Yin is associated with fluids including Blood and elements with qualities that are cold, wet, soft, and slow. A person with more Yin will run cold and like to be covered with blankets, have a soft round body, and be prone to dryness and a desire for warm drinks. When Yin is depleted in the body, the symptoms include insomnia, night sweats, dryness, anxiety, and a restless mind.

Yang is associated with Qi energy and elements with qualities that are hot, dry, hard, and swift. A person with more Yang will tend to run hot, crave constant activity, have a quick mind, and prefer cold foods. When Yang is weak in the body, the symptoms include feeling cold, fatigue, water retention, digestive upset, and a waning libido.

Yin and Yang Deficiency

Yin and Yang imbalance is always rooted in not having enough energy—a state of depletion and weakness. Yin and Yang energies are the strongest when we are young and naturally decline with age. So, it is common to associate Yin and Yang imbalances with signs of aging, including low back pain, insomnia, memory issues, and poor circulation. However, people of all ages can have Yin and Yang imbalances in times of stress, illness, or injury.

Yin and Yang imbalances can be challenging to heal because they are a sign of aging or profound exhaustion. Yin and Yang do not stagnate, and it is not possible to have too much Yin or too much Yang. When there seems to be too much Yin or Yang in the body, it is a reflection of Yin and Yang being out of balance rather than either being in excess. In terms of illness, there is only Yin deficiency and Yang deficiency.

When Yin is deficient, common symptoms are insomnia, difficulty staying asleep, poor memory, dryness, thinning hair, and exhaustion. More severe Yin deficiency leads to deficient heat, which

Yin and yang are the laws of heaven and earth, the great framework of everything, the parents of change, the root and beginning of life and death…

—From the Huang Di Nei Jing Su Wen, an ancient Chinese medicine text looks like night sweats, hot hands and feet at night, anxiety, and mental restlessness.

When Yang is deficient common symptoms are constantly feeling tired, low back pain, swollen ankles, chronic loose stools, and decreased libido. More severe Yang deficiency leads to deficient cold, which presents as feeling cold to the core, waking early in the morning with watery stools, infertility, and decreased sexual function.

Yin and Yang patterns are deeply interconnected, and it is possible to have both Yin and Yang deficiency simultaneously. Yin and Yang deficiency is more common in older folks because they parallel signs of the natural aging process. Yin and Yang deficiency also often results from long-term Qi and Blood deficiency, as seen in people with severe or chronic health concerns. As you read on, note if you are experiencing more than a few symptoms from each pattern. The key here is to determine if these symptoms occur regularly and in a way that negatively affects daily life. Otherwise, see the previous sections on Qi and Blood, for more familiar patterns of illness.

The Yin and Yang of Aging

Unlike in Asian traditions, modern American culture does not hold elders in high esteem. Elders are not sought for council or to share the precious wisdom that only comes with life experience. If anything, they are ignored, infantilized, and forgotten. However, there is no escaping age. The natural waning of energy and vitality affects us all in different ways. Yin and Yang are at their peak when we are born and naturally decline over the course of a lifetime. With age, folks notice a more significant depletion of Yin, Yang, or a combination of the two.

Graceful aging depends on many factors, including the things we put in our bodies. No one herb will increase the length of one's life but understanding the nature of Yin and Yang tonics is one place to start. The folklore of tonic herbs has

YIN + YANG DEFICIENCY SYMPTOMS

YIN DEFICIENCY
—
feeling warm
insomnia
night sweats
anxiety
worry
poor memory
dry mouth
constipation

BOTH
—
exhaustion
low back pain
achy knees
depression
infertility

YANG DEFICIENCY
—
feeling cold
weakness
water retention
apathy
lack of willpower
decreased libido
frequent urination
diarrhea

Asian American Herbalism

always been about cultivating a long life with the sparkle of a wise presence. The goal is not to stay young but to live long and well.

Yin Deficiency

Yin deficiency tends to be chronic with a gradual, lingering nature. This type of illness often occurs after long periods of exertion under stressful conditions, such as when working at a high-pressure job, taking care of young kids or elders, or under the emotional toll of grieving. Yin deficiency symptoms mirror those of menopause, postpartum, burnout, and healing from chronic illness. Yin deficiency can also be seen as part of the natural arc of growing older.

Yin deficiency most frequently affects the Kidney because it is the main organ that produces Yin. When Kidney Yin becomes very weak, it is called Kidney Yin deficiency, and includes all the above symptoms, particularly low back pain, insomnia with night sweats, and waking at night with difficulty falling back asleep. Night sweating from Yin deficiency is due to a deep weakness in which the body can't "hold in" Qi at night, so Yin fluids leak out of the pores as sweat. This dynamic can be addressed with Yin tonic herbs, including the recipes in this section, and the No Sweat Tea recipe (page 91) in the Energetic Healing of Qi section.

Yin deficiency almost invariably presents with some heat, because that is how Yin is burned up, damaged, and depleted. Yin deficiency with heat symptoms, including hot flashes, night sweating to the point of drenching the sheets, dry mouth, and ringing in the ears, is more pronounced in the evening. When this heat aggravates the Mind, it causes emotional distress with more severe insomnia, mental restlessness, uneasiness, anxiety, and worry. Yin deficiency is caused by overworking, old age, emotional strain, lifestyle habits such as excessive sexual activity, and loss of Body Fluids due to high fever, long-term illness, or trauma. Yin deficiency can also result from excessive use of Yang tonic herbs that tend to be warming and stimulating.

Signs of Yin Deficiency:

Experiencing at least three of these symptoms is an indication of Yin deficiency.

- *Tiredness; never feeling well rested*
- *Low back and hip pain*
- *Achy knees*
- *Insomnia with difficulty staying asleep*
- *Night sweats*
- *Poor memory*
- *Anxiety; depression*
- *Lack of willpower and drive*
- *Constipation*
- *Dry mouth and throat*
- *Infertility*
- *Nocturnal emissions; premature ejaculation*
- *Red tongue with a raw texture or peeled coat*

YIN MUSHROOM POWDER

Makes 7 oz (200 g)

INGREDIENTS

2 oz (55 g) white wood ear
   mushroom powder extract

2 oz (55 g) lion's mane
   mushroom powder extract

2 oz (55 g) turkey tail mushroom
   powder extract

1 oz (30 g) reishi mushroom
   powder extract

This Yin Mushroom Powder mix contains three potent medicinal mushrooms that replenish deep energy stores. They have a mild, nutty flavor that mixes well with savory meals, sweet baked goods, and tea lattes. Mushroom powders are potent medicine, which makes them a bit pricy, but they are worth the investment because their medicinal constituents are easy for our bodies to absorb.

In an airtight container, combine the white wood ear, lion's mane, turkey tail, and reishi mushroom powder extracts and mix well. Store away from heat, light, and moisture for up to 12 months.

Use ¼ to ½ tsp of this powder in tea and other drinks, baked goods, and everyday meals. Try it in place of the Blood Tonic Powder in the Floral Black Tea Latte (page 101).

NORI EGG DROP SOUP

Serves 4

INGREDIENTS

4 dried shiitake mushrooms

½ cup (10 g) dried, unprocessed nori seaweed (or 2 nori sheets)

Toasted sesame oil, for brushing nori, plus more for serving

4 cups (960 ml) chicken stock

1 Tbsp soy sauce

1 Tbsp peeled and finely grated fresh ginger

2 large eggs, lightly beaten

1 green onion (green part only), finely chopped

This soup is a simple, nourishing Yin tonic. The eggs and nori work together to build Jing essence and a healthy balance of Yin. Nourishing Yin has a grounding effect on the body and mind by balancing and bringing down the Yang energy. This soup also grounds and brings down Liver Yang rising to ease headaches, a red flushed face, and ringing in the ears. I prefer using dried, unprocessed nori seaweed flakes—sourced from Strong Arm Farms on the Sonoma Coast of California—to increase the Yin-nourishing properties and texture of the dish, but the plain nori sheets that are used to make sushi rolls can be substituted.

In a small bowl, cover the dried shiitake mushrooms with hot water and let soak for about 15 minutes, or until soft and rehydrated. Drain the mushrooms then cut off and discard the stems. Slice the caps into thin strips and set them aside.

Meanwhile, preheat the oven to 200° F (95° C). If using unprocessed nori, arrange the nori in a single layer on a baking sheet and toast in the oven for 2 minutes, or until the nori is crisp and their color has changed from purple to green. Remove from the oven, brush with sesame oil, and use your hands to crumble into ½ to 1 inch (1.25 to 2.5 cm) pieces. If using nori sheets, place the sheets on a baking sheet and toast in the oven for 1 minute, or until crispy and light green in color. Use your hands to tear the sheets into bite-size pieces.

In a medium soup pot, combine the chicken stock, soy sauce, ginger, and toasted nori pieces. Bring to a gentle boil. Once the soup is gently boiling, use chopsticks to stir it clockwise while gently pouring in the lightly beaten eggs. The eggs will form thin ribbons that should set in less than a minute. Serve immediately, topped with chopped green onions and a drizzle of sesame oil.

MARSHMALLOW AND ROSE COLD INFUSION

Makes 4 cups (960 ml)

INGREDIENTS

3 Tbsp dried goji berries

1 Tbsp dried marshmallow root

1 Tbsp dried rosebuds or petals

1 Tbsp dried chamomile flowers

Cold infusions are teas that are made with cool water and steeped for longer periods of time. They are best for extracting nutrients from mucilaginous (slippery) herbs, including marshmallow root, chamomile, and slippery elm bark, which have a gelatinous consistency when steeped in water. Marshmallow root and chamomile are tonics that help bring profound hydration and moisture to the skin and digestive tract. Goji berries and rose benefit Blood by increasing circulation and supplementing body fluids. The rose and chamomile also calm the mind and spirit.

In a 32 oz (1 L) glass jar, combine the goji berries, marshmallow root, rose, and chamomile. Pour 4 cups (960 ml) of cool water over the herbs, cover, and steep at room temperature or in the refrigerator for at least 4 hours and up to overnight. Strain and discard the herbs. Store in the refrigerator for up to 3 days.

The medicinal dose is 1 to 2 cups (240 to 480 ml) twice per day for 1 to 3 weeks. It should be taken slowly over the course of each day.

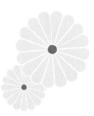

FRESH MULBERRY SWEET TEA

Serves 6

INGREDIENTS

1 cup (140 g) fresh white
mulberries (or ½ cup [60 g]
dried mulberries)

½ cinnamon stick

1 Tbsp honey, plus more as
needed

When fresh mulberries are in season during the summer, this is a wonderful tea to nourish body fluids for constipation brought on by Blood and Yin deficiency. The fresh berries are highly perishable, so you will not find them at the grocery store. However, when you find a local mulberry tree, this tea is a special treat! Mulberry is a Blood and Yin tonic that is especially beneficial for imbalances brought on after periods of burnout and profound exhaustion. Yin- and Blood-deficient exhaustion often leads to issues with insomnia, irritability, fatigue, and general dryness, including dry stools (constipation). Honey is used in this recipe for sweetness and to bring new Qi to the intestines. It's also a traditional remedy to relieve constipation due to Blood deficiency, dryness, and depletion of fluids.

If using fresh mulberries, wash the berries and remove any thick stems. Dried mulberries are ready to use.

In a medium pot, combine the mulberries, cinnamon stick, and 4 cups (960 ml) of water. Bring to a boil then turn the heat to low and simmer uncovered for 20 minutes or until the liquid has reduced by about one-third (there should be approximately 3 cups [720 ml]). Remove from the heat and strain. If using a cheesecloth, squeeze out any extra juice with your hands; if using a colander, press the juice from the berries with the back of a wooden spoon—it's okay if some of the seeds slip through. Discard the mulberries. While the tea is still warm, add honey and stir to dissolve. Serve warm or cold.

The medicinal dose is ½ cup (120 ml) 3 times per day for up to 3 days.

Contraindications: Omit cinnamon during pregnancy. Limit tea if experiencing loose stools or indigestion.

Note: Fresh mulberries should be eaten or prepared immediately, as they spoil quickly once harvested. If needed, store mulberries in a paper towel–lined container in the refrigerator for 1 to 2 days after harvest.

SEAWEED POWDER

Makes 3 oz (85 g)

INGREDIENTS

1 oz (30 g) dried wakame
    seaweed
1 oz (30 g) dried kombu
1 oz (30 g) dulse powder

Sea vegetables are a source of Yin-nourishing medicine from the ocean. Cooking with seaweeds can be intimidating, but this recipe is a simple and useful way to work with a variety of seaweeds. I use this seaweed powder sprinkled as a condiment on rice, grains, salads, and other dishes.

You are likely familiar with wakame (the seaweed floating in miso soup) and kombu, the base of the dashi used to make miso and many other Japanese soups—I often add kombu to the pot when making homemade beans and stocks. Sustainably harvested wakame and kombu are available from quality producers, including Strong Arm Farms in California (see page 313 for sourcing seaweed). A less well-known seaweed is dulse and I love its salty, umami flavor. I purchase dulse that has already been powdered (raw powder, not an extract). This recipe can be made with any combination of these seaweeds.

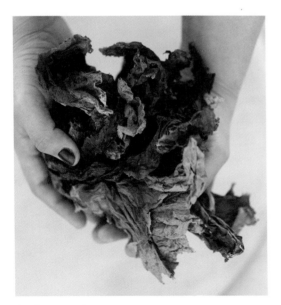

Kombu seaweed

Preheat the oven to 350° F (180° C).

Spread dried wakame and kombu on a baking sheet and bake for 15 minutes, or until the seaweed crumbles and breaks when pressed. Let cool.

Using a ridged suribachi mortar and pestle if possible or a blender, grind the seaweed into a coarse powder. Remove any thick stalks and chunks that do not easily grind into a powder and reserve them for soups and stocks.

Transfer the powder to an airtight container and mix in the dulse powder. Store away from heat, light, and moisture for up to 18 months.

YIN OATMEAL

Serves 2

INGREDIENTS

¼ tsp sea salt

1 cup (100 g) old-fashioned
   rolled oats

3 Tbsp dried mulberries

2 Tbsp raisins

1 small apple or Asian pear,
   cored and diced

1 tsp unsalted butter

½ tsp vanilla extract

½ tsp ground cinnamon

This simple recipe nourishes Yin and increases fluids in the body with everyday foods. Oats are more Yin in nature than rice and are an excellent option for folks with dryness caused by Yin deficiency and heat. The mulberries, raisins, apples, and Asian pear have a hydrating and positive effect on the body fluids. This is especially helpful for people with general dryness that manifests with symptoms including a chronic cough, constipation, dry skin, hair, and eyes. The honey and butter are very moistening and strongly supplement Qi as well. I prefer this oatmeal as a special Yin-nourishing meal rather than a regular breakfast as it can be too sweet for a daily meal.

In a medium pot, add the salt to 3 cups (720 ml) of water. Bring to a boil then turn the heat to medium-low and stir in the oats, mulberries, raisins, and the apple or pear. Simmer, stirring occasionally and adding more water if the oatmeal becomes too thick, for about 10 minutes, or until the oats and dried fruits are soft and plump. Remove from the heat then mix in the butter, vanilla, and cinnamon. Serve immediately.

Contraindication: Omit cinnamon during pregnancy.

Yang Deficiency

Yang deficiency tends to come on quickly with acute, debilitating symptoms. Similar to Yin deficiency in origin, this type of illness often occurs after long periods of stress. It mirrors the symptoms we see in postpartum, burnout, and when healing from chronic illness. Yang deficiency also parallels the natural signs of aging.

Yang deficiency primarily affects the Kidney because it is the source of Yang. Kidney Yang is a warming force in the body, fueled by the inner fire that resides in the Kidney. When it is weak, it is called Kidney Yang deficiency and mainly affects physical strength, endurance, digestion, and sexual function. Kidney Yang transforms fluids in the body and when it is weak, symptoms including frequent urination, edema, and water retention in the legs can arise. If it does not bring vital energy to the brain, Kidney Yang deficiency also causes dizziness and low-grade tinnitus.

Spleen Yang deficiency is another common presentation and shows up as weak muscles, tiredness, depression, and a lack of willpower or direction. Like Qi deficiency, weak Spleen Yang results in an accumulation of dampness. This dampness becomes a vicious cycle by slowing the flow of Body Fluids and Qi, which further weakens the Spleen Yang.

Signs of Yang Deficiency:

Experiencing at least three of these symptoms is an indication of Yang deficiency:

- *Feeling cold, especially in the legs and the back of the body*
- *Exhaustion; constantly feeling tired*
- *Weakness and swelling of the legs*
- *Water retention; puffiness*
- *Abundant clear urination*
- *Urinating at night*
- *Loose stools early in the morning*
- *Diarrhea with undigested food particles*
- *Tinnitus; dizziness*
- *Infertility*
- *Decreased libido*
- *Difficulty achieving and maintaining an erection*
- *Depression; lack of willpower; apathy*
- *A pale, swollen, wet tongue*

If Yang deficiency is not resolved, a more severe presentation is Yang deficiency with cold, which is typical in old age and for people who are burned-out. When Yang becomes significantly depleted, there is insufficient inner heat to move fluids through the body and adequately maintain warmth. This is marked by an increased feeling of cold and fluid retention, or edema, which is dampness that sets in as swollen legs and ankles. A final key symptom is having loose stools, diarrhea with undigested food particles, or "cock's crow diarrhea," meaning that it wakes you at the break of dawn.

Causes of Yang deficiency are poor diet with excessive consumption of cold and raw foods, burnout due to stress and exhaustion, lifestyle habits such as excessive sexual activity, old age, constitutional weakness, chronic illness, and long-term exposure to environmental cold (i.e., cold weather or refrigerated work conditions).

YIN + YANG HERBS

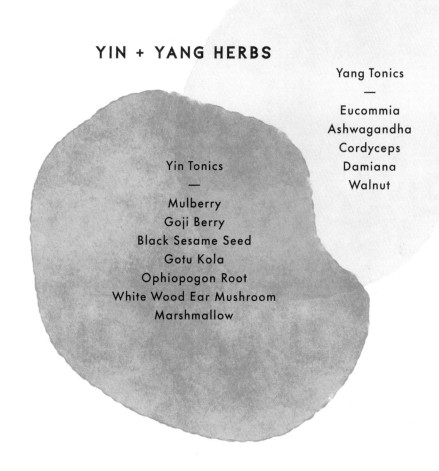

Yang Tonics

—

Eucommia
Ashwagandha
Cordyceps
Damiana
Walnut

Yin Tonics

—

Mulberry
Goji Berry
Black Sesame Seed
Gotu Kola
Ophiopogon Root
White Wood Ear Mushroom
Marshmallow

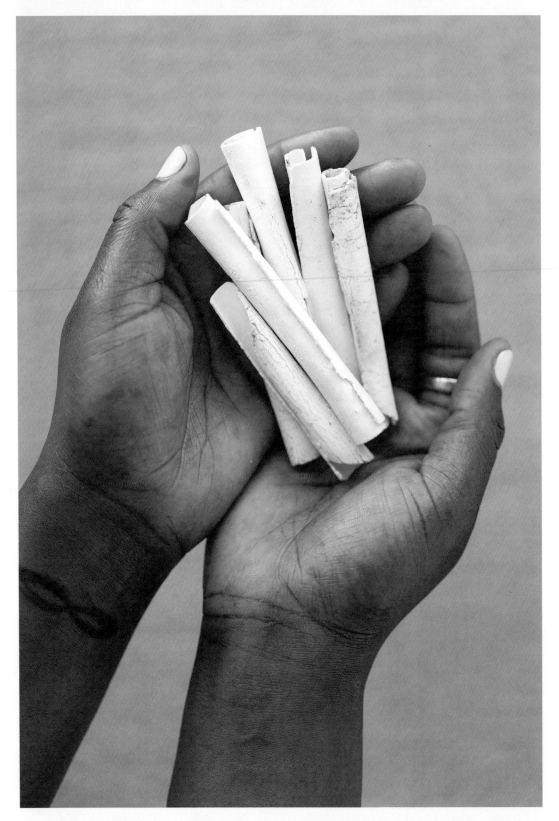

Dried poria
mushroom pieces

YAMA HERBS FOR YIN AND YANG

Makes 2 oz (55 g)

INGREDIENTS

15 dried lotus seeds

½ cup (6 g) dried white wood ear mushrooms

5 in (12 cm) piece dried eucommia bark

3 dried poria pieces, 4 in (10 cm) each

This blend of herbs is of the mountains and forests. Yama means "mountain" in Japanese and reflects where these herbs are grown and their strengthening medicine. It is an earthy mix that balances Yin and Yang energies to warm and revitalize deep stores of energy within. The bark of the eucommia tree is a Yang tonic that strengthens the physical body and helps with aches, pains, and instability. Poria, a mushroom that grows on the roots of pine trees, gently tonifies Qi and clears dampness and water retention that settles in when there is a long-standing Yang deficiency. White wood ear mushroom is a Yin tonic that is used to generate healthy body fluids and benefit circulation. Lotus seed is a Kidney tonic that strengthens Jing and Yin as well.

In an airtight container, combine the lotus seeds, white wood ear mushrooms, eucommia bark, and poria to make one batch of Yama Herbs for Yin and Yang. Store away from heat, light, and moisture for up to 24 months. When preparing multiple batches at once, prefill 3 × 4 in (7.5 × 10 cm) unbleached muslin bags to use as tea bags. Tea bags can also be made by bundling the herbs in a square of cheesecloth and tying them with cotton twine. Each batch of herbs can be infused into large batches of soup like the Medicinal Herb Stock (on page 274).

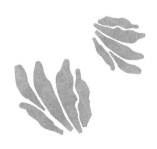

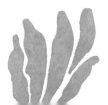

YANG TONIC POWDER

Makes 6 oz (170 g)

INGREDIENTS

2 oz (55 g) cordyceps mushroom
   powder extract

2 oz (55 g) eucommia powder
   extract

2 oz (55 g) astragalus powder
   extract

½ oz (15 g) ashwagandha
   powder extract (optional)

Powdered extracts are my favorite product for people new to herbal medicine. This powder is perfect for increasing energy and balancing hormones including testosterone. It has a mellow flavor that mixes well with tea, coffee, and smoothies. Ashwagandha powder extract can be used in this mix. However, it has a tart flavor that can quickly become overpowering in food and drinks, which is why I list it as optional. For a fun treat, you can mix this powder blend with nutritional yeast and sprinkle it on buttered popcorn.

In an airtight container, combine the cordyceps, eucommia, astragalus, and ashwagandha (if using) and mix well. Store, away from heat, light, and moisture for up to 12 months. Use this powder in tea lattes, coffee drinks, and everyday meals like soup.

Contraindication: This is not recommended during pregnancy due to the ashwagandha.

When to Stop Taking Tonic Herbs

Do not take tonic herbs during the first week of a cold, flu, or infection, because they will strengthen pathogens, including wind, heat, viruses, and bacteria. When sick, it's best to take herbal remedies to treat that specific illness.

SHANTA'S MASALA CHAI

Serves 3

INGREDIENTS

2 whole cardamom pods

2 whole cloves

1 small cinnamon stick

1 cup (240 ml) milk or nondairy
milk alternative

½ in (12 mm) slice of fresh
ginger

1 tsp loose black tea leaves,
such as Assam, Darjeeling, or
Ceylon

1 tsp honey or cane sugar

In my early twenties, I relied on yoga and Ayurvedic herbs to help me heal from debilitating back pain and sciatica. I read about traditional South Asian herbalism and Ayurveda, and took a series of vegetarian Gujrati cooking classes with Shanta Nimbark Sacharoff. This chai is based on the recipe in her book, *Flavors of India: Vegetarian India Cuisine*. The spices in masala chai are warming and energizing. Crushing them releases their volatile oils and makes a more flavorful and fragrant chai. The potent aromatics of the cardamom transform dampness that can accumulate with Yang deficiency. The cloves, cinnamon stick, and fresh ginger warm and move Qi to benefit Yang. And this chai is a traditional way to incorporate herbs into daily drinks. You may substitute 2 teaspoons of garam masala (recipe follows) for the cardamom, cloves, and cinnamon stick.

Using a heavy stone mortar and pestle, lightly pound the cardamom, cloves, and cinnamon into small pieces.

In a small pot, combine the pounded spices with the milk, ginger, and 2 cups (480 ml) of water over medium heat. Watch the pot closely and as soon as the mixture begins to simmer and froth up the sides of the pot, immediately remove it from the heat. Add the black tea, cover, and steep, stirring once, for 2 to 3 minutes. Once the tea is brewed, strain out the spices and tea leaves to prevent the tea from turning bitter and astringent; discard the herbs and tea leaves. Stir in sugar or honey and serve warm.

Contraindication: Omit cinnamon during pregnancy.

GARAM MASALA

Makes 6 oz (170 g)

INGREDIENTS

7 cinnamon sticks

⅓ cup (75 g) whole cardamom seeds (not pods)

¼ cup (30 g) whole cloves

1 Tbsp whole fennel seeds

1 tsp whole black peppercorns

Heat a cast-iron skillet or heavy pan over medium heat. Add the cinnamon, cardamom, cloves, fennel, and peppercorns and roast, tossing or stirring frequently, for 5 minutes, or until fragrant. Take care not to burn the spices. (Alternatively, the spices can also be roasted in a 200° F [95° C] oven for 15 minutes.) Remove from the heat. Once cool, grind to a powder using a heavy stone mortar and pestle or a clean coffee grinder that is only used for herbs and spices. Store in a glass jar away from sunlight for up to two years. Once spices are ground, they start to lose their aromatic properties and keeping them in a cool, dark place slows this process.

Note: This tea is not recommended during pregnancy due to the cinnamon.

DAMIANA ROSE TEA

Makes 4 oz (115 g) loose-leaf tea

INGREDIENTS

3 oz (85 g) loose black tea leaves (optional)

1 Tbsp dried damiana leaves

1 Tbsp dried rosebuds or petals

1 Tbsp dried lemon verbena leaves

Honey or cane sugar, for serving

Reflecting the uplifting, energizing nature of Yang, this tea eases stress, tension, and everyday pains. Black tea is a warming, energizing, strong base to carry a variety of herbs and flowers. Damiana leaves are a Yang tonic and an herbal aphrodisiac to improve libido. The rose in this recipe benefits the flow of energy in the body and has a unique effect on the Heart, which processes all emotions. Lemon verbena is an uplifting, sweet, and fragrant leaf, but leaves that have a citrus scent quickly lose their aroma once dried, so the freshness of the lemon verbena is key to the flavor of this tea blend. This recipe also works as an herbal tea by omitting the black tea.

In an airtight container, combine the black tea, damiana, rose, and lemon verbena. Store away from heat, light, and moisture for up to 12 months.

To make a cup of tea, place 1 tsp of the tea in a teapot and pour 1 cup (240 ml) of simmering water (180° F [80°C]) over the tea. Cover and steep for 3 minutes before straining. Pour the tea into a mug, add honey or sugar, and enjoy.

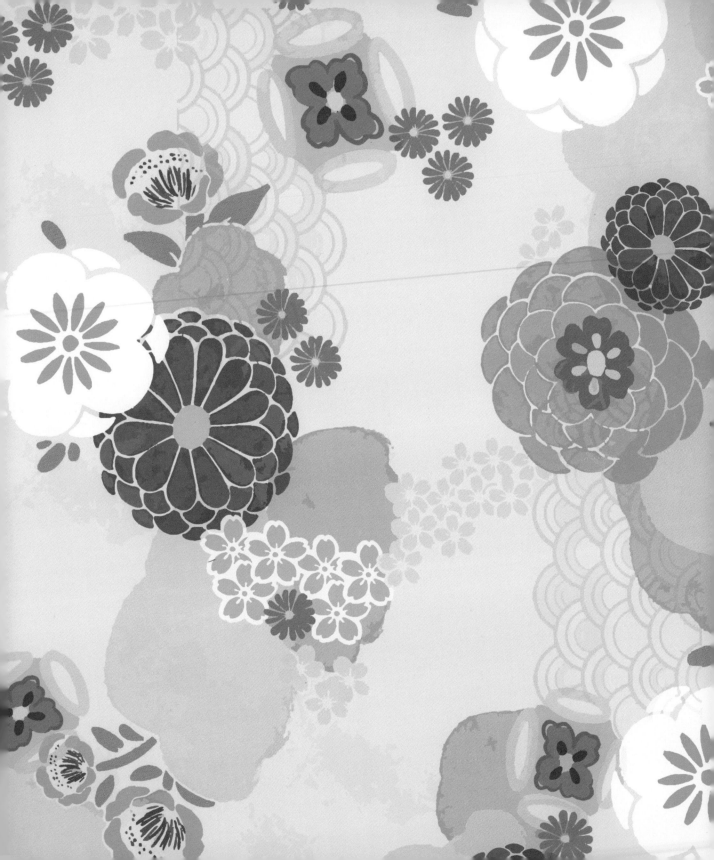

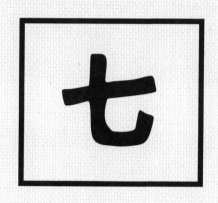

CHAPTER SEVEN

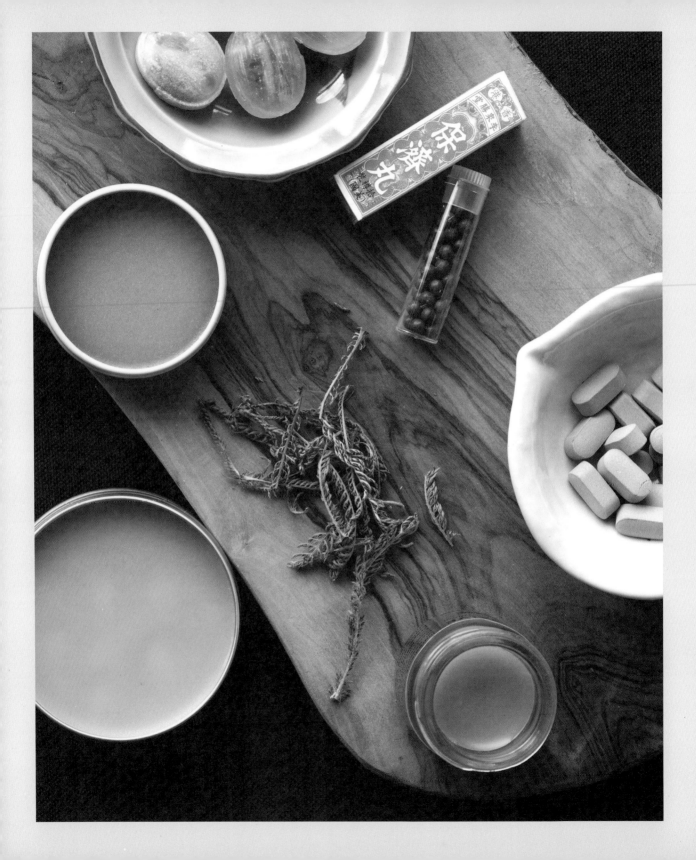

EVERYDAY AILMENTS

The struggle of living with bouts of low energy and poor vitality is very real. Improving energy and vitality is one of the most requested issues that people come in for help with at my clinic. Often these dips are due to daily stressors at work, drama in our personal lives, issues with hormone imbalance, chronic illness, and physical pain. I believe it is also the result of living in our modern world and all the emotional and economic stress that saps our deep energy reserves. Combined with a poor diet, sedentary lifestyle, and a lack of community, our modern lifestyle can leave us overworked and under-energized.

It's common to think of vitality and energy as the same. But energy refers to the strength and momentum that we carry in our daily activities, while vitality is the capacity for mental clarity and a general sense of well-being. In both cases, herbs can improve the quality of one's day-to-day life, cultivating strong and healthy Qi. This section will give you key takeaways for incorporating specific herbs, recipes, and my favorite qigong posture to increase your energy and vitality.

VITALITY AND ENERGY

Vitality

One key aspect of vitality is mental clarity and the capacity to focus and concentrate. Focus and concentration are often related to the brain's health but are also connected to the health of the Spleen Qi. Energetically, the Spleen rules the intellect; when it's healthy, it is easy to focus, memorize new material, and think clearly. If the

Spleen is weak, the intellect dulls, and focus, concentration, and memory are impaired. The root cause of this imbalance is often unhealthy lifestyle choices combined with periods of intense study and sustained mental focus, such as intense social media and screen time.

This cycle of cognitive and intellectual burnout is often a source of suffering for students and people with high-pressure jobs and lives. In these cases, there is a lot of potential to strengthen vitality by incorporating tonic herbs into daily meals and drinks. Qi tonic herbs immediately increase overall vitality, while Blood tonics gradually address the root causes of illness by replenishing energetic organs including the Spleen. Green tea, gotu kola, and ginkgo biloba are traditional herbs used across many Asian cultures to address vitality by increasing Qi and Blood and enhancing microcirculation in the brain.

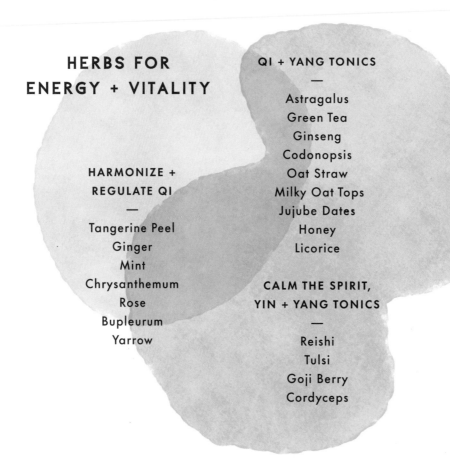

HERBS FOR ENERGY + VITALITY

HARMONIZE + REGULATE QI
—
Tangerine Peel
Ginger
Mint
Chrysanthemum
Rose
Bupleurum
Yarrow

QI + YANG TONICS
—
Astragalus
Green Tea
Ginseng
Codonopsis
Oat Straw
Milky Oat Tops
Jujube Dates
Honey
Licorice

CALM THE SPIRIT, YIN + YANG TONICS
—
Reishi
Tulsi
Goji Berry
Cordyceps

Asian American Herbalism

HANA BANCHA GREEN TEA

Makes 4 oz (115 g) loose-leaf tea

INGREDIENTS

3 oz (85 g) loose bancha green
tea leaves

1 Tbsp dried chrysanthemum
petals

10 dried chrysanthemum
flowers

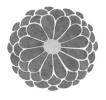

Bancha, a green tea enjoyed daily in Japan, is made from late-harvested tea leaves and stems. It has a refreshing crisp flavor that is energetically cool and beneficial for vitality. I blend bancha green tea with dried chrysanthemum to echo and increase green tea's cooling and Qi-balancing properties. This combination gently eases stress, relieves tension headaches, improves mental clarity, reduces inflammation, and clears toxins and dampness. "Hana" means flower in Japanese. With this recipe, I use the chrysanthemum petals that fall to the bottom of the herb jar and add whole dried chrysanthemum flowers because they are simply beautiful. This tea is named in honor of my great grandma Hana Sonoda Kaku.

In an airtight container, combine the bancha green tea, chrysanthemum petals, and chrysanthemum flowers. Store away from heat, light, and moisture for up to 12 months.

To make a cup of tea, place 1 tsp of the tea in a teapot and pour 1 cup (240 ml) of barely simmering water (170° F [75° C]) over the tea. Cover and steep for 1 to 2 minutes before straining. If desired, re-steep by pouring fresh, simmering water over the tea for a second cup. Drink immediately.

Note: Green tea develops a bitter flavor when steeped for too long or with water that is too hot. The right flavor should be green, fresh, and soft.

FORAGED GINKGO TEA FOR FOCUS

Serves 2

INGREDIENTS

¼ cup (10 g) fresh yellow ginkgo
   leaves
2 Tbsp fresh mint leaves
1 Tbsp fresh rosemary leaves

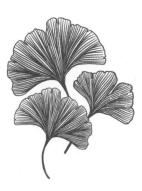

The downtown where I live in Northern California is peppered with ginkgo trees. Their unmistakable fan-shaped leaves are harvested in the late summer when they turn golden yellow and have been used for generations to benefit the brain, memory, and circulation. Ginkgo leaf, mint, and rosemary invigorate Qi to enhance memory and overall brain health. Mint and rosemary are easy to find in many gardens and markets year-round. And as always, only take what you need when foraging herbs from public spaces. This recipe calls for fresh herbs, but it can be made with dried herbs as well. The ratio is four parts ginkgo leaves to two parts mint and one part rosemary.

Gently rinse the ginkgo, mint, and rosemary in cool water and remove any woody stems. Place the fresh herbs in a teapot or glass jar and pour 2 cups (480 ml) of boiling water over the herbs. Cover and steep for 5 minutes. Strain and serve immediately.

   If using dried herbs, place 1 tsp of the Foraged Ginkgo Tea for Focus in a teapot for every 1 cup (240 ml) of water. Pour boiling water (200° F [95° C]) over the herbs, cover, and steep for 5 to 10 minutes. Drink immediately.

Contraindication: Ginkgo slows blood clotting and may also cause bleeding if taken with fish oil supplements, ibuprofen, naproxen, aspirin, or blood thinning medication.

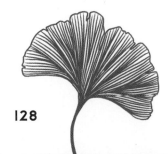

Asian American Herbalism

Energy

In life, there is a natural ebb and flow of energy over the course of each day, week, season, and lifetime. Thus, the strength of one's daily energy is experienced differently at times due to the wide range of human experiences. Stress, hormones, illness, mental health, and the changing of the seasons all affect this ebb and flow. The key to understanding your energy is consistency and balance. When your energy feels inconsistent or extreme, helpful herbs will harmonize Qi and move stagnation.

Some of the questions you may ask yourself to better understand your energy and vitality include: How do you feel throughout the day? Is your energy consistent? Does it decrease after eating? Does it dip in the afternoon? Do you feel well rested when you wake up in the morning? Is your vitality currently impacted by hormone cycles or stress?

Irregular Energy

In a healthy system, one's energy is strongest in the morning and gradually wanes as bedtime approaches. Energy should be consistent and sustained. However, irregular energy cycles can be common in folks who otherwise have seemingly strong energy throughout the day. This includes waking up feeling unrested, energy that dips in the afternoon or after eating a meal, and a high energy level in the evening hours. Irregular energy specifically indicates Qi stagnation affecting the energetic Liver. Healing herbs, such as tangerine peel, tulsi, mint, chrysanthemum, and ginger, address irregular energy by harmonizing Qi and clearing stagnation. If you're inclined to use caffeine to increase and sustain your energy, I recommend green tea over other stimulants because of its unique energetic quality as a medicinal plant to sustain energy and increase mental clarity and discernment.

Low Energy

Experiencing low energy is often due to overexertion from working long hours and not getting adequate rest. This almost always coincides with an irregular diet and lifestyle choices to cope with the stressors (i.e., drinking alcohol, scrolling social media for hours, etc.). Low energy that dips in the afternoon, after eating a meal, or that is accompanied by a depressed feeling indicates a Qi deficiency that affects the energetic Spleen and Kidney. In these cases, tonic herbs are incredible gifts of the earth that can slowly rebuild deep energy stores. They should be taken over time (for at least three months) to be effective. Qi tonic herbs include mugwort, astragalus, reishi mushroom, ginseng, ashwagandha, goji berries, and cordyceps.

Vitality and energy are greatly affected by caffeine, stimulant drugs such as Adderall, and cocaine. Like an energetic credit card, stimulants cash in on instant energy by drawing from the deep energy reserves. As such, herbs that replenish and benefit Qi are profoundly valuable to offset and heal from the effects of caffeine and stimulants.

COOL QI HERBAL TEA FOR ENERGY

Makes 2 oz (55 g) loose-leaf tea

INGREDIENTS

½ cup (20 g) dried astragalus

½ cup (10 g) dried mint

½ cup (6 g) dried chrysanthemum flowers

½ cup (14 g) dried nettle

This is a cooling herbal tea blend that balances and strengthens Qi energy. Cooling tea blends are ideal for folks who generally run hot (day or night) and have spontaneous sweating, irritability, red skin, and a red tongue. Astragalus is a Qi tonic herb that has a unique balancing effect on the body and mind. Mint and chrysanthemum cool heat and move stagnant Qi, which can cause mental and physical tension. Nettle has a salty nature that benefits the Kidney energy to restore the deep reserves of Qi and Blood.

In an airtight container, combine the astragalus, mint, chrysanthemum, and nettle. Store away from heat, light, and moisture for up to 12 months.

To make a cup of tea, place 1 tsp of the tea in a teapot and pour 1 cup (240 ml) of boiling water (200° F [95° C]) over the tea. Cover and steep for 5 minutes before straining. If desired, re-steep by pouring fresh, boiling water over the tea for a second cup. Drink immediately or store in the refrigerator for 1 to 2 days.

The medicinal dose is 1 cup (240 ml) per day for 3 days or as needed. It should be taken slowly over the course of each day.

Contraindication: Omit nettles in cases of cardiac or renal failure.

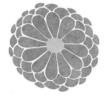

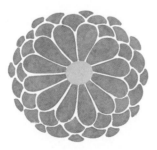

WARMING UPLIFT HERBAL TEA

Makes 4 oz (115 g)
loose-leaf tea

INGREDIENTS

½ cup (20 g) dried astragalus

½ cup (55 g) dried goji berries

½ cup (55 g) dried tangerine peel (or one 1 in [2.5 cm] piece fresh tangerine peel per cup of tea)

1 knob of fresh ginger, thinly sliced for serving (optional)

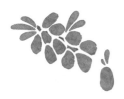

This herbal tea blend increases energy and lifts Qi in the body and mind. Warming tea blends like this one are desirable for folks who run cold, are prone to water retention (damp and edema), rarely sweat, experience cold hands and feet, and have a pale, swollen tongue. Astragalus is a Qi tonic herb that lifts sinking energy in the body and mind. A common manifestation of sinking energy is depression or feeling down. Astragalus is magic for lifting the spirits and healing this dynamic. Fresh ginger and tangerine peel both move stagnant Qi and soothe digestive upset that is common for folks with Qi deficiency. Goji berries naturally sweeten this tea blend and benefit both Qi and Blood.

In an airtight container, combine the astragalus, goji berries, and dried tangerine peel; if using fresh tangerine peel, wait to add it. Store away from heat, light, and moisture for up to 12 months.

To make a cup of tea, place a slice of fresh ginger and 1 tsp of the tea in a teapot. If using fresh tangerine peel, add a 1 in (2.5 cm) piece to the teapot as well. Pour boiling water (200° F [95° C]) over the tea and herbs. Cover and steep for 5 minutes before straining. If desired, re-steep by pouring fresh, boiling water over the tea and herbs for a second cup. Drink slowly over the course of each day. Store in the refrigerator for up to 2 days and warm before drinking.

The medicinal dose is 1 cup (240 ml) twice per day for 3 days or as needed.

ASHWAGANDHA GARAM DOOTH — WARM SWEET HERBAL MILK

Serves 3

INGREDIENTS

3 cups (720 ml) milk or
nondairy milk alternative

3 tsp ashwagandha powder (or
3 whole dried 3 in [7.5 cm]
ashwagandha roots)

2 whole cardamom pods, lightly
crushed

2 Tbsp sliced almonds

2 Tbsp raisins

1 Tbsp dried mulberries

Pinch of ground cinnamon

1 tsp honey or maple syrup, for
serving (optional)

I learned this recipe in the kitchen of Shanta Nimbark Sacharoff while studying Ayurvedic medicine. Ashwagandha is a traditional herb from India and South Asia that lends itself well to warm milk tea. It is a balancing tonic herb that calms the mind and balances the nervous system. While it can be found as an herbal powder extract at many health foods stores, in recent years, I've also found small-scale farms and CSAs in California offering freshly dried ashwagandha root. Either the powder or freshly dried root can be used in this recipe. The dried fruits and almonds add sweetness to this drink.

In a small saucepan, combine the milk, ashwagandha, cardamom, almonds, raisins, mulberries, and cinnamon over low heat. Warm, stirring frequently to ensure the milk does not scorch or burn, for about 10 minutes, or until fragrant. Remove from the heat and let cool for 3 minutes. Taste for sweetness and add honey or maple syrup (if using). Strain, pour into 3 mugs, and serve.

Contraindication: This is not recommended during pregnancy due to the ashwagandha and cinnamon.

Gathering Qi from Heaven and Earth – Qigong for Vitality and Energy

Qigong is a classical Chinese medicine practice of movement, meditation, and breath work. I had the honor of learning qigong with Daju Suzanne Friedman, and her teaching profoundly influenced my understanding of the energetics within the human body and mind. The Gathering Qi from Heaven and Earth is a standing posture that grounds our energy. The intention is to replenish energy and vitality by drawing Qi from the natural world. It is a balancing posture that reflects your actual energy in the moment. If you feel energized after this meditation, you can take that energy into the rest of your day. However, if it makes you sleepy, it is a sign that you need to rest!

Steps for the Qigong Meditation:

1. Find a comfortable standing position and feel your body grounded.

2. Your feet should be shoulder-distance apart, and your knees slightly bent. Roll your shoulders back, and let your arms hang naturally by your sides. This is called wuji posture.

3. Following your natural breath, take a moment to come into the space, into the moment.

4. And with each breath, start to relax the body and mind.

5. Release the chest and throat, the jaw, tongue, and eyes. Soften the belly, fingers, and toes.

6. As you inhale, extend your arms out to the sides of your body with the palms facing the ground. The arms come up and over the head in a big sweeping motion. Visualize the Qi from the natural world drawing into the palms of your hands. The first half of this motion draws in Qi from the earth, and the second half draws in Qi from the sky.

7. As you exhale, draw the hands down from overhead with the palms facing the ground. With the fingertips facing each other, the hands push downward and over the front of the body. Visualize the Qi you gathered from the earth and sky washing over your body.

8. Repeat this cycle three to six times, following the rhythm of your deep breath. Repeating movements in multiples of three has a strengthening and healing effect.

ANXIETY AND DEPRESSION

Anxiety and depression are experienced individually but are also illnesses of our modern-day collective wellness. At the root of this suffering is the fact that we live in an oppressive society ruled by capitalism and colonialism. A multitude of human suffering has always existed; however, we are now more aware of it through the internet and social media. The dire state of climate collapse, systemic racism, pandemic disease, war, and human suffering are at the forefront of our collective consciousness. In this light, anxiety and depression are reasonable human responses to the complex issues of our time. Ultimately, we want to change the underlying conditions that lead to stress on our bodies and minds. However, we also need strategies to take care of ourselves while processing these issues in real time. I believe returning to our roots with culturally relevant healing practices and earth-based medicine is part of this healing.

Many modern-day health concerns are directly connected to mental health. I often find that people with anxiety and depression are highly creative and capable individuals living a life that is deeply out of balance. Depression has a sinking energy that can be experienced as

HERBS FOR ANXIETY + DEPRESSION

NERVINES
—
Chamomile
Lavender
Lemon Balm
Oat Straw
Milky Oat Tops
Rosemary
Skullcap

HEART TONICS
—
Hawthorn Rose
Mimosa Tree Bark + Flower
Motherwort
Passion Flower

BALANCE + UPLIFT THE SPIRIT
—
Astragalus
Lemon Verbena
Honeysuckle
Tangerine Peel

Asian American Herbalism

loneliness, hopelessness, and numbness. With anxiety, there is a spiraling, edgy discomfort in the body and mind. They both share an overwhelming sense that one's emotional and spiritual needs are not being met. Energetically this is connected to the health of the energetic Heart, which is the center of all emotional processing. For healing, I look to Heart herbs, including rose, hawthorn, motherwort, passionflower, oats, and mimosa tree flowers and bark. Taking herbs for anxiety and depression is only one part of supporting mental health. Therapy, exercise, community, time in nature, and pharmaceutical medications can all be essential parts of a wellness plan. Be sure to consult a medical provider when trying new herbs and coping strategies for anxiety and depression.

Anxiety

Anxiety is a feeling of uneasiness, fear, overwhelm, and a general sense of unbearable pressure. It is a normal, temporary mind-body state that occurs with stress or in times of intense difficulty. However, when short-term anxieties are left unaddressed, they can become a debilitating and chronic illness. In the body, anxiety prompts heart palpitations, sweating, imbalanced feelings of heat or coldness, insomnia, breathing issues, and pain. There is often a marked inability to turn off the mind, calm the body, maintain focus, or gain mental clarity. Debilitating cycles of anxiety energetically occur when there is a depletion of Qi and Heart Blood. This depleted state is akin to being ungrounded, like an unanchored boat.

Over time, anxiety in the body and mind will lead to Heat that rises up to the head and brings an uncomfortable, oppressive edge. The tongue is a reliable way to check for Heat in your body—look for any redness, pain, or sores on the tip of the tongue, which indicate Heart heat. Effective herbs for addressing day-to-day anxiety are often the simplest—such as nervines like chamomile, lemon balm, milky oat tops, and lavender that calm the nervous system. Anxiety rooted in significant burnout of Qi and Blood deficiency is addressed by long-term use of tonic herbs to restore energetic balance. For this purpose, a three-month course of Qi and Blood tonic herbs can include any combination of astragalus, mugwort, white peony root, longan fruit, goji berry, ginseng, dang gui, and jujube dates.

NERVINES

—

Nervines are herbs that heal our nerves. They tone, balance, and strengthen the nervous system to address anxiety, depression, stress, and tension. They can be taken as needed with immediate effect, such as milky oat tops for panic or skullcap for insomnia. But I find them to be most effective when taken over time. There is a cumulative effect to their medicine that heals the deeper emotional underpinnings of anxiety and depression. Nervines are essential medicine for our overstimulated modern-day culture and include chamomile, lavender, lemon balm, milky oat tops, oat straw, rosemary, and skullcap.

FRESH LEMON BALM WATER

Serves 6

INGREDIENTS

3 sprigs fresh lemon balm,
about 5 in (12 cm) each

Lemon balm is my go-to garden herb to offset stress and overwhelm. As an herb in the nervine category, it works to heal and balance the nervous system over time. In our modern, fast-paced culture, who doesn't need that? Lemon balm has a very mild, gentle nature and must be taken over time to have a substantial effect. This, combined with its sweet lemon scent and ability to soothe frayed nerves, crying, teething, belly aches, and overstimulation, makes it especially wonderful and safe for children.

Lemon balm is one herb that I recommend people try to grow themselves. The fresh herb is substantially more effective for easing anxiety because it quickly loses its delicate essential oils once dried. And as a member of the mint family, it is easy to grow and will return each year with little fuss.

In a pitcher or large glass jar, combine the lemon balm with approximately 6 cups (1.4 L) of cool water. Steep at room temperature for 1 to 4 hours (the herbs will infuse more quickly on warmer days). To quicken the process, gently muddle or crush the sprigs and leaves with the back of a wooden spoon. Once the water is ready, you will taste the subtle lemon flavor. The leaves can remain in the pitcher as you drink the infused water over a day or two. Store in a pitcher or glass jar in the refrigerator for 1 to 2 days.

CALM HEART, COOL MIND TEA

Makes 2 oz (55 g) loose-leaf tea

INGREDIENTS

1 cup (20 g) dried tulsi
½ cup (10 g) dried rose petals
¼ cup (7 g) dried oat straw
2 Tbsp dried milky oat tops
2 Tbsp dried honeysuckle

For many years I taught seasonal wellness workshops at Tara Firma Farms in Petaluma, California, and formulated this tea specifically for summer classes. Although it can be enjoyed any time of year, summer is the season for healing the Heart. Seasonal connection to the organs represents a window of time ripe for energetic healing. This Heart-centered herbal tea blend harmonizes the Heart Qi and calms anxiety. Tulsi is a quintessential adaptogenic herb, because it balances the nervous system to bring equilibrium to the body-mind. Rose speaks to the Heart energy, the center of all emotional processing and healing. Honeysuckle moves stagnant Qi, cools Heat, and clears toxins to release toxic emotional holding patterns. And milky oat tops and oat straw help buffer the nervous system from stress to help ease emotional strain.

In an airtight container, combine the tulsi, rose, oat straw, milky oat tops, and honeysuckle. Store away from heat, light, and moisture for up to 12 months.

To make a cup of tea, place 1 heaping tsp of the tea in a teapot and pour 1 cup (240 ml) of boiling water (200° F [95° C]) over the tea. Cover and steep for 10 minutes before straining. Drink immediately.

The medicinal dose is 1 cup (240 ml) twice per day for 3 days or as needed.

Contraindications: This tea is not recommended during pregnancy, or when pregnancy is possible, due to the tulsi. Tulsi is also not recommended in cases of diabetes due to its effect on regulating blood sugar.

CALM HEART TEA LATTE

Serves 2

INGREDIENTS

2 tsp Calm Heart, Cool Mind Tea (page 137)

1 tsp dried lemon verbena

1 cup (240 ml) milk or nondairy milk alternative

1 tsp honey (optional)

Ground cinnamon, for serving

A satisfying recipe for both tea and coffee drinkers, this tea latte uses the Calm Heart, Cool Mind Tea (page 137). I enjoy delicious, fun recipes like this, as a way to incorporate herbal medicine into daily life. Keeping the medicine interesting is key for enjoyment and consistency in taking herbs. The Calm Heart, Cool Mind Tea is a Heart-nourishing blend to ease anxiety. The addition of lemon verbena, particularly when it is locally grown, adds a natural sweetness and a lovely flavor. Milk and honey have Yin-nourishing properties that have a stabilizing effect on an anxious mind. This recipe is all about connecting to the Heart within you and to the heart of herbalism.

Place the tea and lemon verbena in a teapot and pour 1 cup (240 ml) of boiling water (200° F [95° C]) over the tea. Cover and steep for 10 minutes before straining. In a blender or using a frother, blend the milk and honey (if using) for about 10 seconds, or until frothy and just incorporated. Pour the tea into mugs, top with the frothed milk and cinnamon, and serve.

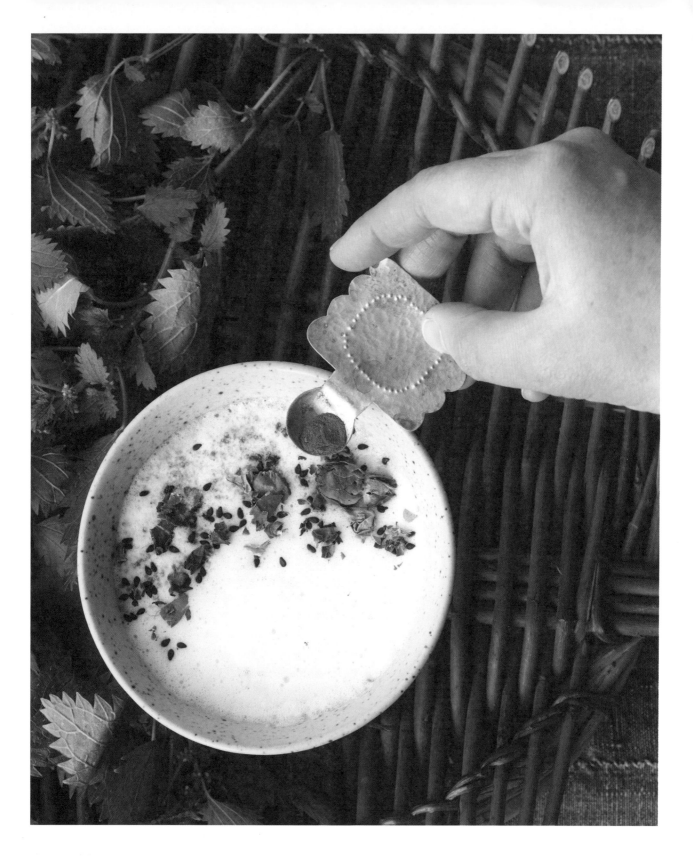

HEART-CENTERED SHIO BATH OR FOOT SOAK

Yields 1 bath or foot soak

INGREDIENTS

3 cups (60 g) dried rose petals

3 cups (80 g) fresh rose
  geranium or geranium, cut
  into 2 in (5 cm) pieces

Peel of 1 fresh tangerine (or
  lemon or other citrus fruit)

2 cups (400 g) Epsom salt

¼ cup (50 g) baking soda

10 to 20 drops lavender or rose
  essential oil (optional)

A Heart-centered shio bath is a beautiful remedy when healing an anxious or tender Heart. Shio is "salt" in Japanese. When the energetic Heart is overwhelmed, the mind becomes restless, anxious, worried, and unable to relax. Rose and rose geranium heal the energetic and physical heart. These herbs are called for when there are heart palpitations or fullness and discomfort in the chest. Epsom salts contain magnesium, a vital mineral for proper nerve and muscle health—including the heart muscle. Magnesium is more quickly depleted in times of stress, and adding Epsom salt to one's bath is a safe way to replenish this mineral. The heat of a warm bath also enlivens stagnant Qi and fluids by increasing circulation. Tangerine peel moves stasis in the body and is particularly helpful for folks with cold extremities. Cold fingers and toes are a sign that circulation of Blood, lymph, and Qi is stagnant. This is because Qi energy, like blood, transitions and changes direction at the extremities.

This recipe may be modified for a foot soak. Foot baths are especially therapeutic as Heart medicine because they draw excess energy from the mind, face, and upper chest and bring that energy down to the gut. This allows a person to get out of their head and become more in tune with their instincts.

For a bath: Bring 4 cups (960 ml) of water to a rapid boil then remove from the heat. Add the rose, rose geranium or geranium, and tangerine peel then cover the pot with a lid, and steep for 15 minutes while drawing a very warm bath.

When the bath is ready, strain the herbs from the bath "tea" then add the tea, along with the Epsom salt and baking soda, to the bath water. For an extra-lovely scent, drop in essential oils while in the bath—their volatile oils release and evaporate quite quickly. Soak for 20 minutes for a full therapeutic effect. ↗

For a foot soak: Follow the same instructions for boiling water and steeping the herbs. Fill a large basin or bucket with warm water to soak the feet and ankles comfortably. Add the bath tea, just 1 cup (200 g) of Epsom salt, the baking soda, and essential oils. Sit in a comfortable chair and soak your feet for 20 minutes for a full therapeutic effect.

Depression

In the clinic, I find that a common cause of depression is anger directed at the self. Over time, this internalized anger and repressed emotion affects the energetic Liver and causes Qi stagnation with symptoms that create irregularity in the body and mind—mood swings, mental restlessness, agitation, headaches, insomnia, digestive upset, and sores on the sides of the tongue. In these cases, healing herbs, such as lemon balm, bupleurum, aged tangerine peel, dang gui, yarrow, fresh ginger, mint, and chrysanthemum, harmonize the Qi dynamic and move the Liver Qi specifically. The emotional strain of depression always has a damaging effect on the energetic Heart, because the Heart is the center of emotional processing. Thus, herbs that speak to the Heart, such as rose, hawthorn, motherwort, mimosa tree bark and flower, and passionflower, are also healing for depressive states.

Depression is often experienced as a heavy, mental sinking—like foggy dampness that settles over and clouds the mind. This dynamic of Qi sinking with dampness leads to a dulling of the senses, delayed reactions, difficulty with recall, and in severe cases, mania and psychosis. Over time, this dynamic causes Qi to sink, which is felt in the body as exhaustion, numbness, a down-bearing pressure, or a sinking feeling in the gut. In these cases, aromatic herbs that transform damp, including poria, pearl barley, cleavers, plantain, and bee balm, are key. Astragalus is my favorite herb to draw the energy up and secure the exterior boundary (Wei Qi) to create a safe space to find equilibrium while undergoing deep healing and transformation.

HEARTBREAK SUN TEA — A TEA FOR EMOTIONAL DIGESTION

Makes 4 oz (115 g) loose-leaf tea

INGREDIENTS

½ cup (10 g) dried rose petals

½ cup (20 g) dried astragalus

½ cup (55 g) dried goji berries

¼ cup (7 g) dried oat straw

2 Tbsp dried violet leaves

2 Tbsp dried motherwort leaves

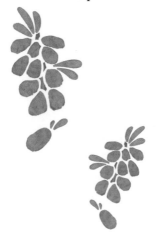

When I was growing up, my mom made sun teas under the blazing hot Sacramento sun. I would watch as the tea bags released their magic in swirls of color, transforming glass pitchers of water into tea. Summer is the ideal time to utilize the warmth of the sun to make sun teas, or solar infusions. This tea blend combines uplifting and balancing Heart herbs that aid the processing or digesting of emotional strain. Rose is a classic Heart medicine that eases emotional strain and the processing of a wide range of emotions. Astragalus and goji berries are uplifting tonic herbs that alleviate depression and strengthen energetic boundaries to protect against absorbing negative energy from others. Oat straw has magnesium and calcium, which benefits the heart muscle and calms anxiety. Violet clears heat and toxic holding patterns that can accumulate under challenging times and manifest as irritability, skin rashes, and nightmares. Motherwort is a healing herb that carries a healing mother earth energy that is supportive in times of burnout and loneliness.

In an airtight container, combine the rose, astragalus, goji berries, oat straw, violet, and motherwort. Store in an airtight container away from heat, light, and moisture for up to 12 months.

To make a sun tea, fill a pitcher or large glass jar with 3 cups (720 ml) of cool water and 3 heaping Tbsp of the tea. Cover loosely and steep outside in direct sunlight for 4 to 6 hours. Once ready, you will notice that the infusion has taken on a slight color and will taste of rose and sweet goji berries. Strain well and drink warm or chilled. Store in a glass jar in the refrigerator for up to 2 days.

Contraindication: Omit motherwort during pregnancy.

CHAMOMILE COLD INFUSION

Makes 3 cups (720 ml)

INGREDIENTS

1 Tbsp dried or fresh chamomile

1 Tbsp dried or fresh rose petals

1 tsp dried marshmallow root

1 knob of fresh ginger, peeled
    and thinly sliced

Chamomile is quintessential flower medicine—gentle enough for children yet potent enough for healing significant illnesses. Flower medicine is resilient, and if you grow chamomile in the right conditions, it will thrive and spread all around the garden. Although dried chamomile is terrific medicine, the flavor of fresh chamomile is sweet like an apple and worth sourcing from your local farmers and flower growers.

Chamomile is particularly effective for easing depression and related physical symptoms, including pain, insomnia, and digestive upset. When combined with fresh ginger, the gentle down-bearing energy of chamomile helps to bring on delayed periods and eases menstrual cramps that are caused by depression and anxiety (Qi stagnation). The addition of rose speaks to the energetic Heart and supports its ability to process and heal from difficult emotions. Chamomile, rose, and marshmallow root are all mucilaginous (slippery) herbs, which means that when extracted in a cold infusion, they release a gelatinous quality that is deeply hydrating and soothing. This is a wonderful tea to have on warm days.

In a pitcher or large glass jar, combine the chamomile, rose, marshmallow, and ginger with approximately 3 cups (720 ml) of cool water. Steep at room temperature for 2 to 4 hours (the herbs will infuse quicker on warmer days). Once ready, you will notice that the infusion has taken on a slight color and a viscous consistency from the herbs. Strain well and drink the cool, infused water over the course of a day or two. Store in a glass jar in the refrigerator for 1 to 2 days.

To make a cup of tea, place 1 tsp of the tea in a teapot and pour boiling water (200° F [95° C]) over the tea. Cover and steep for 10 minutes before straining. Drink immediately.

OPEN HEART ELIXIR

Makes 2 to 3 cups (480 to 720 ml)

INGREDIENTS

1 cup (20 g) dried rosebuds or petals

½ cup (60 g) dried mimosa tree bark (or mimosa flowers)

½ cup (60 g) dried hawthorn berries

2 Tbsp dried schisandra

2 cups (480 ml) 80 to 100 proof brandy

1 cup (240 ml) raw honey

Elixirs are traditional remedies that extract herbal medicine with a blend of alcohol and honey. This elixir recipe was crafted with the summer in mind and is meant to be enjoyed as an aperitif or subtle Heart-opening medicine. Rose and mimosa tree bark lead this Heart-centered blend. They are used in traditional Chinese medicine for their uplifting and joyful energy. Hawthorn berries address heartache's physical and emotional manifestations by gently opening and supporting the Heart's energy. Astringent schisandra draws energy inward and strengthens boundaries to create a safe space to heal and process emotion in times of loss, grief, numbness, and all the manifestations of a broken heart.

In a 4 cup (960 ml) glass jar, combine the rose, mimosa, hawthorn berries, and schisandra. Pour the brandy over the herbs, filling the jar three-quarters of the way full. Add honey to the jar until the mixture is 1 in (2.5 cm) from the top of the jar (you may not need to use all of it). Reserve the extra alcohol for topping off the mixture as the herbs absorb the liquid during the first week of tincturing. Cover with a plastic or a nonreactive lid (or line metal lids with parchment paper or plastic wrap). Label the jar with the date and ingredients. Store away from heat, light, and moisture and gently shake the mixture every 1 to 3 days.

After 4 weeks, use cheesecloth or fine-mesh sieve to strain the elixir; discard the herbs. The final elixir is stable at room temperature and can be stored in a clean glass jar away from heat, light, and moisture for up to 3 years. You can tell if an elixir has spoiled by changes in smell or taste, or any visible signs of mold or fermentation.

Elixirs are taken as a medicinal tonic and a social drink, so the dose varies from a few drops to a small liquor glass. For acute heartache, take 1 tsp twice a day for at least 3 days or as needed. Otherwise, share with family and friends as a digestif or in a cocktail.

Contraindication: This elixir is not recommended during pregnancy due to the mimosa tree bark.

MIMOSA FLOWER TEA FOR A CHEERFUL SPIRIT

Serves 1

INGREDIENTS

1 Tbsp dried mimosa flowers

Mimosa flower is called *he huan hua* in Chinese Mandarin, which translates to "collective happiness flower." It calms the mind by moving stagnant Liver Qi and harmonizing energy within the body and mind. Mimosa is a wonderful medicine for healing depression or anxiety that causes a feeling of tightness in the chest, pain, irritability, restlessness, forgetfulness, and insomnia. Like most flower medicine, its effect is mild and gentle and should be taken over time for the full benefit.

Place the mimosa flowers in a teapot and pour 1 cup (240 ml) of boiling water (200° F [95° C]) over the flowers. Cover and steep for 10 minutes before straining. Drink immediately.

The medicinal dose is 1 cup (240 ml) twice per day for up to 1 month.

Contraindication: This tea is not recommended during pregnancy due to the mimosa flowers.

STRESS

In response to modern-day stress and overstimulation, there is a growing cultural shift away from the glorification of hyper-productivity and always being tired. Every day we are immersed in technology and media of various forms. Our access to limitless information is a heavy weight to carry, and we are expected to take in, process, and digest data at an unnatural pace. It's become an addiction that disturbs our sleep cycles and biological rhythms.

I believe this culture of exhaustion is rooted in a loss of connection with ourselves and to the rhythms of the natural world. How readily we forget to check in with the celestial lights in our sky and the light that glows within. We've lost the meaning and purpose of darkness, downtime, and intimacy. We're in desperate need of learning how to reconnect with our humanity and our place in the natural world. It is time to reconnect, and herbs and healing traditions help us to do just that (see the Meditation for Connecting to the Natural World on page 155).

Qi Stagnation

Stress stagnates the Qi and drains energy from the mind-body. It has a direct effect on the energetic Liver, and when the Liver Qi stagnates, it causes tightness in the center of the body, such as cramps or sharp pains in the rib cage or tension in the middle of the spine. This Liver Qi stagnation can lead to symptoms that affect the upper part of the body—think headaches, jaw clenching, shortness

HERBS FOR STRESS

LIVER QI HERBS
—
Chrysanthemum
Bupleurum
Tangerine Peel
Dandelion
Ginger
Nettle

CALM THE SPIRIT
—
Tulsi
Chamomile
Lavender
Lemon Balm
Oat Straw + Milky Oat Tops
California Poppy
Reishi Mushroom
Passionflower

COOLING HERBS
—
Honeysuckle
Mint
Yarrow
Violet
Red Clover
Burdock Root

of breath, hiccups, belching, sighing, and redness in the face. On the other hand, Liver Qi stagnation can affect the lower body with issues in the gut, such as irregular digestion, gas, bloating, diarrhea, constipation, menstrual cramps, frequent urination, hip pain, and water retention. So, the first step in addressing stress is herbs that unwind and unbind the energetic Liver and Qi energy. My favorite herbs for this are chrysanthemum, mint, dandelion, and fresh ginger.

Understanding the Nervous System

The nervous system includes the brain, spinal cord, and the nerves that travel to every part of the body. Within the nervous system at large, the autonomic nervous system (ANS) is specifically responsible for automatic and unconscious actions of the body and mind. The ANS has two primary modes that complement one another—the sympathetic nervous system and parasympathetic nervous system.

The parasympathetic system is active during rest, after eating, digestion, elimination, and sexual arousal. Healthy parasympathetic activation allows for rest, healing, and recalibration of the body-mind. Therefore, herbs and practices that bring the body into a parasympathetic restful state are key for recovery. Meditation, qigong, yoga, acupuncture, massage, and time in nature are parasympathetic healing practices. My favorite herbs for this purpose are milky oat tops, oat straw, lemon balm, chrysanthemum, and adaptogens such as tulsi.

The sympathetic nervous system is activated by stress, and our reaction to it is the fight-flight-freeze response. It is the way our mind-body registers threats to our safety and pushes us to survive and get through difficult situations. When the sympathetic nervous system is activated, stress hormones, including cortisol and adrenaline, are released. In a healthy state, stress hormones are released for a short period, and then the body recovers by reentering a parasympathetic state. However, modern-day culture creates imbalanced states where stress hormones are being released around the clock, and this is the cause of many modern-day illnesses.

ADAPTOGENS
—

Adaptogenic herbs help the body adapt to stress by increasing the body's resilience to physical, emotional, and environmental stressors. Adaptogens restore healthy physiological rhythms, such as sleep (circadian rhythm), hormones, digestion, and metabolism.

Just as exercise is needed to build endurance and stamina in the physical body, herbs for stress need to be taken consistently over time to recalibrate the mind-body-spirit. It is a process to unlearn the chaotic patterns of everyday life and to support the mind and body in relearning how to fully experience how to operate with ease and grace. Herbs: astragalus, ashwagandha, eleuthero, licorice, reishi, rhodiola, schisandra, and tulsi.

EARTHLING TEA

Makes 1 oz (30 g) loose-leaf tea

INGREDIENTS

1 cup (20 g) dried tulsi

½ cup (6 g) dried chrysanthemum

¼ cup (5 g) dried lemon balm

2 Tbsp dried milky oat tops

2 Tbsp dried oat straw

Honey, for serving (optional)

Ground cinnamon, for serving (optional)

1 knob of fresh ginger, thinly sliced for serving (optional)

Herbs connect us to the earth and to our humanity. This herbal tea blend represents grounding, life-affirming energy. Tulsi is an adaptogenic herb treasured in Ayurvedic and South Asian medicine and wellness traditions. While it is one of my go-to herbs for healing the effects of stress, it also has the capacity to bring equilibrium to the mind and body. When available, freshly dried tulsi is recommended for the best flavor. Lemon balm has the power to bring you back into your body and ease the tension that shows up as anxiety. Chrysanthemum is a cooling herb that moves stagnant Qi and clears toxic mental and physical patterns. Nutrient-dense milky oat tops and oat straw calm edginess by healing and soothing the nervous system. This tea blend has a delicate earthy flavor that plays well in many recipes. For sweet tea, add a touch of honey and cinnamon. For a warming tea, add a slice of fresh ginger.

In an airtight container, combine the tulsi, chrysanthemum, lemon balm, milky oat tops, and oat straw. Store away from heat, light, and moisture for up to 12 months.

To make a cup of tea, place 1 heaping tsp of the tea in a teapot and pour 1 cup (240 ml) of boiling water (200° F [95° C]) over the tea. Cover and steep for 5 to 10 minutes before straining. Add honey, cinnamon, and fresh ginger (if using) and drink immediately.

Contraindications: This tea is not recommended during pregnancy, or when pregnancy is possible, due to the tulsi. Tulsi is also not recommended in cases of diabetes due to its effect on regulating blood sugar.

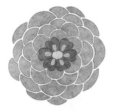

Asian American Herbalism

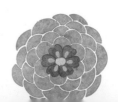

TULSI ROSE TEA LATTE

Serves 2

INGREDIENTS

1 tsp dried tulsi

1 tsp dried rosebuds or rose petals

1 tsp dried chamomile

1 cup (240 ml) milk or nondairy milk alternative

1 tsp honey (optional)

Ground cinnamon, for serving

Dried rose petal, for serving

This light and flavorful herbal tea blend makes a comforting and stress-reducing tea latte. Tulsi is an adaptogen that balances the nervous system and stress response. Chamomile calms the mind and eases stress that is held in the body. Rose speaks to the energetic Heart and addresses emotional strain. Milk and milk alternatives nourish Yin and body fluids which grounds one's energy and buffers the mind-body from stressors.

In a teapot, combine the tulsi, rose, and chamomile and pour 1 cup (240 ml) of boiling water (200° F [95° C]) over the tea. Cover and steep for 10 minutes before straining. In a blender or using a frother, blend the milk and honey (if using) for about 10 seconds, or until frothy and just incorporated. Pour the tea into mugs then top with the frothed milk, a sprinkle of cinnamon, and a dried rose petal and serve.

Contraindications: This tea is not recommended during pregnancy, or when pregnancy is possible, due to the tulsi. Tulsi is also not recommended in cases of diabetes due to its effect on regulating blood sugar.

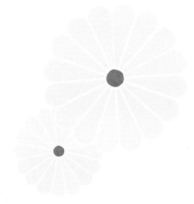

BONSAI HERBAL TEA

Makes 3.5 oz (100 g) loose-leaf tea

INGREDIENTS

½ cup (55 g) dried goji berries

½ cup (6 g) dried chrysanthemum

½ cup (10 g) dried mint

¼ cup (7 g) dried nettle

2 Tbsp dried dandelion leaf

2 Tbsp dried honeysuckle

This is a minty and lightly sweet herbal tea blend to move Qi stagnation, reduce heat, and nourish the Blood. Mint, chrysanthemum, and honeysuckle are cooling herbs that release stagnant Qi that shows up as irritability, tension, and stress. Chrysanthemum and goji berries are a classic herbal pair to nourish Blood and are traditionally used to address allergies and red eyes. Dandelion and nettle also benefit Blood and prevent Qi stagnation. I think of it as a complement to the traditional Chinese formula Xiao Yao Tang (translated as "Free and Easy Wanderer").

The energy of this tea is like the scene in the movie *The Karate Kid*, when Mr. Miyagi throws his fists in the air and yells, "BANZAI!!" Banzai is a Japanese exclamation that means "ten thousand years" as a wish for long life. It is used like a cheer or send-off—creating a big, happy, free feeling. Growing up, my grandpa Hiroshi Yamamoto would yell this to us whenever we drove away from his home, and I always thought he was saying, "BONSAI!!" as in the tree. It is now a favorite memory and the reason behind the name of this tea blend.

In an airtight container, combine the goji berries, chrysanthemum, mint, nettle, dandelion, and honeysuckle. Store in an airtight container away from heat, light, and moisture for up to 12 months.

To make a cup of tea, place 1 tsp of the tea—make sure to include chrysanthemum and goji berries—in a teapot and pour 1 cup (240 ml) of boiling water (200° F [95° C]) over the tea. Cover and steep for 5 to 10 minutes before straining. Drink immediately.

Contraindication: Omit nettles in cases of cardiac or renal failure.

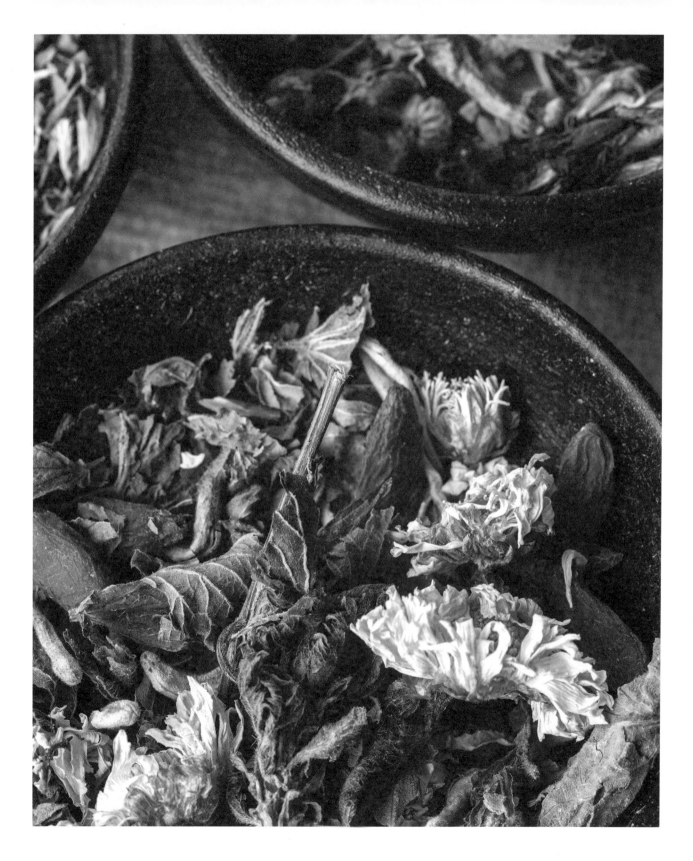

EASY DOES IT TEA

Makes 2 oz (60 g) loose-leaf tea

INGREDIENTS

½ cup (14 g) dried oat straw

½ cup (14 g) dried nettle

¼ cup (9 g) dried horsetail

¼ cup (5 g) dried lemon balm

¼ cup (5 g) dried marshmallow leaf

¼ cup (7 g) dried chamomile

Easy Does It Tea allows the body and mind to handle daily stress with more grace. This medicinal blend has a cumulative effect that is meant to be taken regularly to balance and fortify the nervous system over time. Oat straw, nettle, and horsetail are rich in calcium and minerals to heal long-term stress and damage to the nervous system. Lemon balm lifts the spirit and eases nervous tension. Marshmallow leaf and chamomile have a mucilaginous (slippery) quality that hydrates frayed nerves and softens the emotional toll of long-term stress.

In an airtight container, combine the oat straw, nettle, horsetail, lemon balm, marshmallow leaf, and chamomile. Store in an airtight container away from heat, light, and moisture for up to 12 months.

To make a cup of tea, place 1 heaping tsp of the tea in a teapot and pour 1 cup (240 ml) of boiling water (200° F [95° C]) over the tea. Cover and steep for 10 minutes before straining. Drink immediately.

Contraindication: Omit nettles in cases of cardiac or renal failure.

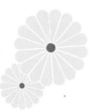

OAT INFUSION FOR STRESS AND OVERWHELM

Makes 3 cups (720 ml)

INGREDIENTS

¼ cup (7 g) dried oat straw

¼ cup (7 g) dried milky oat tops

One of the first signs of spring is the oats that line every country road and fill fields all over our Northern California town. This recipe was written with these rolling, abundant oat fields in mind. The oat straw and the milky oat top are nutrient dense, with B vitamins, calcium, and magnesium to benefit the nervous system, mind, and body. The oat straw heals long-term, chronic stress in the body, while the milky oat tops are more effective at addressing acute stress. You can use oat straw and milky oat tops interchangeably in this recipe, depending on what you have on hand, but I prefer to include both parts of this plant.

In a 4 cup (960 ml) glass jar, combine the milky oat tops, oat straw, and 3 cups (720 ml) of simmering water (180° F [80°C]). Always take care when adding hot water to glass jars. It should never be boiling otherwise the jar can crack. Loosely cover the top of the jar and steep for 20 to 30 minutes before straining. Store in the refrigerator and drink over the course of the next 2 days. In times of intense stress or when healing from burnout, make this infusion once weekly for 3 months.

Foraging and Harvesting Oats

Oats are not only for oatmeal. The oat plant produces three medicinal parts—the oat straw (stem), the milky oat top (immature seed), and the oats (mature seed). You will know that the green, milky oat tops are ready to harvest when they produce a drop of white "milk" when squeezed. Milky oat tops and oat straw that are freshly harvested and still green in color need less of a steep to impart their medicine. Just be sure to harvest away from the roadside, vineyards, or fields sprayed with pesticides.

Note: To dry freshly harvested oat straw and milky oat tops, tie them in ½ in (12 mm) bundles and hang upside down in a dry place for 5 to 10 days. Once dried, the oat straw stalks will easily break in half. Pull off the milky oat tops from the oat straw then use scissors or shears to cut the oat straw into ½ in (12 mm) pieces.

MILKY OAT BATH

Yields 1 bath

INGREDIENTS

½ cup (14 g) dried oat straw
and/or milky oat tops

1 cup (100 g) old-fashioned
rolled oats

¼ cup (7 g) dried lavender or
dried rose petals (5 g)

1 cup (127 g) coconut milk
powder

¼ cup (50 g) baking soda

This herbal milk bath is a play on the fragrant, opaque mineral baths from Japan. Oats are renowned for adding softness, nourishment, and moisture to the body, inside and out. Just as oatmeal baths are a classic remedy for dry, itchy skin, an oat infusion is a remedy for dry, irritated energy. Simmering and steeping the milky oat tops and oat straw draws out their medicinal properties. Although you can add a variety of flowers or herbs to a bath tea, the addition of lavender or rose has particularly calming and Heart-warming effects. Rolled oats, coconut milk powder, and baking soda soften and hydrate the skin. The lesson of this bath is to take time to be held in softness and grace.

In a medium pot, bring the oat straw and/or tops and 4 cups (960 ml) of water to a boil. Reduce heat and gently simmer for 15 minutes and then remove from heat. Add the oats and the lavender or rose, cover the pot with a lid, and steep for 15 minutes while drawing a very warm bath.

When the bath is ready, strain the herbs and oats from the bath "tea" then add the bath tea, along with the coconut milk powder and baking soda to the bath water. Soak for 20 minutes for a full therapeutic effect.

Asian American Herbalism

Guided Meditation for Connecting to the Natural World

Meditative practices are one of the most important tools for easing stress and overwhelm. These practices can be active (yoga, qigong, tai chi, walks in nature) or still (acupuncture, massage, meditation). I enjoy guided meditations because they bring my busy, distracted mind to a place of stillness. To try this yourself, prepare by recording the meditation and playing it back to yourself or by having a friend read it aloud to you. I've written the mediation as I would say it aloud, with pauses between each line. When ready, find a comfortable place to lie down or recline and dedicate a good twenty minutes for resting after the guided meditation has been read. Remove distractions and noises and create a space where you can fully tap into the moment and release the stress and tension of the day.

Meditation:

→ Find a comfortable reclined position and feel your body fully supported.

→ Following your natural breath, take a moment to come into the space, into the moment.

→ And with each breath and exhalation, start to soften and release the body.

→ Soften the belly, fingers, and toes.

→ Release the chest and throat, the jaw, tongue, and eyes.

→ Visualize your body as it is, with roots from your back drawing down toward the earth.

→ Visualize branches, like the branches of a tree, reaching from the front body up to the sky.

→ Allow each of these connections to tap into the energy of the natural world, so that with each breath, each inhalation, the Qi from the natural world effortlessly fills you up.

→ As you breathe fully and naturally, visualize that this energy is the color gold.

→ And this golden energy lights up your spine and fills your torso and chest.

→ The golden energy reaches the fingers and each toe.

→ It washes over your brain and fills your entire body, so much so that it begins to radiate from you.

→ Imagine that the golden Qi is so vital that it forms an energetic bubble just a few inches off your skin, like a boundary. A protection.

→ With this in place, begin to let go. Allowing thoughts, sensations, even little movements to pass right through you.

→ As you settle in, breath by breath. Again and again.

COLD, FLU, AND ALLERGIES

Colds, the flu, and allergies are just a fact of life—no one is immune to catching seasonal illnesses or falling ill. Head and chest colds are such a part of the human condition that many herbal remedies for these ailments, passed down through generations, are found in the kitchen. The comfort of grandma's chicken soup, made with thyme, oregano, garlic, and onion, comes to mind.

Asian American herbalism refers to all head colds and allergies as wind invasions. Wind invasions happen when pathogens from the natural world enter the body due to changes such as seasonal transitions or when the weather becomes unseasonably warm or cold. This concept of pathogens, which includes wind, cold, heat, damp, and dryness, is discussed in-depth in the Energetics of Illness chapter (page 61).

Wind invasions are acute illnesses that come on quickly and last up to a week. When wind invasions are unchecked, they can travel deeper into the body and develop into chest colds with cough, congestion, exhaustion, and flu-like symptoms that can last for weeks. This is where herbal medicine comes into play—not only for prevention but also for keeping illnesses from progressing deeper into the body and becoming more severe.

Wind Invasions – Head Colds

Although we are all susceptible to head colds, the frequency and severity are connected to the health of the Lung and the strength of the Wei Qi (defensive Qi). Wei Qi is an energy that extends from the surface of the muscles to the exterior of the skin. It forms an energetic boundary around the body that prevents disease by warding off pathogens, such as wind, cold, heat, bacteria, viruses, and allergens. This energetic boundary also protects against negative and draining energy from other people (for more on causes of illness, see page 72). Healthy Wei Qi is a major factor in determining whether someone catches a head cold and indicates the strength of one's immune system.

Depending on the weather and season, wind invasions can break through the body's defenses (Wei Qi) to cause illness. Wind invasions are treated with specific herbs depending on if the wind invasion coexists with heat symptoms (wind-heat) or cold symptoms (wind-cold). Understanding wind-heat versus wind-cold is key for effectively treating a head cold with herbal medicine.

Head colds due to wind-heat present with fever, sore throat, restlessness, throbbing headache, sweats, red skin rashes, and cough with yellow or dark phlegm. Wind-heat is treated with cooling herbs, such as mint and honeysuckle. Wind-cold illness comes with cold symptoms including chills with mild fever, scratchy throat, stiff neck, body aches, headaches, congested nose, lack of sweating, and cough with white or clear phlegm. Head colds due to wind-cold are treated with warming herbs, such as fresh ginger and green onion. The following section will cover herbs and remedies for treating wind invasions and how to prevent them from becoming chest colds.

HERBS FOR WIND INVASION

WARM
—
Cinnamon
Shiso
Green Onion
Fresh Ginger

COOL
—
Mint
Elder
Yarrow
Thyme
Sage
Mulberry
Chrysanthemum
Feverfew

COUGH + PHLEGM:
—
Mullein
Marshmallow
Loquat Leaf
Elecampane
Apricot Kernel
Cherry Bark

WIND HEAT VS. WIND COLD

WIND HEAT
—
fever > chills
sore throat
thirst
sweats
irritability
congestion with yellow
or green phlegm

WIND COLD
—
chills > fever
scratchy throat
body tension
headache
sneezing with clear phlegm

How to Treat a Head Cold by Releasing the Exterior

Releasing the exterior is both a folk remedy and herbal category in traditional Chinese medicine. Release-the-exterior herbs push pathogens, including wind, out of the body and past the exterior of the body or past the Wei Qi layer.

These herbs are often diaphoretic, meaning that they remove pathogens by sweating them out. As a folk remedy, releasing the exterior is done by consuming tea and resting for the first few days of an illness to treat and prevent it from going deeper. See page 158 for instructions on releasing the exterior.

How to Not Get Sick – Three Tea Blends for Wind Invasions

A warm cup of herbal tea is a timeless remedy across all cultures for when you feel an illness coming on. Head colds develop quickly, so I prefer teas made with things that can be found at the market or in the garden. These teas can be one herb, such as mint for a wind-heat sore throat or fresh ginger to kick the body chills of a wind-cold invasion. The recipes that follow have many ingredients, but they can all be simplified by using any one herb or a combination of those listed. When preparing these tea blends, follow the instructions on How to Treat a Head Cold by Releasing the Exterior below.

RELEASING THE EXTERIOR

HOW TO TREAT A HEAD COLD

—

This method can prevent a head cold by sweating out the Wind pathogens. Start with an herbal tea recipe for wind invasion. Choose an appropriate recipe for either wind heat or wind cold symptoms. Place 1 heaping tsp of herbal tea in a teapot for every 1 cup (240 ml) of water. Pour boiling water (200° F [95° C]) over herbs and cover. Steep for ten minutes, strain, and drink 2 cups (480 ml). Bundle up in bed to induce a light sweat. Sleep and take another 1 cup (240 ml) of the warmed tea when you wake up. Repeat this method once per day for up to three days.

To speed up the process, take a hot shower or bath before bed (keep hair dry to prevent a chill). The heat from the hot shower will help to induce a sweat. This method can restore good health rather quickly but if symptoms persist or worsen after three days then other remedies may be necessary.

ELDERFLOWER AND MINT TEA FOR GENERAL WIND INVASION

Makes 2 cups (100 g) loose-leaf tea

INGREDIENTS

1 ¼ cups (22 g) dried mint

½ cup (30 g) dried elderflower

¼ cup (10 g) dried yarrow flower

1 knob of fresh ginger, peeled and thinly sliced for serving

We all know the feeling in those first few hours when you're starting to come down with something. This early-stage head cold is considered a wind invasion, but there is often no clear predominance of wind-heat versus wind-cold symptoms (for examples of wind-heat vs. wind-cold, see page 156). This is a foolproof tea for those times, and the mint makes it tastes especially good. Mint, elderflower, and yarrow are release-the-exterior herbs that help the body to release wind by sweating it out. Fresh ginger is a warming herb that balances the recipe in case of wind-cold symptoms, including chills, body aches, clear runny nose, and headache. Note that you can increase the amount of mint or ginger to make the tea more palatable, because yarrow and honeysuckle have a bitter aftertaste.

In an airtight container, combine the mint, elderflower, and yarrow flower. Store away from heat, light, and moisture for up to 12 months.

To make a cup of tea, place 1 slice of fresh ginger and 1 heaping tsp of the tea in a teapot and pour 1 cup (240 ml) of boiling water (200° F [95° C]) over the ginger and tea. Cover and steep for 5 to 10 minutes before straining. Follow the instructions on How to Treat a Head Cold by Releasing the Exterior on page 158.

Contraindication: This tea is not recommended during pregnancy due to the yarrow.

THYME AND SAGE TEA FOR WIND-HEAT

Makes 1 ¼ cups (50 g) loose-leaf tea

INGREDIENTS

½ cup (30 g) dried thyme

¼ cup (5 g) dried sage

¼ cup (4 g) dried calendula flowers

¼ cup (10 g) dried yarrow flowers

Many common kitchen herbs have antibacterial and antiviral properties—think thyme, oregano, sage, and garlic. This tea blend is great for times when a head cold catches you off guard because it uses herbs that you can find at local markets and maybe even your garden. Thyme, sage, and yarrow are cooling herbs that release-the-exterior for wind-heat symptoms, including fever, cough, yellow phlegm, and sore throat. Thyme specifically benefits the Lung, and sage protects against dehydration by reducing severe fever sweats. Calendula is a wild card addition that eases body aches and painful sinuses by moving Qi. I learned this recipe from my friend Abby Rappoport, at a seasonal wellness workshop she taught on strengthening the immune system.

In an airtight container, combine the thyme, sage, calendula, and yarrow. Store away from heat, light, and moisture for up to 12 months.

To make a cup of tea, place 1 heaping tsp of the tea in a teapot and pour 1 cup (240 ml) of boiling water (200° F [95° C]) over the tea. Cover and steep for 5 to 10 minutes before straining. Follow the instructions on How to Treat a Head Cold by Releasing the Exterior on page 158.

Contraindications: This tea is not recommended during pregnancy due to the yarrow, or while breastfeeding because the sage will reduce or stop the flow of breast milk. It is also not recommended during pregnancy due to the calendula's Blood moving properties.

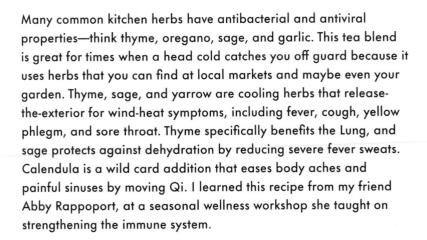

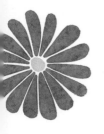

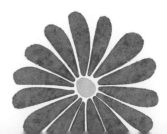

GREEN ONION AND GINGER TEA FOR WIND-COLD WITH NAUSEA

Makes 4 cups (960 ml)

INGREDIENTS

4 green onions, roots removed and cut in half

1 knob of fresh ginger, cut into 3 pieces

5 fresh or dried green shiso leaves (optional)

This traditional Chinese herbal tea recipe treats head colds with herbs from your local Asian market. The use of warming herbs, including ginger and green onion, is key for treating wind-cold symptoms, including chills, headache, and sinus congestion with a runny nose. Shiso leaves, also known as perilla, settle the stomach and should be added to the mix when there is nausea or an upset stomach. Fresh shiso is easy to grow and can be found in Asian markets. Fun fact: shiso is traditionally taken to prevent seafood poisoning, and the decorative plastic green leaf in to-go sushi boxes represents a shiso leaf.

In a small pot, bring the green onions, ginger, shiso, and 4 cups (960 ml) of water to a boil. Cover, reduce the heat, and gently simmer for 10 minutes.

Follow the instructions on How to Treat a Head Cold by Releasing the Exterior on page 158.

Contraindication: Omit shiso in cases of diabetes.

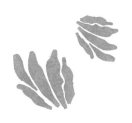

Gua Sha to Ward Off Early-Stage Head Colds

Growing up, I was not allowed to go to bed with wet hair for fear of catching a cold. My mom now tells me that she never knew exactly how or why it worked; she just knew that it did. Decades later, I've come to learn that we keep the back of our heads and neck protected, warm, and dry to prevent wind invasions. Wind invasions enter the body through the skin, and we are particularly vulnerable to this at the back of the neck. There are even acupuncture points on the back of the neck named for their ability to treat wind. They have names like wind pool (feng chi) at Gallbladder 20 and wind mansion (feng fu) at Du 16.

Gua Sha is a scraping massage and folk healing method that has been used in homes in China, and across the Asian diaspora for many generations. Gua Sha along the back of the neck prevents head colds by releasing the exterior to remove wind pathogens from the body, which has the same effect as the release-the-exterior herbs in the previous tea recipes. When someone comes into my clinic with a head cold, I immediately think to gua sha the back of their neck. And this is how you do it at home:

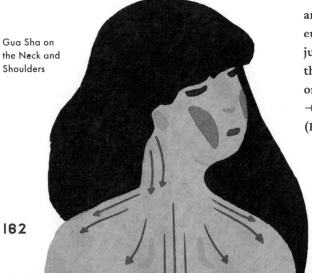

Gua Sha on the Neck and Shoulders

→ You will need a body oil and a gua sha tool (i.e., olive oil and a porcelain soup spoon or gua sha stone, which are readily available online).

→ While you can technically do this yourself, having someone else do gua sha for you on the back of your neck and shoulders is best because they can apply an intense pressure that is difficult to achieve on your own.

→ Lightly apply oil to the skin from the back of the neck to the shoulders.

→ Using the gua sha tool with medium pressure, scrape the tool down the back of the neck using long strokes. From the base of the skull, draw the tool down to the upper back and the top of the shoulders. The direction is always down and out to the sides.

→ There shouldn't be any pain. If there is, apply more oil and less pressure. Avoid gua sha directly on the vertebrae or bones.

→ The treatment takes one to two minutes. Oftentimes, gua sha will cause a pink, red, brown, or purple color to develop on the surface of the skin. This is safe, and it is an indication of stagnation or trapped wind! It is more like a painless hickey than a bruise. When this happens, continue the treatment until the color stops developing or for up to 30 seconds.

→ Afterward, treat the skin as if it is "open" and protect it from extremely windy and cold environments for two days. For example, do not jump into a cold swimming pool. I like to keep the area covered with a bandanna, long hair, or a hoodie.

→ For more in-depth information, see page 283 (Healing Practices).

ELDERBERRY SYRUP

Makes 3 cups (720 ml)

INGREDIENTS

½ cup (60 g) black elderberries

6 dried astragalus slices, each about 3 in (7.5 cm)

5 whole cloves

1 cinnamon stick

1 tsp elecampane

5 sticks dried licorice

4 in (10 cm) piece fresh tangerine peel (or 1 Tbsp dried tangerine or other citrus peel)

1 knob of fresh ginger, chopped in half

1 tsp vanilla extract (¼ vanilla bean)

1 to 2 cups (240 to 480 ml) raw honey (see note)

2 Tbsp 80 proof brandy or vodka (optional)

Elderberry Syrup is one of the most popular herbal remedies for supporting a healthy immune system in Western herbalism. It is a preventative medicine that's most effective when taken regularly during cold and flu season or at the start of an illness. Studies show that elderberry can reduce the duration of a cold or the flu by up to four days. And as a bonus, the sweet flavors are a hit with kids.

This recipe is my Asian American twist on a classic elderberry syrup with the addition of astragalus, licorice, ginger, and tangerine peel. Elderberries and astragalus are two of my favorites and some of the most effective herbs for boosting the immune system. However, elderberries are quite cold, so the warmth of cinnamon and cloves is essential for balance in this recipe. Elecampane root and licorice work synergistically as expectorants, which means that they help remove congestion and stubborn phlegm. Licorice, tangerine peel, and ginger harmonize and move Qi to keep energy healthy and strong. The vanilla is also a harmonizer that brings all the flavors together.

In a medium pot, combine the elderberries, astragalus, cloves, cinnamon, elecampane, licorice, tangerine peel (if using dried), ginger, and 4 cups (960 ml) of water. Partially cover and bring to a gentle simmer. Keep an eye on the mixture to ensure it does not boil, as the medicinal strength is weakened under a rapid boil. Continue to simmer gently for 20 to 40 minutes, or until the liquid is reduced by about half then remove from the heat, add the fresh tangerine peel (if using) and stir in the vanilla. Steep for 5 minutes then use cheesecloth or a fine-mesh sieve to strain. Let the mixture cool to room temperature then stir in the honey and brandy or vodka (if using). Store in a glass jar in the refrigerator for up to 2 months. The more honey and liquor added, the longer it will keep. →

Elderberry Syrup (continued)

The medicinal dose is ½ to 2 tsp for kids and ½ to 1 Tbsp for adults, taken once daily. When sick, take that dosage every 2 to 4 hours until symptoms clear or for 3 to 4 days.

Note: For a thick syrup, increase the honey so that it is equal to the elderberry liquid (i.e., 2 cups liquid to 2 cups honey).

Contraindication: Omit cinnamon during pregnancy. Omit licorice in cases of kidney disorders, hypertension, and congestive heart failure.

Allergies

Allergies are wind invasions that come on seasonally due to allergens such as pollen, grass, mold, and chemicals. Like head and chest colds, allergies are caused by wind pathogens and weak Wei Qi. To prevent allergies, Qi tonic herbs, such as astragalus and mugwort, are taken over time (for at least three months) to strengthen healthy Wei Qi. And then, there are herbs, including nettle, chrysanthemum, goji berry, magnolia bud, and thyme, to address specific allergy symptoms, such as red, irritated eyes, sinus congestion, sneezing, runny nose, fatigue, mental clarity, and general malaise. The recipe for Bonsai Herbal Tea (page 150) and the recipes in the previous section on head colds are also effective for allergies.

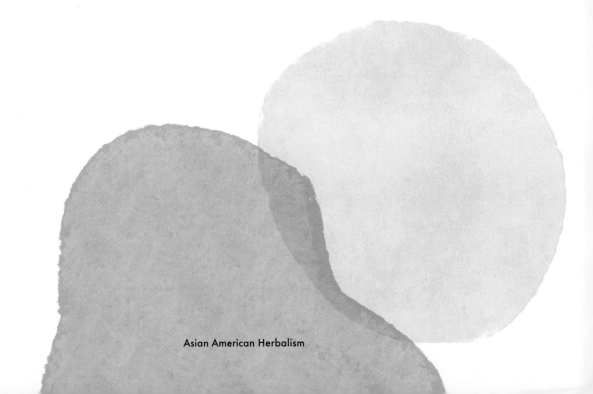

MAGNOLIA BUD TEA FOR ALLERGIES AND SINUSITIS

Makes 2 cups (100 g) loose-leaf tea

INGREDIENTS

1 cup (80 g) dried magnolia flower buds

½ cup (10 g) dried shiso leaf

½ cup (7 g) dried chrysanthemum

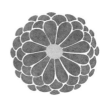

When you stand under a magnolia tree, you are in the presence of the ancients. With fossils dating back 20 million years, magnolia is a bridge to the distant past, but it's also a significant healing plant. From bark to bud to flower, the magnolia tree gifts us with medicine that heals us to our very core. Magnolia balances the movement of Qi from the Lungs to the gut, transforms phlegm, and calms the mind.

The magnolia flower buds used in this tea are great for allergies, congestion, and inflamed and infected sinuses (sinusitis). Magnolia flower buds open nasal passages and treat wind-cold symptoms, including congestion and sneezing. Collect the firm, unmarked fuzzy buds if harvesting them yourself—you'll find them in the early spring before the flowers bloom. Shiso leaf and chrysanthemum are also well suited for treating allergies because they reduce damp (congestion) and clear inflammatory heat toxins.

In an airtight container, combine the magnolia, shiso, and chrysanthemum. Store away from heat, light, and moisture for up to 12 months.

To make a cup of tea, place 1 heaping tsp of the tea in a teapot and pour 1 cup (240 ml) of boiling water (200 F [95 C]) over the tea. Cover and steep for 5 to 10 minutes before straining.

For chronic allergies, drink 1 to 2 cups (240 to 480 ml) daily right before allergy season or at the first sign of allergies. Continue as needed. Follow the instructions on How to Treat a Head Cold by Releasing the Exterior on page 158.

Contraindication: Omit shiso in cases of diabetes.

HERBAL EYE COMPRESS FOR IRRITATED EYES

Makes 2 cups (480 ml)

INGREDIENTS

¼ cup (3 g) dried
  chrysanthemum
1 Tbsp dried goji berries
A cotton washcloth or piece of
  cotton flannel

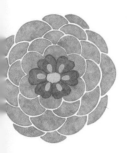

Herbal pairs, or dui yao, have a synergistic energy that strengthens their medicine when used together. Chrysanthemum and goji berries are my favorite herbal pair, and are traditionally used to heal red, irritated eyes. They address both the Qi (chrysanthemum) and the Blood (goji berry) of eye ailments when taken as a tea or used as an eye compress. As a wash, chrysanthemum and goji berry can be used for all eye inflammations regardless of if they're due to allergies or an infection. Note that antibiotic eye drops and ointments only clear up bacterial infections and do not address allergies or viral infections.

My children both had ongoing eye infections for the first year of life, so I would prepare an herbal eye compress to soothe and gently speed up the healing process. Make the compress by soaking a small towel in the herbal wash and gently holding it over the affected eye. Always use caution when working with the eyes and never apply pressure for the risk of damaging the retina. Be sure to wash hands well when working with infected eyes and to not cross-contaminate as infection from one eye can spread to the other.

In a glass jar, combine the chrysanthemum, goji berries, and 2 cups (480 ml) of simmering water (180° F [80°C]). Always take care when adding hot water to glass jars. It should never be boiling otherwise the jar can crack.

Cover and steep for 15 minutes before straining with cheesecloth or a fine-mesh sieve to remove all the plant material. Cool and store in a glass jar in the refrigerator for up to 2 days. ↗

To prepare the eye compress, take a small washcloth and soak it with the herbal tea. While lying down, gently place the soaked fabric on the affected eye. Never put any pressure on the eyeball and do not pour the herbal tea directly into the eyes. Apply for 10 to 15 minutes, 2 to 3 times a day until symptoms subside or for up to 5 days.

Note: If both eyes are affected, use different cloths to avoid cross-contaminating.

Variations

—

Mulberry Leaf Eye Wash for Red Hot Eyes: For eyes that are notably red, hot, and infected, add ¼ cup (5 g) dried mulberry leaf to the eye compress recipe and follow the instructions.

—

Quick Green Tea Eye Compress for Sore Eyes: Make a cup of green tea and reserve the wet tea bag. Once cool, place the tea bag on the affected eye, following the instructions in the eye compress recipe.

Chest Colds, Flu, Cough and Congestion

Chest colds can linger for weeks with fever, cough, congestion, exhaustion, and flu-like symptoms. When this happens, it is vital to sleep as much as possible, hydrate, and take herbs, such as the Breath Work Tea (page 169) and the Thyme Steam for Cough and Congestion (page 170). When a chest cold develops into something deeper, phlegm and profound dehydration can cause various problems, including chronic cough, recurring sinus infections, insomnia, irritability, and loss of voice. The following recipes are effective for healing the Lungs and keeping chest colds from becoming more severe.

ON FEVERS

Fevers are a sign of illness. They are the immune system's way to fight off, to literally burn off, disease. Acute fevers should run their course in three to four days and simple at-home remedies can alleviate discomfort using cooling and release-the-exterior herbs. Herbs address fevers in this way to support the body's natural healing process rather than suppressing it. Release-the-exterior herbs that vent fevers are cooling in nature and include mint, ginger, yarrow, elderflower and elderberry, chrysanthemum, and thyme. If you have any concerns, contact your doctor immediately to rule out infection or fevers above 104°F (40°C) for adults and 101°F (38°C) for kids.

BREATH WORK — A LUNG SUPPORT TEA

Makes 3 cups (100 g) loose-leaf tea

INGREDIENTS

1 cup (40 g) dried marshmallow root

½ cup (7 g) dried mullein leaves

½ cup (10 g) dried mint (or dried lemon balm)

½ cup (30 g) dried elderflower

¼ cup (7 g) dried nettle

¼ cup (5 g) dried tulsi

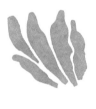

Every autumn, our community in Northern California braces for fire season, dreading the dark, smoky days that obscure the sun and fall heavy on our lungs. In 2017, the Tubbs fires devastated my hometown in Sonoma County, creating unforgettable community trauma. This herbal tea blend was formulated with fire season in mind, and it is appropriate for taking during and after smoke exposure.

I've also come to use this formula as a general Lung-support tea. It is a balanced blend of herbs to heal the Lungs, support immunity, and clear heat toxins from the system. Marshmallow leaf soothes and hydrates delicate lung tissue. Mullein is a natural expectorant that helps the lungs to cough up phlegm, mucus, and toxins. Mint and elderflower cool the body to clear wind-heat and inflammation. They also benefit the immune system and support strong, healthy Qi. Nutrient-dense tulsi and nettle nourish and balance from within. This tea is also supportive in times of transition, letting go, and grief (for the emotional energy of the Lung, see page 64). It's also soothing and delicious as an herbal iced tea with lemonade.

In an airtight container, combine the marshmallow, mullein, mint, elderflower, nettle, and tulsi. Store away from heat, light, and moisture for up to 12 months.

To make a cup of tea, place 1 heaping tsp of herbal tea in a teapot and pour 1 cup (240 ml) of boililng water (200° F [95° C]) over the tea. Cover and steep for 10 minutes before straining. Drink immediately.

The medicinal does is 1 cup (240 ml) twice per day for 3 days or as needed.

Contraindications: Omit tulsi in cases of diabetes, during pregnancy, or when pregnancy is possible. Omit nettles in cases of cardiac or renal failure.

THYME STEAM FOR COUGH AND CONGESTION

Makes 1 steam

INGREDIENTS

1 to 2 drops thyme essential oil

2 drops eucalyptus essential oil

1 drop oregano essential oil

This is one of the top ten herbal recipes I use at home. It is particularly effective for kids with croup or any deep, rattling coughs that are worse at bedtime. Steams hydrate delicate lung tissue and sinuses to expel stubborn phlegm from the airways. Phlegm is a condensed form of dampness that tends to be thick and has a dirty or toxic quality. People who run damp will be more susceptible to phlegm and congestion.

While there are two variations for this recipe, I prefer using essential oils in a cool-mist humidifier because it can be hard to handle the intensity of a steam pot when you're ill. Effective for all kinds of coughs, thyme calms the respiratory system and helps the lungs to cough up phlegm and stubborn congestion. Oregano and eucalyptus enhance thyme's antiseptic properties and help open the lungs to receive the medicine. These essential oils are commonly found at many health foods stores.

Add thyme, oregano, and eucalyptus essential oils to a cool-mist humidifier and fill with cold water. Adjust the amount of essential oil so that the scent is not so strong that it is bothersome. Diffuse near the bedside while the person naps and overnight during sleep. Repeat 1 to 2 times per day for up to 5 days.

LOST VOICE HYDRATION TEA

Makes 2 cups (480 ml)

INGREDIENTS

3 whole dried boat seeds

1 Tbsp dried goji berries

½ tsp honey or sweetener
(optional)

Healthy Qi and Yin fluids are essential for a strong and clear voice. Losing one's voice is a sure sign that all the energetic resources have taken a hit. This recipe is for restoring voice loss due to overuse or when recovering from a fever or chest cold.

Boat seeds look like hard, brown nuts, but once soaked in water, they bloom into a clear, white, jellyfish-looking flower. They can be found at Asian markets or online by their Mandarin Chinese name, pang da hai. They are particularly effective in bringing back a weak voice or healing a raspy voice due to Yin deficiency after a cold or the flu. Boat seeds can be taken alone, but I prefer to add goji berries and honey to add sweetness to the tea and increase the nourishing properties.

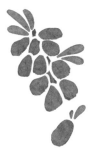

In a large glass jar, combine the boat seeds, goji berries, and 2 cups (480 ml) of simmering water (180° F [80°C]). Always take care when adding hot water to glass jars. It should never be boiling otherwise the jar can crack. Let soak for 10 minutes, or until the boat seeds are fully bloomed. Don't strain the tea and stir in the honey or sweetener (if using). Drink slowly over the course of a day.

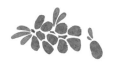

LOQUAT COUGH SYRUP

Makes 3 cups (700ml)

INGREDIENTS

4 cups (70 g) fresh loquat leaf,
   cut and loosely packed, or
   2 cups (20 g) dried loquat leaf

6 loquat fruits, halved and
   seeded

2 in (5 cm) knob of fresh ginger,
   quartered

1 cinnamon stick

3 cups (720 ml) honey

2 tsp vanilla extract

Loquat trees grow readily in my mother's garden. She loves these trees and enjoys giving transplants to friends, using the fallen leaves for garden mulch, and harvesting the leaves so that I can make cough syrup. The dark-green serrated leaves and peachy-yellow fruit make for a beautiful and medicinal addition to any garden.

This cough syrup recipe is a spin on the classic loquat cough syrups you can find in Asian markets and herb shops. Loquat leaf treats lung conditions due to Lung heat and dampness, with symptoms that include a deep cough, congestion with clear or yellow phlegm, sore throat, and dry mouth. Loquat leaf is bitter and cooling, so it is most effective for coughs that are accompanied by or that started with a fever. It should not be used in cases of illness marked by vomiting and no present fever. Loquat cough syrup is traditionally made using only the leaves; however, I add fresh loquat fruit for flavor when it's in season in my mother's garden.

When harvesting loquat leaves, pick mature dark green leaves that are even in color without any moldy, dark spots. Remove any thick stems and use scissors to cut the leaves into 1 to 2 in (2.5 to 5 cm) pieces. Dried loquat leaves can easily be found online, but depending on where you live, fresh loquat leaves can be found locally. The fresh loquat fruit can be substituted with an Asian pear (cut and quartered).

In a large pot, bring the loquat leaves and fruit, ginger, cinnamon, and 12 cups (2.8 L) of water to a boil. Turn the heat down to medium, stir, and gently boil, uncovered, for 45 minutes, or until the liquid has reduced by half (6 cups [1.4 L]). Remove from the heat and use a cheesecloth-lined colander or fine-mesh sieve to strain. Discard the spent leaves and herbs. Pour the liquid back into the pot and return to a gentle boil. Continue gently boiling for 25 minutes, or until reduced by half (3 cups [720 ml]). Remove from the heat. ↗

While the syrup is still warm, add equal parts honey to the liquid mixture (3 cups [1 L]) and stir until well incorporated. Let cool completely then add the vanilla. Store in glass jars in the refrigerator for up to 4 weeks or freeze in a freezer-safe container for up to 3 months. The cough syrup can also be canned for long-term storage.

Note: Loquat leaves have tiny hairs that irritate the throat and must be removed by straining the liquid very well through cheesecloth or a fine-mesh sieve.

Contraindications: Omit cinnamon during pregnancy.

Variation

—

Loquat Cough Syrup for Congestion: Add the following herbs at the same time as the loquat leaves in the above recipe. Asian pear heals and moistens the Lung. Elecampane root and licorice work together as natural expectorants to help the body cough up stubborn congestion in the lungs.

1 Asian pear (or another pear variety), cored and quartered
2 tsp dried elecampane root
20 sticks dried licorice

Contraindication: Omit cinnamon during pregnancy. Omit licorice in cases of kidney disorders, hypertension, and congestive heart failure.

SKIN CONDITIONS

The skin is our largest organ and our protective exterior boundary. It is the bridge between our inner world and the outside environment. It senses, communicates, and determines how we perceive the world. The skin holds us in and reflects our internal health.

Vital, glowing, plump skin is a sign of good internal health. Skin ailments, on the other hand, reflect an internal imbalance. For example, redness and bumps on the cheeks indicate stomach issues, including food sensitivities. Itchy, red rashes that come and go (urticaria) are a sign of heat and Blood deficiency. Cold sores, herpes, and shingles can be linked to an underlying Liver Qi stagnation with damp heat. Pimples and oozing cuts and bumps show our body's capacity to fight infection. And a bloody scrape and scab show our body's capacity to heal.

A dermatologist once told me that the key to healing skin is to not mess with it too much. However, there is undoubtedly an instinct to touch the skin. It is hard not to fixate on redness, swelling, dryness, changes in texture, irritation, itchiness, pain, pimples, bumps, and other irregularities. We use herbal remedies not only to expedite healing but also to give us ways to tend to skin issues in a minimally invasive way.

In Asian American herbalism, we address skin issues internally and at the skin's surface. At the most basic level, an herbal salve is a balm that can soothe both the skin and a busy mind. Yarrow and clay masks are great for drying excess oil and dampness at the skin's surface, while herbal teas address these excesses from the inside out. Lemon balm oil tends to external cold sores and herpes outbreaks, while traditional Chinese medicine formulas including Xiao Yao Tang balance the internal Qi stagnation.

HERBS FOR HEALTHY SKIN

SOOTHING
—
Chrysanthemum
Calendula
Chickweed
Lemon Balm
Plantain
Red Clover

EXTERNAL
—
Arnica
Comfrey
Mullein Flowers
Lavender
Oat Straw and
Milky Oat Tops
Rice Bran

INVIGORATING
—
Gentian
Dandelion
Yarrow
Violet
Safflower
Burdock Root

MUGWORT AND NUKA BATH FOR SMOOTH SKIN

Makes 1 bath

INGREDIENTS

¾ cup (80 g) rice bran

¼ cup (15 g) dried mugwort leaves

¼ cup (50 g) baking soda

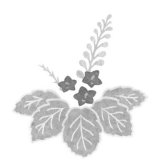

"Nuka" is the Japanese word for rice bran and it is used in baths to balance and hydrate the skin. This formula is soothing and hydrating like an oatmeal bath. It also calms inflammation and reduces redness and itchiness from insect bites and poison ivy. Rice bran water can be used to wash hair as well. Mugwort has an invigorating nature and was traditionally used as a skin wash to treat various ailments, including eczema and itchiness. The Milky Oat Bath (page 154) is another hydrating bath option.

Place the rice bran and mugwort leaves in the center of a piece of cheesecloth or cotton fabric that measures at least 6 × 6 in (15 × 15 cm) and tie it into a bundle with string so that the rice bran stays intact.

Draw a very warm bath and add the rice bran bundle and baking soda to the bath water. Gently squeeze the bundle as it absorbs the water. The rice bran will start to dissolve, and the milky liquid will make the bath water softer and slightly yellow in color. Soak your body for 20 minutes for a full therapeutic effect.

Variation

—

Compress method: Prepare the rice bran in a cheesecloth or fabric bundle as described above. Heat 8 cups (2 L) of water until simmering (180° F [80°C]). Remove from the heat and steep the rice bran bundle in the water for at least 15 minutes. Occasionally squeeze the bundle gently to help the rice bran dissolve and release a milky liquid. Dip a washcloth in the rice bran water and gently press the rice bran water into any dry, itchy skin, irritations, or bug bites, or use as a hair rinse.

CALENDULA SUN OIL FOR HEALTHY SKIN

Makes 1½ cups (360 ml)

INGREDIENTS

1 cup (16 g) dried calendula

2 cups (480 ml) safflower oil

This is an herb-infused oil that brings together the healing powers of calendula, safflower, and the sun. Calendula is arguably the best flower medicine for healing the skin and has been documented as medicine since Ancient Egypt.

When you pick fresh calendula flowers, you will notice that they leave a sticky resin on your fingers. This resin contains antiseptic properties to prevent infection and promote healthy skin; it also provides skin healing for cuts, scrapes, dry skin, rashes, and irritations. Safflower oil is my favorite carrier oil because it is rich in linoleic acid (an omega fatty acid), which moisturizes, improves the skin's natural barrier, and prevents break outs. Safflowers are also used in traditional Chinese medicine for their blood-moving properties. Safflower and calendula both stimulate the circulation of Blood, lymph, and Qi, which is perfect for inflammation just below the skin's surface, such as with bruises, swollen joints, hemorrhoids, and swelling in the chest, armpits, and groin. This recipe uses a sun oil or solar infusion technique because there is something undeniably magical about oil that is infused under the warm glow of the sun.

To prepare the calendula flowers, place them in a blender and pulse 10 to 20 times until broken down into smaller pieces.

In a 2 cup (480 ml) glass jar, combine the calendula and about 1¼ cups (300 ml) of the safflower oil. There should be 1 to 2 in (2.5 to 5 cm) of oil covering the top of the herbs, so they do not spoil. Save the remaining oil to top off the herbal mixture as the herbs absorb the oil. Cover tightly and place the jar in a sunny window or a warm spot to infuse for 2 to 4 weeks. Gently shake the mixture every few days and top off with oil as needed to keep the flowers fully submerged. ↗

Using cheesecloth or a fine-mesh sieve, strain the oil, squeezing out as much oil as possible with your hands or the back of a wooden spoon. Pour the strained oil into a clean glass jar, being careful not to pour off any water or plant materials that may settle at the bottom of the oil. Discard the remaining water and plant materials as they will spoil the finished oil. Label the jar with the date and ingredients. Store away from heat, light, and moisture for up to 1 year.

Variation

—

Quick stovetop method: This recipe can be made quickly by heating the herbal oil on a stovetop or crockpot (for more on infused oils, see page 292).

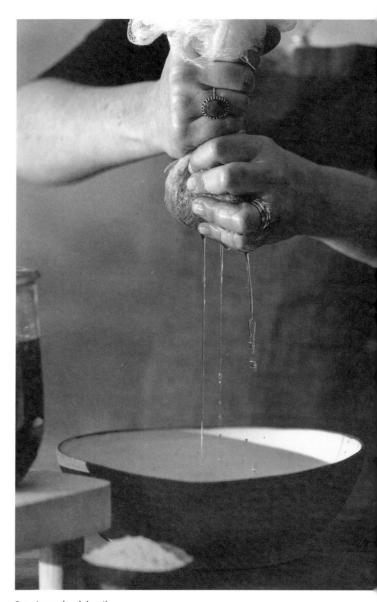

Pressing calendula oil

FIRST AID OIL

Makes 1½ cups (360 ml)

INGREDIENTS

1 cup (16 g) dried calendula

2 Tbsp dried comfrey leaves

2 Tbsp dried yarrow leaves

2 Tbsp dried violet flowers and
leaves

2 Tbsp dried plantain leaves

2 cups (480 ml) safflower oil

This First Aid Oil is a variation on the Calendula Sun Oil in the previous recipe. It is an antiseptic herb-infused oil that prevents infection and promotes healing for cuts, scrapes, bumps, blisters, and broken skin. Comfrey and plantain, with their strong abilities to clear heat and reduce inflammation, are two of the best herbs for healing bumps, bruises, and cuts. Yarrow and violet clear damp heat and prevent infection from setting into cuts and scrapes. To treat a cut or bruise, apply this oil three times daily. If using a bandage, change the dressing at the same time.

Follow the Calendula Sun Oil recipe (page 176), but add the herbs listed here, along with the calendula. Follow the instructions for making a slow-infused oil or use the quick stovetop method. This oil can be used on its own or made into a First Aid Salve (page 179).

Comfrey is only used for the skin and topical herbal medicine. In modern-day practice, it is not taken internally or used on deep wounds because studies have shown that it can be toxic to the liver when ingested due to pyrrolizidine alkaloids.

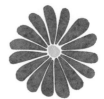

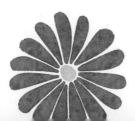

Asian American Herbalism

FIRST AID SALVE

Makes 9 oz (255 g)

INGREDIENTS

1 cup (240 ml) First Aid Oil
(page 178)

1 oz (30 g) beeswax, grated

10 drops tea tree essential oil
(optional)

This First Aid Salve is my go-to remedy for minor cuts, scrapes, bumps, bites, blisters, and broken skin. Salves have greater staying power on the skin due to the use of thickening agents such as beeswax. This salve effectively prevents infection, reduces inflammation, and speeds up skin healing. Calendula, comfrey, and plantain are some of the best herbs for healing skin from cuts, scrapes, and minor wounds. Violet is used in traditional Chinese medicine to clear damp heat, which we see in cases of low-grade infection when there is skin that is red and swollen. I add tea tree oil as a natural antiseptic and preservative; however, lavender or rosemary essential oils will also work. This salve replaces the antibiotic ointments that we grew up with and is free of petroleum. To treat a cut or bruise, apply this salve once or twice per day. If using a bandage, change the dressing at the same time.

In a small pot, carefully warm the First Aid Oil over low heat. Add the beeswax and stir until just melted into the oil. Remove from the heat and add essential oil (if using). Immediately pour the mixture into clean, dry containers and let cool. Label the jar with the date and ingredients. Once the salve is cool and hardened, secure the containers with a lid and store away from heat, light, and moisture for up to 1 year. (For more on making salves, see page 293.)

LEMON BALM OIL FOR COLD SORES AND HERPES

Makes 1½ cups (360 ml)

INGREDIENTS

9 sprigs fresh lemon balm, about
5 in (12 cm) each (or 1 cup
[20 g] dried lemon balm)

2 cups (480 ml) olive oil

Lemon balm is an excellent antiviral herb. A simple infused oil is a great way to lessen painful outbreaks of viral herpes, including cold sores and shingles. It can be used directly on sores, and when used regularly, it may reduce future outbreaks. This oil can also be made into a salve or lip balm and used liberally on the lips (see page 293, for how to make a salve). Burdock Root Bitters (page 202) can also relieve nerve pain before and during herpes outbreaks. And Fresh Lemon Balm Water (page 136) is another way to layer this cooling, antiviral medicine into your daily routine.

If working with fresh lemon balm, remove the leaves from the stems and reserve. In a 3 cup (720 ml) glass jar, combine the lemon balm and enough olive oil to completely cover the herbs. There should be 1 to 2 in (2.5 to 5 cm) of oil covering the top of the herbs, so they do not spoil. Save the remaining oil to top off the herbal mixture as the herbs absorb some of the oil. Cover tightly and place the jar in a sunny window or a warm spot to infuse for 2 weeks. Gently shake the mixture every few days.

Using cheesecloth or a fine-mesh sieve, strain the oil, squeezing out as much oil as possible with your hands or the back of a wooden spoon. Pour the strained oil into a clean glass jar, being careful not to pour off any water or plant materials that may settle at the bottom of the oil. Discard any remaining water and plant materials as they will spoil the finished oil. Store away from heat, light, and moisture for up 1 year.

Long Dan Xie Gan Tang

This classic TCM formula clears damp heat from the Liver with a mix of herbs, including the cold, bitter gentian. At the first sight of a cold sore or herpes outbreak, I recommend taking this formula in pill form for one week. Due to the draining nature of the formula, it is key to follow it up with Blood and Qi tonic herbs. My go-to is one week of Xiao Yao Tang, which moves Liver Qi and nourishes Blood and Qi.

TWO LEAF TEA FOR TOXIC SWELLING

Makes 3 ¼ cups (75 g)
loose-leaf tea

INGREDIENTS

1 cup (16 g) dried
 chrysanthemum, preferably
 yellow flowers
1 cup (20 g) dried mulberry leaf
1 cup (10 g) dried loquat leaf
3 Tbsp dried honeysuckle
 flowers

Simplicity is sophistication in herbalism. This tea blend uses chrysanthemum, mulberry leaf, and loquat leaf, three very common traditional Chinese medicine herbs for treating low-grade infections due to wind-heat. This simple yet elegant tea is strong enough to drain out heat toxins, which can present as hot skin sores, cystic acne, painful pimples, herpes/cold sores, and low-grade infections. Yellow chrysanthemum is especially good for treating skin ailments with heat, toxins, and wind; however, white chrysanthemum is a fine substitute. Despite what their name suggests, dried honeysuckle flowers have a bitter flavor. Bitter is key for draining toxic heat, but if too much is added, it makes the tea difficult to drink. Loquat leaves have hairs that irritate the throat, so be sure to use a tea bag or fine-mesh sieve when straining this tea.

In an airtight container, combine the chrysanthemum, mulberry, loquat, and honeysuckle. Store away from heat, light, and moisture for up to 12 months.

To make a cup of tea, place 1 heaping tsp of the tea in a teapot and pour 1 cup (240 ml) of boiling water (200° F [95° C]) over the tea. Cover and steep for 10 minutes before straining. Drink immediately.

The medicinal dose is 1 cup (240 ml) twice per day for 3 days or as needed.

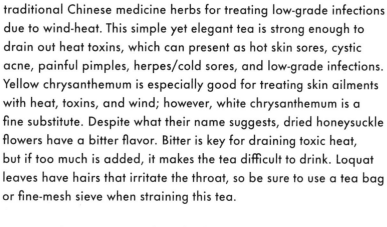
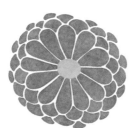

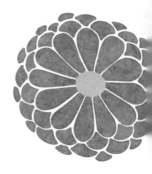

PAIN

Pain begins and ends in the head. Pain sensations are chemical/neurological messages traveling between the body and the brain via the nervous system. Thus, pain is perceived, regulated, aggravated, prolonged, and healed in the mind. Herbal medicine can alleviate many different types of pain by bringing the body and mind into greater balance. And our capacity to recover from pain speaks to the incredible power of the mind and body connection.

Pain is not the cause, but the result, of imbalance. It is our body's way of communicating, sometimes quite loudly, that something needs our attention. Pain tells us when to stay off an injured knee and when the body needs rest. Even though we have over-the-counter pain killers to provide immediate relief, herbalism is a tool that addresses both the pain and the underlying issue. Herbalism can offer pain relief in many ways, including:

- Calming the nervous system to interrupt the pain cycle.
- Massage and healing touch to move stagnation and comfort the nerve endings in the skin.
- Balancing energetics that underlie painful sensation, such as cooling the heat of inflammation and warming and stimulating areas that are stagnant.

Successful holistic treatment for injury combines herbal medicine (internally and externally), massage, exercise, and movement therapy.

HERBS FOR PAIN

COOLING
—
Dandelion
Burdock Root
Mint
Red Clover
Feverfew
Sage
White Peony Root
Motherwort
Calendula

WARMING
—
Mugwort
Ginger
Turmeric
Cinnamon
Frankincense
Safflower
Tangerine Peel
Dang Gui
Eucommia

NEUTRAL
—
Myrrh
Horsetail
Licorice

Asian American Herbalism

Energetics of Pain

Stagnant Qi

Qi stagnation is the most common cause of pain that I treat in my clinic. This type of pain feels like a dull pressure or cramping pain that comes and goes. This pain is often due to emotional strain and stress that comes on slowly and without a noticeable traumatic event. An example is low back pain that becomes a muscle spasm for seemingly no reason. The pain we don't see is often ignored until it becomes debilitating, which is much more difficult to heal. I always say that the longer an injury has existed, the longer the course of herbs is needed for healing. Qi stagnation pain is also related to lingering physical injuries that have set in like a deep bruise. This prolongs the healing process of minor injuries, such as a strained muscle or twisted ankle.

Wind and Arthritic Pain

Arthritic pain is caused by degeneration and damage to the cartilage and bone of the joints. Energetically this pain is due to internal wind that affects the muscles, joints, and acupuncture meridians—this is known as wind obstruction syndrome. This wind is different from the wind-heat/wind-cold that causes cold and flu. It is a wind that lies deep in the body and creates a variety of uncomfortable sensations—stiffness, rigidity, muscle contractions, sudden pain, pain that moves around, and severe pain in specific joints.

Common examples are:

- Knee, elbow, and wrist pain from athletic injuries and repetitive stress.
- Finger stiffness and rigidity due to rheumatoid arthritis.
- Neck, shoulder, and spinal pain due to inflammation and old injuries.

Pain Assessment

Pain is an ailment that we often cannot see and that changes over time; thus, identifying and following pain patterns is a valuable part of the healing process. A simple pain assessment keeps track of healing progress and helps identify the most effective healing methods. Questions about pain can be quite in-depth, and a complete intake follows the OPQRST mnemonic:

Onset

How long has this pain been going on, and when did it start?

Provocation

What makes it better or worse? If heat takes away the pain, warming herbs and heat therapy will help. If activity and movement make the pain worse than rest, gentle massage, and tonic herbs are appropriate. Also, note that pain that remains unchanged over time may signal a deeper underlying issue that a medical provider should check.

Quality of Pain

How would you describe the pain now and as it changes over time? Sharp, burning, pulsating, or constant pain is a sign of excess. Dull pressure, numbness, and heavy pain that comes and goes is a sign of deficiency.

Region

Where is the pain located, and does the pain move? Pain radiating or shooting across a body area indicates a pinched nerve.

Scale

The pain scale is 1–10, with 10 being the most extreme pain. This is used to chart the progress of pain and to gauge whether healing treatments are effective or not.

Time

Is it more painful during the day or at night? Pain that is worse upon waking and improves with physical activity is an excess pain. Pain that increases in the evening or is aggravated by physical activity is a deficiency pain. Pain that is only present at night may be related to Yin deficiency (for more on Yin and Yang deficiency, see page 105).

Stages of Healing

Healing from traumatic injuries to soft tissue, such as sprains, strains, deep bruises, and repetitive stress injuries, occurs in three stages. Understanding the stages of healing is key because it provides guidelines for applying various healing techniques.

The first stage of healing lasts up to one week and is a time of acute injury. It is marked by swelling, redness, heat, and pain due to inflammation. Treatment during this time relies on cooling the area to reduce inflammation and relieve pain. Rest is key during this time because it allows the body's immune system to heal the area and prevents accidental reinjury. Healing treatments should be gentle and include salves, liniments, and herbal teas. Soaks, compresses, and massage should be avoided at this time because they can worsen inflammation by increasing circulation to the area.

The second stage of healing lasts for up to one month. It is a time when the initial pain, swelling, and bruising have fully developed and are beginning to subside. Healing treatments are very important during this stage to prevent stagnation. When the initial inflammation and swelling have subsided, massage and more invigorating therapies can be introduced to increase circulation to the area above and below the injury. Salves, liniments, soaks, compresses, and internal herbal teas should be used consistently during this time.

The third stage of healing begins one month after the initial injury and can continue for years. Treatment during this time is key for preventing and healing chronic injury. This stage is marked by low-grade pain, stiffness, and achiness. Healing treatments focus on moving stagnation, increasing circulation, breaking down adhesions and scar tissue, relaxing tense holding patterns in the surrounding muscles, and removing pathogens that may have set in (i.e., wind, damp, heat, cold). Healing ways, including massage and gua sha, liniments, soaks, compresses, and internal herbal teas, should be used regularly and as needed during this time.

STAGES OF HEALING

FOR SPRAINS, STRAINS, DEEP BRUISES, AND REPETITIVE STRESS INJURIES

1

The first week of the injury. Marked by swelling, redness, heat, and pain due to inflammation. Treatment cools the area to reduce inflammation and relieve pain. Rest and gentle healing with salves, liniments, and herbal teas.

2

The first two to four weeks of injury. Pain, swelling, and bruising fully develop and begin to subside. Healing treatments prevent stagnation from setting in by increasing circulation to the area with salves, liniments, soaks, compresses, and herbal teas.

3

One month after the injury occurs and beyond. Healing prevents chronic injury by moving stagnation, relaxing muscle, and clearing pathogens like damp and wind. Includes more vigorous massage, gua sha, liniments, soaks, and herbal teas.

MENDER TEA FOR BONE AND SOFT TISSUE HEALING

Makes 2 cups (55 g) loose-leaf tea

INGREDIENTS

½ cup (14 g) dried oat straw
½ cup (5 g) dried red clover
½ cup (18 g) dried horsetail
½ cup (14 g) dried nettle

Bones are covered by long sheaths of connective tissue called periosteum that help the bones grow, heal, and seamlessly connect to the muscles and joints. Thus, herbal medicine for bone and soft tissue healing is one and the same! This tea blend heals musculoskeletal ailments by providing vital minerals and nutrients. Nutrient-dense red clover increases circulation to reduce inflammation and clear Blood and Qi stagnation. Nettles are like an herbal multivitamin with many nutrients, including iron and calcium. Their salty nature speaks to Kidney energy, which also has an energetic influence on the bones. Oat straw is a nervous system healer, high in calcium and magnesium, that also eases chronic stress held in the body. And the high silica content in horsetail is renowned for bone healing.

In an airtight container, combine the oat straw, red clover, horsetail, and nettle. Store away from heat, light, and moisture for up to 12 months.

To make a cup of tea, place 1 heaping tsp of the tea in a teapot and pour 1 cup (240 ml) of boiling water (200° F [95° C]) over the tea. Cover and steep for 10 minutes before straining. Drink immediately.

The medicinal dose is 1 to 3 cups (240 to 720 ml) per day for at least 2 weeks.

Contraindication: Omit nettles in cases of cardiac or renal failure.

NERVE TONIC TEA

Makes 3 cups (190 g) loose-leaf tea

INGREDIENTS

1 cup (134 g) dried rose hips

½ cup (15 g) dried lemongrass

½ cup (10 g) dried lemon balm

½ cup (14 g) dried oat straw and/or milky oat tops

½ cup (14 g) dried nettle

1 tsp ground cinnamon powder

This tasty tea blend calms the nervous system and heals musculo-skeletal ailments and injuries from the inside out. All sensation, including pain, is perceived by a network of nerves that cover the entire body. Even after a broken bone, muscle strain, or deep bruise has long healed, there can be residual pain from the surrounding nerves. Rose hips are used traditionally to reduce pain and stiffness due to arthritis and after medical procedures. Lemongrass and lemon balm calm the nervous system and gently increase the circulation of Blood, Qi, and lymphatic fluid. Oat straw and milky oat tops are well-known nerve tonics and, when taken over time, heal and strengthen the integrity of the nervous system. Nettle is a nutrient-dense powerhouse herb that brings both physical and energetic healing to mind and body.

In an airtight container, combine the rose hips, lemongrass lemon balm, oat straw and/or milky oat tops, nettle, and cinnamon powder. Store away from heat, light, and moisture for up to 12 months.

To make a cup of tea, place 1 heaping tsp of the tea in a teapot and pour 1 cup (240 ml) of boiling water (200° F [95° C]) over the tea. Cover and steep for 10 minutes before straining. Drink immediately.

The medicinal dose is 1 to 3 cups (240 to 720 ml) once per day for at least 2 weeks.

Contraindications: Omit cinnamon during pregnancy. Omit nettles in cases of cardiac or renal failure.

CINNAMON DECOCTION FOR COLD PAINS

Makes 4 cups (960 ml)

INGREDIENTS

5 cinnamon sticks

3 in (7.5 cm) knob of fresh
    ginger, quartered

5 sticks dried licorice

Peel of 1 fresh tangerine

Honey or sweetener, for serving

Warmth is what makes us human and our health depends on a proper balance of warmth. Pain is often due to cold that has invaded the body from the outside world. Cold pains are stagnations that block the free flow of Qi and Blood, and they feel different depending on where they settle in the body. In the muscles and joints, cold pains can be felt as stiffness, tightness, contraction, or a dull ache. In the abdomen, cold pain can come on as an intense stomach pain with cramping, diarrhea, or vomiting. And menstrual cramps that are improved with a heating pad are often due to cold.

In all cases, this pain is better with warming herbs and heat therapies, including moxibustion, baths, and soaks. The herbs in this tea blend work together to warm and stimulate circulation to stop the pain and move stagnation. Due to its blood-moving properties, do not use this tea during pregnancy.

Using your hands or a mortar and pestle, break the cinnamon sticks into ½ in (12 mm) pieces.

In a large pot, bring the cinnamon sticks, ginger, licorice, and 8 cups (2 L) of water to a boil. Turn the heat to low and simmer with the lid cracked for 30 minutes, or until the liquid has reduced to about 4 cups (960 ml). Remove from the heat then strain the herbs with a slotted spoon and discard. Add the tangerine peel, cover, and steep for 15 minutes while the decoction cools. Serve with honey or sweetener.

The medicinal dose is 1 cup (240 ml) every 4 hours until nausea subsides for up to 2 days. The decoction may be taken slowly over the course of each day. Store in glass jars in the refrigerator for up to 3 days.

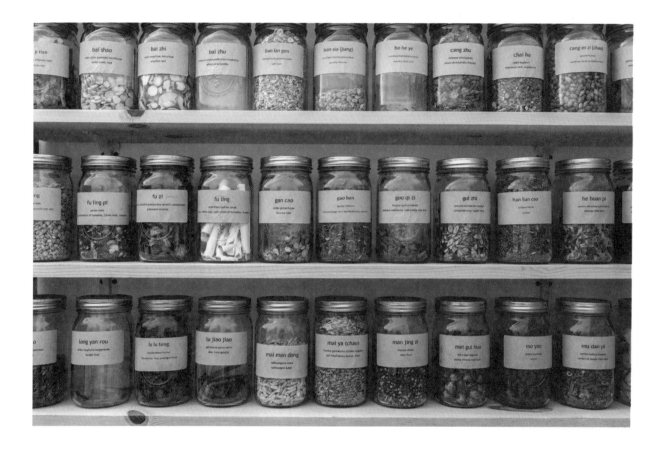

Variation

—

Add one 5 in (12 cm) piece dang gui to increase Blood moving and circulatory properties for deep bruises, joint injuries, and fractured bones. Dang gui heals pains that are rooted in cold and stagnation. It also facilitates the healing process by nourishing Blood and soft tissue injuries. This variation is also appropriate for menstrual cramps and pain.

Contraindication: This tea is not recommended during pregnancy due to the cinnamon.

FRESH GINGER COMPRESS

Makes 1 ginger compress

INGREDIENTS

4 in (10 cm) knob of fresh
  ginger, grated

The versatility of ginger in food and medicine across many Asian healing traditions is unparalleled. It is, without question, my mother's favorite herb, and she swears by simply eating the pickled ginger that comes with sushi to alleviate pains anywhere in the body. Modern studies agree with my mom and show that ginger has anti-inflammatory properties that reduce pain and swelling of arthritic joints.

In this recipe, the ginger is placed directly on the body as a compress to stimulate the circulation of Blood, lymph, and body fluids. Increased circulation works to ease pain by calming inflammation and drawing toxins out of the joints and connective tissues. Ginger compresses can be used to heal everyday pains, including menstrual cramps, gas, arthritis, joint pain, and muscle spasm in the low back and hips. As a caution, keep ginger compresses away from the face and groin because the spicy volatile oils can irritate delicate skin. Stop using immediately if any skin irritation or uncomfortable redness appears.

To prepare the ginger, grate it using a grater or food processor. Put the grated ginger in a piece of cheesecloth and tie the cheesecloth to make a large tea bag.

In a large pot, bring 10 cups (2.4 L) of water to a boil. Turn the heat to low, add the ginger in the cheesecloth tea bag, and simmer for 1 hour. Remove from the heat and let cool until the water is still very hot but is cool enough to touch without burning the skin. There will be a strong ginger aroma. ↗

Use the ginger tea bag as a compress and apply it directly to the body. Alternatively, you can make a hot towel compress by dipping a cotton washcloth or fabric into the ginger water. With either method, wring out the towel/tea bag and gently apply it to the area of the body you wish to treat. Cover the compress with a dry towel to retain heat. Refresh and replace the warm ginger compress every 5 to 10 minutes until the skin becomes warm and rosy pink. This usually takes 2 to 3 cycles.

This compress can be done daily or as needed until the pain subsides. Save the ginger water and bundle by storing them in the refrigerator for up to 3 days.

Note: Steam soaks should not be used to treat fresh injuries that are still swollen, because the heat can increase inflammation at this point and cause more pain.

MUGWORT WARMING MASSAGE OIL

Makes 1½ cups (360 ml)

INGREDIENTS

3 in (7.5 cm) knob of fresh ginger, very thinly sliced

½ cup (30 g) dried mugwort leaves

10 licorice slices, each about 2 in (5 cm)

5 dang gui slices, each about 4 in (10 cm)

1 cinnamon stick

2 cups (480 ml) fractionated coconut oil (or unrefined coconut oil)

Healing massage with warming herbal oils is deeply comforting. This oil infuses warm, invigorating herbs, including mugwort, fresh ginger, and cinnamon, and smells lovely—I swear by this formula for gua sha and cupping massage at my clinic. For external use only, it should be gently massaged into the skin for five to ten minutes to draw the herbal medicine deep into the skin. Oiling the abdomen eases issues with the gut, such as gas and cramping pain. It can be used as a massage oil for aches, pains, and muscle spasms along the entire back, from the shoulders down to the hips. It is effective for arthritic joint pain, particularly for stiffness that worsens in cold, damp weather. And finally, it is a hydrating yet non-greasy body oil.

Mugwort is the star of this recipe because it is used for the same reason it's used in moxibustion—to alleviate pain by dispersing cold and stagnant energy (for more on moxibustion, see page 283). Dang gui and licorice are used topically for their strong ability to move stagnant Qi and Blood that shows up as cramping pain, swelling, inflammation, numbness, and discomfort. Mugwort also works to treat pain associated with emotional and traumatic holding in the body. I've found that healing from physical pain also requires mental and emotional healing.

I like to use fractionated coconut oil because it's a dry oil that absorbs quickly into the skin and stays liquid at room temperature for ease of use. If you plan to make this oil into a salve, such as Wow Gao (page 194) or don't mind a semisolid final product, you can use unrefined coconut oil instead. ↗

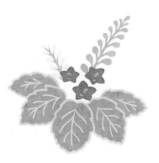

Place the ginger slices on a towel-lined plate and let dry out
for a day.

In a double boiler, combine the ginger, mugwort, licorice,
dang gui, and cinnamon. Cover with the coconut oil and slowly
warm over medium-low heat for 30 to 60 minutes, or until the
oil begins to take on the scent of ginger and cinnamon. If tiny
bubbles appear, turn the heat down or remove from the heat.
Do not simmer or overheat the oil—it will turn the oil rancid
and fry the herbs. Remove from the heat and cool until just cool
enough to handle. Using cheesecloth or a fine-mesh sieve, strain
the oil, pressing the herbs to extract as much oil as possible.
Let the oil to cool to room temperature then pour into clean glass
jars, being careful not to pour off any water or plant materials
that may settle at the bottom of the oil. Discard the remaining
water and plant materials as they will spoil the finished oil.
Store away from heat, light, or moisture for up to 1 year.

Note: Use a pot made of enamel, glass, stainless steel, or other nonreactive
material (not aluminum).

WOW GAO — HEALING MASSAGE SALVE

Makes 9 oz (255 g)

INGREDIENTS

1 cup (240 ml) Mugwort
Warming Massage Oil
(page 192) or another carrier
oil

1 oz (30 g) beeswax, grated or
pastilles

10 drops tea tree essential oil
(optional)

Salves are called gao in Mandarin Chinese. A salve is a simple preparation of oil and beeswax applied to the skin to promote healing. Wow Gao was originally formulated to be used for gua sha and healing massage on painful, achy joints. Its warming and Blood-moving properties are great for pain with stiffness that is aggravated in cold weather. Wow Gao can be used like moxa, a heat therapy (page 283), and applied liberally on the body for achy hips, low back pain, and menstrual cramps.

In a small pot, warm the Mugwort Warming Massage Oil over low heat until tiny bubbles form, but do not allow it to boil. Add the beeswax and stir until just melted into the oil. Remove from the heat and add 10 drops of essential oil (if using). Immediately pour the mixture into clean, dry containers and let cool. Label the jar with the date and ingredients.

Once the salve is cool and hardened, secure it with a lid and store away from heat, light, and moisture for up to 1 year. For tips on making salves, see page 293.

KICK-ASS LINIMENT FOR PAIN

Makes 3 cups (720 ml)

INGREDIENTS

½ cup (45 g) dried red sage root

¼ cup (7 g) dried comfrey leaves

2 dang gui slices, each about
  4 in (10 cm)

2 Tbsp dried safflower

1 Tbsp frankincense resin

1 Tbsp myrrh resin

6 sticks dried licorice

1 cinnamon stick

4 cups (960 ml) rubbing alcohol
  or 100 proof vodka

Liniments are used in many martial arts traditions to support the healing of joints, ligaments, tendons, muscles, and connective tissue such as fascia. These alcohol-based preparations effectively heal deep within the body by penetrating the skin layer and drawing the herbal medicine deep into the connective tissue and muscle. In this liniment recipe, I use red sage root as the primary herb to promote blood flow, dispel stagnation, and clear heat and inflammation. I also use it because I can source it locally in the San Francisco Bay Area. The other Blood movers in this mix are safflower, dang gui, frankincense, and myrrh. Frankincense and myrrh are a synergistic herbal pair that increase blood circulation to relax painful joints and ease pain by clearing Blood stagnation. Comfrey is renowned for its ability to heal both superficial skin and more profound injuries. And licorice and cinnamon relieve pain by moving Qi stagnation.

In a 4 cup (960 ml) glass jar, combine the red sage root, comfrey, dang gui, safflower, frankincense, myrrh, licorice, and cinnamon. Pour the rubbing alcohol or vodka over the herbs, filling the jar three-quarters of the way full. There should be a 2 in (5 cm) space between the herbs and the top of the jar. Reserve the extra alcohol for topping off the mixture as the herbs absorb the liquid during the first week of tincturing. Cover with a plastic or nonreactive lid (or line metal lids with parchment paper or plastic wrap) and label the jar with the date, ingredients, and "for external use only." Store away from heat, light, and moisture and gently shake the mixture every 1 to 3 days. →

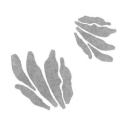

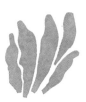

After 4 weeks, use cheesecloth or a fine-mesh sieve to strain the liniment; discard the herbs. Store in a clean glass jar away from heat, light, or moisture for up to 6 years. You can tell if an alcohol-based preparation has spoiled by changes in smell or taste, or any visible signs of mold or fermentation.

For an acute injury, massage the liniment into the injured area for 15 minutes, 3 times daily. Continue until the initial pain and inflammation resolves. For chronic injuries, apply daily or as needed.

Note: It is important to source frankincense and myrrh from reputable herb suppliers because of issues with the exploitation of human labor and the overharvesting of resources (see Resources on page 312 for herb companies).

How to Gua Sha a Painful Joint

Before acupuncture school, I worked as a physical therapy aide helping patients with their workouts and applying ice and heat packs. I remember watching the physical therapist use a hard, plastic tool to scrape injured joints to the point where the patients would grimace with discomfort. However, they always came back for more because it effectively reduced pain by breaking down scar tissue, adhesions, stiffness, and inflammation. Soon after, I learned that this technique was a take on gua sha.

In my clinic, I regularly use gua sha techniques for joint pain in the elbow, wrist, knee, ankle, and foot. Gua sha is both a healing treatment and a way to visually see where the injury lies. As you gua sha, the areas of injury will become red, purple, or pink, which is the sha, or marks, of stagnation. Gua sha draws this stagnation up to the surface, and in doing so it increases circulation so that healthy Qi and the immune system can heal the area. This is how you do it at home (for more in-depth gua sha instructions, see page 284):

- You will need a body oil and a gua sha tool (i.e., olive oil and a porcelain soup spoon or gua sha stone that can be bought online).
- Lightly apply oil to the affected joint and the area around it within a 5 in (12 cm) radius. For example, with knee pain, you will also oil the lower thigh and upper calf.
- Starting just above the painful joint and using medium-light pressure, scrape the gua sha tool down in long strokes. Work on the muscles and soft tissue and stop the gua sha at any bony prominences. Skip the bony areas and continue to gua sha the muscles and soft tissues below the joint.
- There will be some tenderness, like a deep massage. If it feels painful, apply more oil and less pressure. It is painful and unproductive to gua sha over bone—do not do that.
- A pink, red, brown, or purple color may develop on the skin. This is safe, and it is an indication of stagnation! It is more like a painless hickey than a bruise.
- The treatment takes 1 to 2 minutes.
- The joints tend to be very tender and cannot take heavy-handed treatment. The best course of treatment is frequent, gentle sessions.
- Afterward, treat the skin as if it's "open" and protect it from extremely windy and cold environments for two days. For example, do not jump into a cold swimming pool.

DIGESTION AND ELIMINATION

If you want to understand the current state of your health, observing your digestion and elimination will tell you everything. Proper digestion and elimination are the cornerstones of health because they represent our capacity to receive energy and assimilate nutrients from the natural world. The consistency of daily elimination shows us, quite literally, how well we're able to get rid of waste and release things that are not serving us well. This applies to both the physical and the energetics of the body.

Digestion begins with the intake of food and drink and follows a profound and sophisticated process within the body that ends with the elimination of wastes through bowel movements and urination. The natural rhythm of digestion can be interrupted through illness, injury, stress, food sensitivities, food poisoning, poor eating habits, and lack of proper nourishment. I find that mental and emotional stress is the main cause of poor digestion and elimination. And energetically, these issues manifest in different ways. Let's consider the digestive system in three parts: digestion, bowel movements, and urination.

HERBS FOR DIGESTION

MOVE	NOURISH
Burdock Root	Plantain
Ginger	Hemp Seed
Cardamom	Mulberry
Tea	Honey
Mugwort	Sesame Seed
Fennel	Marshmallow
Corn Silk	Walnut
Chinese Hawthorn	
Senna	CALM
	Korean Mint
DETOX	Tulsi
Honeysuckle	Licorice
Shiso	Chamomile
Dandelion	Citrus Peel
Cleavers	Umeboshi
Jasmine	Lemon Balm
	Calendula

Healthy Digestion and Indigestion

The movement of Qi guides healthy digestion. When the Qi is not balanced, indigestion arises and causes issues with appetite, gas, belching, and acid reflux. If left unhealed, indigestion will negatively affect everything from energy and sleep to pain and mental health.

Everyone experiences bouts of indigestion, but how it shows up for each individual tells us a lot about the balance and movement of Qi within. This is so important to an in-depth understanding of one's health that I talk extensively about digestion with every single patient that comes through my clinic. During the health intake, I ask about various aspects of digestion and consider how they fall into three main categories: Qi deficiency, Qi stagnation, and food stagnation.

Qi Deficiency Indigestion

Symptoms of gas, bloating, low appetite, irregular appetite, loose stools, and diarrhea are all signs of Qi deficient indigestion. There can also be inconsistent daily energy and dips in energy after eating. Herbs for healing include Qi tonics, Qi harmonizers, and warming and damp clearing herbal remedies. Long-term Qi deficiency indigestion often leads to Qi stagnation.

Qi Stagnation Indigestion

These cases include many Qi deficiency symptoms and a stuck feeling in the torso and gut. Qi stagnation indigestion includes symptoms that shoot upwards (i.e., acid reflux, belching, nausea, vomiting), push downwards (i.e., painful gas, loose stools, diarrhea with undigested food particles), and things that are marked by irregularity (i.e., slow bowel movements, alternating between loose stools and constipation). Herbs for healing include invigorating herbs that move Qi to create calm and balance within.

Food Stagnation Indigestion

This commonly manifests with sluggish, uncomfortable, and even painful digestion and is often due to overindulgence and eating food that is difficult to digest (i.e., processed, greasy, fried, too sweet, too cold). Herbs for healing include damp clearing, invigorating, and cooling herbal remedies.

Store-Bought Digestive Remedies

Bitters

Digestive bitters are alcohol tinctures made with bitter herbs (for a recipe, see page 202). They have been used for generations and in many cultures to benefit digestion. Nowadays, they are often sold as a cocktail ingredient, so you can find them in many grocery stores and bottle shops.

Curing Pills or Po Chai Pills

Found in all Asian markets and herb shops, these over-the-counter pills are sold as a general digestive aid. They are also effective as a hangover cure because they clears dampness and stagnation due to overindulgence.

Digestive Enzymes

General digestive enzymes are helpful before a rich, heavy meal or a potluck-type event. Lactase enzymes for lactose intolerance are common digestive enzymes found at most drug stores and markets. Digestive enzymes are also found in foods such as papaya, which contains the enzyme papain, and pineapple, which contains bromelain. They're so effective for aiding digestion that bromelain and papain are sold in the supplement sections of some markets and pharmacies.

Probiotic Foods and Supplements

Probiotic foods and supplements are key for maintaining a healthy balance of bacteria in the gut. In many cultures, probiotic foods were taken at every meal, and I remember eating homemade Japanese-style pickles, tsukemono, and miso-ginger condiments growing up. I believe that food-based probiotics are much more effective than pills and supplements. However, a diversity of probiotic sources is essential for healthy digestion, and you can achieve this by trying different fermented foods and supplement brands.

ZEN BELLY TEA

Makes 2 ½ cups (80 g)
loose-leaf tea

INGREDIENTS

1 cup (30 g) dried Korean mint
   (huo xiang)
½ cup (10 g) dried peppermint
½ cup (12 g) dried marshmallow
   leaf
¼ cup (5 g) dried lemon balm
¼ cup (15 g) dried licorice

Zen Belly is a delightful, after-meal tea blend that encourages healthy digestion. Korean mint (huo xiang) and peppermint are carminative herbs, which means that they benefit digestion by moving Qi to ease gas, bloat, and indigestion. Licorice synergizes with the minty-anise flavors of the mints and relieves crampy stomach pains by relaxing the smooth muscle in the intestines and balancing the Qi dynamic. Marshmallow leaf and lemon balm are added to hydrate the digestive tract and calm the mind-body aspects of digestion.

This tea blend has a naturally sweet anise flavor reminiscent of pastis aperitifs from the Mediterranean. As a teenager, I studied abroad in Nîmes, France, and lived with a lovely, bohemian family. There I witnessed a slower lifestyle centered around time spent with family and friends in the garden and kitchen. The Chouleur family introduced me to their region's healing flavors, including the sweetness of anise, the bitterness of digestifs, and the astringent depth of red wine. Living there expanded my understanding of how food and drink can be medicine.

In an airtight container, combine the Korean mint, peppermint, marshmallow, lemon balm, and licorice. Store away from heat, light, and moisture for up to 12 months.

To make a cup of tea, place 1 heaping tsp of the tea in a teapot and pour 1 cup (240 ml) of boiling water (200° F [95° C]) over the tea. Cover and steep for 10 minutes before straining. Drink immediately.

Contraindication: Omit licorice in cases of kidney disorders, hypertension, and congestive heart failure.

GENMAICHA GREEN TEA WITH UMEBOSHI

Makes 1 cup (240 ml)

INGREDIENTS

1 tsp loose genmaicha green tea
leaves

1 umeboshi plum and pit

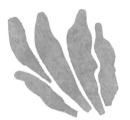

*Contraindication: Umeboshi should
not be taken to stop diarrhea due
to food poisoning or acute illness
because it will slow the system from
clearing the infection.*

I grew up watching my grandma drink green tea with an umeboshi plum every day, and at ninety-seven years old, she still enjoys it this way. This recipe is a tribute to this precious memory. A simple digestive tea with only two ingredients—umeboshi and genmaicha green tea—it heals indigestion due to Qi deficiency.

Umeboshi is a fermented or pickled Japanese plum-like fruit called ume. Once the ume are harvested and dried, they are soaked in vinegar with shiso leaves and aged. Ume nourishes Yin and balances body fluids. Because of its nourishing and sour nature, it helps to alleviate chronic diarrhea caused by deep depletion (Qi deficiency). You can use as much or as little as you prefer. Grandma uses part of an umeboshi plum and sometimes only a pit leftover from making onigiri. Occasionally, she adds the juice, although there isn't much juice available.

Green tea also helps the body drain damp heat from the belly, which shows up as indigestion, gas, loose stools, weight gain, and water retention. Genmaicha green tea is a hearty green tea and can handle a longer steep than other, more delicate green teas. And a purposeful 3 to 4 minute steep brings out the bitter and astringent properties that clear up any damp heat.

Place 1 tsp of the genmaicha green tea in a teapot and pour 1 cup (240 ml) of simmering water (180° F [80° C]) over the tea. Cover and steep for 3 to 4 minutes before straining. Add as much or as little of the umeboshi plum and pit to the tea. Drink the tea slowly as the umeboshi infuses into the tea. If desired, re-steep by pouring fresh, simmering water over the tea for a second cup.

Note: Many umeboshi plums contain artificial food coloring and preservatives. Clearspring umeboshi are organic and dye-free umeboshi (see Resources on page 312).

BURDOCK ROOT BITTERS

Makes 3 cups (720 ml)

INGREDIENTS

2 Tbsp dried burdock root

2 Tbsp dried dandelion root

2 Tbsp dried orange peel (or the peel of a fresh tangerine)

3 in (7.5 cm) knob of fresh ginger, quartered

1 Tbsp whole fennel seeds

10 whole cardamom pods

4 cups (960 ml) 80 proof vodka or brandy

Digestive bitters are alcohol tinctures made with bitter herbs, such as burdock root, chamomile, dandelion, and gentian. They have been used for generations and in many cultures to benefit digestion, especially after a heavy meal. The bitter flavor has a strong effect on digestion by stimulating the intestines and the production of saliva, bile, and gastric juices. It also influences the pancreas, which helps regulate blood sugar and appetite. Energetically, bitters have a draining quality that removes food stagnation, heat, and dampness from the body. Orange peel further invigorates Qi and dries up damp in the stomach to resolve diarrhea due to Qi stagnation. This formula also features carminative herbs, including fennel, cardamom, and ginger to relieve indigestion, gas, and bloat.

In a 4 cup (960 ml) glass jar, combine the burdock root, dandelion, orange peel, ginger, fennel, and cardamom. Pour the vodka or brandy over the herbs, filling the jar three-quarters of the way full. There should be a 2 in (5 cm) space between the herbs and the top of the jar. Reserve the leftover alcohol for topping off the mixture as the herbs absorb the liquid during the first week of tincturing. Cover with a plastic or nonreactive lid (or line metal lids with parchment paper or plastic wrap) and label the jar with the date and ingredients. Store away from heat, light, and moisture and gently shake the mixture every 1 to 3 days.

After 4 weeks, use cheesecloth or a fine-mesh sieve to strain the bitters; discard the herbs. Store in a clean glass jar away from heat, light, or moisture for up to 6 years. You can tell if an alcohol-based preparation has spoiled by changes in smell or taste or visible signs of mold or fermentation.

Take ½ to 1 tsp before meals to stimulate the digestive system. For a digestive drink, mix with sparkling water and a fresh aromatic herb garnish (i.e., citrus peel, lemon balm, basil, thyme).

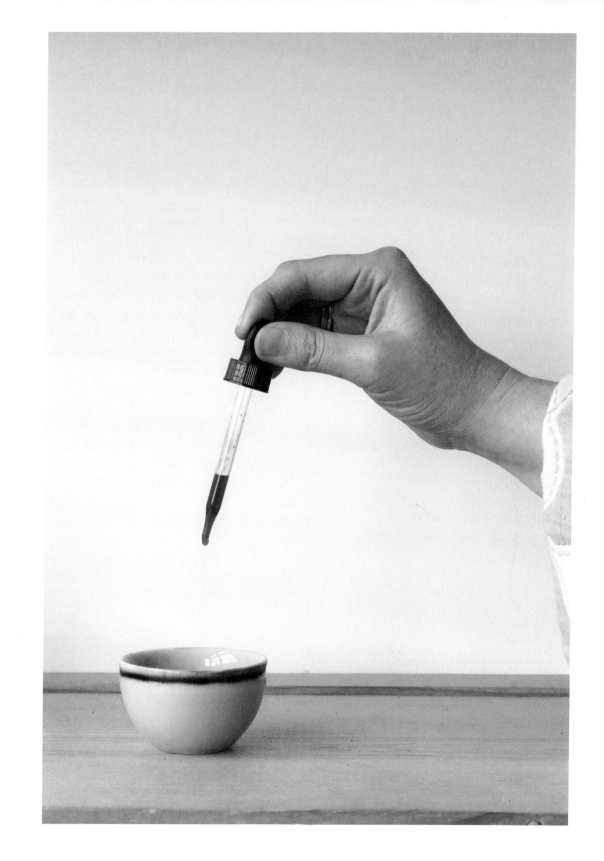

Everybody Poops

Everybody poops and consistency is the name of the game. Regular, healthy bowel movements are necessary for cleaning out day-to-day waste and toxins from the body. Healthy bowel movements happen once or twice a day, ideally in the morning hours, and have the form and consistency of a ripe banana. Unhealthy bowel movements generally fall into two categories: diarrhea and constipation. However, the energetics are a bit more complex and tell us specific information about what is going on within.

Constipation

This is a condition when bowel movements are slow, impacted, difficult, or occur less than once per day. Sluggish stools mean that cellular waste and toxins are sitting in the intestines. This increases inflammation and is particularly detrimental to hormonal balance and pain in the body. Energetically this is commonly due to Blood deficiency and Qi stagnation.

Blood Deficiency Constipation

Bowel movements are dry and slow, with impacted stools that are difficult to push out. Healing herbs, such as Blood tonics, Yin tonics, and cooling and hydrating herbs, are key.

Qi Stagnation Constipation

Bowel movements occur irregularly with pebbly, impacted, and hard stools. When Qi stagnation is severe, constipation and diarrhea may alternate. Herbs for healing include invigorating herbs that move Qi and create calm and balance within.

Diarrhea

Bowel movements tend to be loose, soft, unformed, liquid, and with undigested food particles. This type of imbalance causes irritation and inflammation in the digestive tract lining. Stools being eliminated quickly prevents the body from assimilating key nutrients and fluids. Energetically this occurs due to Qi deficiency or toxic heat.

Qi Deficiency Diarrhea

Bowel movements are loose and frequent. In severe cases, they can be liquid with undigested food particles. Hemorrhoids are a sure sign of chronic Qi deficiency affecting the bowels. Healing herbs will firm up the bowel movements and slow the frequency, and they include Qi tonics, Qi harmonizers, and warming and damp clearing herbs.

Toxic Heat Diarrhea

Bowel movements are affected by bacteria and viral infections, food poisoning, emotional stressors, and inflammatory bowel disease. Bowel movements tend to be aggressive and uncomfortable, with diarrhea and burning. The episodes pass once the toxins have been purged from the body. Herbs for healing will help the infection pass and reduce inflammation, and they include damp clearing, invigorating, cooling, and reducing herbs.

MUGWORT TEA TO WARM THE BELLY

Makes 2 cups (480 ml)

INGREDIENTS

1 Tbsp dried mugwort leaves

1 knob of fresh ginger, thinly sliced

This tea will warm the belly and heal chronic bellyaches and loose stools. Long-term cases of thin, loose, or watery stools are a sign of Qi or Yang deficiency. There may also be some cold trapped in the intestines causing gas, abdominal pain, and urgent bowel movements. This is very different from an occasional sour stomach or food poisoning, and knowing the difference is key to supporting the root cause of discomfort. Mugwort and ginger are herbs that invigorate the belly to move out coldness and stagnation, and warm to strengthen the Qi dynamic. For deeper healing, see how to use moxibustion on the lower abdomen on page 283.

In a large teapot or glass jar, combine the mugwort and ginger. Bring 2 cups (480 ml) of water to a simmer (180° F [80°C]) and pour over the herbs. Always take care when adding hot water to glass jars. It should never be boiling otherwise the jar can crack. Cover and steep for 10 minutes before straining. Drink immediately.

For acute diarrhea, drink ½ cup (120 ml) of tea every 30 minutes until abdominal pain subsides. Belching or passing gas is a sign that the tea is working. For chronic cases, drink 1 cup (120 ml) of tea daily in the first part of the day for up to 1 week. Follow up with moxibustion treatment on the lower belly on acupuncture points Ren 4–6 (see instructions on page 288).

FLOWER TEA TO HARMONIZE AND DETOXIFY THE MIDDLE

Makes 4 cups (960 ml)

INGREDIENTS

2 Tbsp loose black tea leaves, preferably oolong

1 Tbsp dried rose petals

1 Tbsp dried tangerine peel (or the peel of 1 fresh tangerine)

1 tsp dried jasmine flowers

Pinch of dried honeysuckle flowers (about 10 flower threads)

Pinch of dried calendula petals

Honey, for serving (optional)

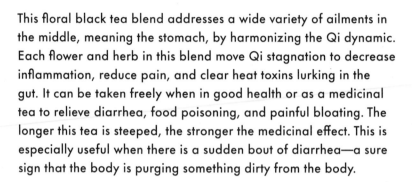

This floral black tea blend addresses a wide variety of ailments in the middle, meaning the stomach, by harmonizing the Qi dynamic. Each flower and herb in this blend move Qi stagnation to decrease inflammation, reduce pain, and clear heat toxins lurking in the gut. It can be taken freely when in good health or as a medicinal tea to relieve diarrhea, food poisoning, and painful bloating. The longer this tea is steeped, the stronger the medicinal effect. This is especially useful when there is a sudden bout of diarrhea—a sure sign that the body is purging something dirty from the body.

In a large teapot or glass jar, combine the black tea, rose, tangerine, jasmine, honeysuckle, and calendula and pour 4 cups (960 ml) of simmering water (180° F [80°C]) over the herbs. Take care when adding hot water to glass jars. It should never be boiling otherwise the jar can crack. Cover and steep for 3 minutes before straining. Sweeten with honey (if using) and drink slowly throughout the day.

For acute indigestion or food poisoning, drink ½ cup (120 ml) of tea every 30 minutes until abdominal pain subsides. An initial increase in bowel movements, vomiting, belching, or passing gas is a sign that the tea is working. For chronic cases of toxic heat in the gut, drink 1 to 2 cups (240 to 480 ml) of tea daily for up to 1 week or as needed.

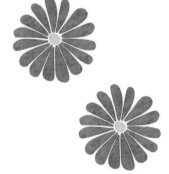

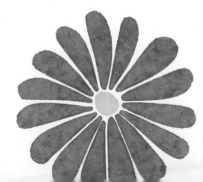

REST AND DIGEST TEA

Makes 4 oz (115 g) loose-leaf tea

INGREDIENTS

1 cup (30 g) loose chamomile tea leaves

¾ cup (15 g) dried marshmallow leaf

½ cup (60 g) dried orange peel

½ cup (10 g) dried lemon balm

¼ cup (10 g) dried marshmallow root

Pinch of dried calendula petals

Honey, for serving (optional)

1 knob of fresh ginger, sliced thin for serving (optional)

There is a second brain in the gut called the enteric nervous system. This network of nerves travels from the esophagus to the anus and plays a major role in digestion and mental health. The gut-brain connection of the enteric nervous system is a scientific way to understand what we already know from experience—the mind and mental health play a big part in proper digestion.

This tea blend works to calm both the mind and the digestive tract. Chamomile is the quintessential herb for this purpose. Like marshmallow leaf and root, it has a mucilaginous (slippery) quality that hydrates the mucous membranes of the gut to heal Blood deficiency constipation. Orange peel, lemon balm, and calendula move Qi to work out stress in the body and mind.

In an airtight container, combine the chamomile tea, marshmallow leaf, orange peel, lemon balm, marshmallow root, and calendula. Store away from heat, light, and moisture for up to 12 months.

To make 4 cups of tea, put 2 Tbsp of the tea in a pitcher or large glass jar and cover with 4 cups (960 ml) of cool water. Stir and cover with a dish towel or loose lid. Steep at room temperature for 1 to 4 hours before straining. Once ready, the tea will turn yellow and smell like chamomile. Store in the refrigerator for up to three days.

Drink the tea over the course of 1 to 2 days, adding honey and a slice of ginger (if using).

ROLL OUT TEA FOR CONSTIPATION

Makes 3 cups (330 g)
loose-leaf tea

INGREDIENTS

1 cup (80 g) dried licorice slices

½ cup (55 g) dried goji berries

½ cup (80 g) hemp seeds

½ cup (60 g) dried orange peel

¼ cup (30 g) whole fennel seed

3 cinnamon sticks, crushed or
    broken into ½ in (12 mm)
    pieces

1 Tbsp senna leaf (optional; only
    for severe constipation)

Honey, for serving (optional)

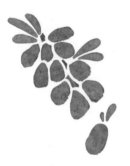

The power of herbs really shines through when it works to relieve painful, stubborn constipation! This kind of difficulty can be caused by extreme situations such as narcotic medications, but more often, it comes on over time due to poor diet, stress, dehydration, and Qi stagnation.

Licorice harmonizes Qi and relieves crampy stomach pains by relaxing the smooth muscle in the intestines. The smooth muscle acts automatically and facilitates the movements of digestion (peristalsis) in the gut. Moving the body, gentle exercise, and massaging the belly can also help the smooth muscles to move properly. Orange peel, fennel seed, and cinnamon are moving and warming herbs that increase movement in the gut energetically. In contrast, goji berries, hemp seeds, and honey lubricate the bowels to relieve constipation caused by dryness and lack of fluids. I only use senna leaf in cases of severe constipation that are not responding to anything else, because it will cause intense (sometimes painful) contractions in the smooth muscle of the intestines to purge bowel movements.

In all cases of constipation, it is important to follow up with Blood tonic herbs (see page 98 for examples) to nourish fluids after taking herbs that drain and exhaust the body. For long-term relief, lifestyle and dietary factors should be addressed to heal the root causes of the imbalance. ↗

Asian American Herbalism

In an airtight container, combine the licorice, goji berries, hemp seeds, orange peel, fennel, cinnamon, and senna leaf (if using). Store away from heat, light, and moisture for up to 12 months.

To make a cup of tea, combine 1 tsp of the tea and 1 cup (240 ml) of water in a small pot. Bring to a boil, reduce heat, and simmer covered for 10 minutes before straining. Sweeten with honey (if using).

The medicinal dose is ½ cup (120 ml) every hour until the bowel moment feels complete. Repeat daily for up to 1 week.

Contraindications: This tea is not recommended during pregnancy due to the cinnamon. It is not recommended in cases of kidney disorders, hypertension, and congestive heart failure due to the licorice. Use caution when using senna leaf; it may cause stomach cramping for sensitive folks.

Urination

Even after taking rounds of antibiotics and making various lifestyle changes, many folks live with chronic, nagging symptoms of bladder irritation. Urinary issues include hesitant or urgent urination, discomfort, pressure, and feeling like the bladder isn't empty. Healthy urination is pale yellow, free from discomfort, and should feel in balance with daily water intake.

With chronic urinary issues, there is usually a lot of heat present. This heat can show up physically (i.e., red skin, feeling hot, sweating) and mentally (i.e., insomnia, anxiety, irritability). Heat affecting the urinary system includes urination that is burning, frequent, urgent, irritated, and dark. It can also turn into urinary tract infections. Energetically there is a connection between the Heart and Urinary Bladder, so anxieties that reside in the Heart often impact issues with urination. Emotional stressors, hormone imbalance, hygiene, and hydration always influence urination. Diet is also important when healing from urinary issues. Stay away from damp, heat-forming foods, including alcohol, sweets, processed foods, hot spices, fatty meats, and fried foods.

Consistency and a strong dose are key when taking herbs to prevent recurrent flare-ups of urinary tract infections and cystitis (bladder inflammation). In all cases of potential infection, continue taking the herbal remedies for at least three days after symptoms have resolved to address any residual bacteria and toxins. Seek medical treatment immediately if symptoms worsen or if they do not completely resolve after five days. These types of infections can be dangerous and life-threatening. Severe symptoms include fever, inability to urinate, and discomfort or pain in the lower abdomen and back. Immediately seek medical treatment if you experience any of these symptoms or if there is any question about safety.

CALM AND CLEAR PEE TEA

Makes 4 cups (90 g) loose-leaf tea

INGREDIENTS

1 cup (30 g) dried cleavers

1 cup (24 g) dried plantain leaves

½ cup (12 g) dried blessed thistle

½ cup (10 g) dried marshmallow leaf

½ cup (10 g) dried lemon balm

Unsweetened cranberry juice, for serving (optional)

This herbal tea blend contains a balanced mix of herbs to calm the bladder, drain damp heat, and move Qi to prevent stagnation in the pelvic organs. Cleavers are an invigorating, diuretic plant that moves stagnant fluids in the body and assists in the elimination of damp heat by urination. Plantain and blessed thistle work together to strongly clear damp heat. Plantain and marshmallow leaves nourish Yin and protect body fluids that are key to balancing the draining effect of the other herbs. Lemon balm is an antiviral that benefits the immune system and calms any emotional components of the imbalance. Adding unsweetened cranberry juice to the final tea offsets the grassy flavor of this blend and increases the efficacy of preventing UTIs. For folks with recurring UTIs, this tea can be taken as desired or a few times per week.

In an airtight container, combine the cleavers, plantain, blessed thistle, marshmallow leaf, and lemon balm. Store away from heat, light, and moisture for up to 12 months.

To make a cup of tea, place 1 heaping tsp of the tea in a teapot and pour 1 cup (240 ml) of boiling water (200° F [95° C]) over the tea. Cover and steep for 10 minutes before straining. Drink immediately. If desired, re-steep once by pouring fresh, simmering water over the tea and herbs for a second cup. Add ¼ cup (60 ml) of unsweetened cranberry juice (if using) to each cup of tea for extra prevention of UTIs.

CORN SILK TEA

Makes 4 cups (960 ml)

INGREDIENTS

2 ears of fresh, raw corn

Whenever you have fresh corn silk—the stringy fibers between the corn and husk—on hand, this tea can be taken for recurring urinary issues. Corn silk treats urinary issues by increasing urination to drain damp-heat stagnation. It also benefits Qi stagnation issues including a general feeling of discomfort and pressure in the pelvic region. And on an energetic level, corn silk benefits the Kidney and Heart, which both have a role in the processing of urination physically (Kidney) and emotionally (Heart).

Prepare corn silk by husking the corn; reserve the corn for another use. Put the corn silk and 4 cups (960 ml) of water in a small pot and bring to a boil. Turn the heat to low, cover, and simmer for 10 minutes. Strain and store in the refrigerator.

The medicinal dose is 3 to 4 cups (720 to 960 ml) per day for at least three days after symptoms have resolved, and up to one week.

THE MENSTRUAL CYCLE

For people who have a menstrual cycle, understanding the physiology and energetics can give so much insight into overall health. The menstrual cycle is ruled by the endocrine system, which is about the hormones. Hormones are the body's chemical messengers, affecting nearly everything in the body, including energy, sleep, blood pressure, stress response, mental health, sexual function, and lifelong development. Thus, herbal medicine that balances the hormones of the menstrual cycle has a ripple effect that benefits overall wellness.

An Average Menstrual Cycle

There is no generic normal for the menstrual cycle (the cycle). However, understanding what an average, healthy cycle looks like helps put your own natural rhythms into context.

The cycle is a series of hormonal cascades that start with the first period (menarche) and end with menopause. Each cycle lasts twenty-four to thirty-five days and begins with the first day of the period. The period (menses) is the shedding of the uterine lining, which typically lasts about four days but can range from two to seven days.

MENSTRUAL CYCLE HERBS

TONICS + STRENGTHEN
—
Raspberry Leaf
Motherwort
Nettle
Alfalfa Leaf
Lotus Seed
Black Wood Ear Mushroom

INVIGORATE
—
Motherwort
Mugwort
Dandelion
Ginger
Yarrow
Citron
Cinnamon
Daikon
Chrysanthemum

BALANCE
—
Vitex
Dang Gui
White Peony Root
Licorice
Rose
Chamomile
Oat Straw and Milky Oat Tops

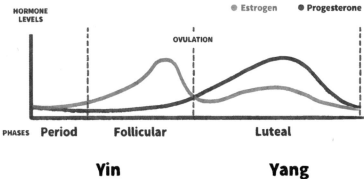

HORMONE LEVELS

● Estrogen ● Progesterone

OVULATION

PHASES **Period**   **Follicular**   **Luteal**

Yin Yang Period
Cycle Chart

Yin   **Yang**

After the period, the follicular phase begins. It is named after the follicle or egg that develops during this time. Estrogen is the dominant hormone of this phase and is akin to Yin. It slowly builds and peaks around day fourteen of the cycle. The peaking of estrogen prompts ovulation, which is the release of an ovum (egg) from the ovary.

After ovulation, the luteal phase begins. It is named after the corpus luteum, which means "yellow body" in Latin, and is a little scar on the ovary left over from ovulation that secretes the hormone progesterone. Progesterone is the dominant hormone of the luteal phase and is akin to Yang. Progesterone gradually builds during this phase and causes the body to retain water, slows digestion, and increases body temperature. The luteal phase lasts for about two weeks. Progesterone peaks during this phase and gradually decreases to bring on the period, unless, of course, there is a pregnancy. In that case, the corpus luteum continues to supply progesterone until the placenta takes over near the end of the first trimester.

Menstrual Cycle Irregularities

Menstrual cycle irregularities can be caused by many factors, including birth control, endocrine disorders (i.e., endometriosis and polycystic ovarian syndrome), environmental endocrine disruptors, disordered eating, extreme physical activity, fibroids, pelvic inflammatory disease, sexually transmitted infections (STIs), pregnancy, and breastfeeding. It is important to understand and rule out any underlying issues when taking herbs for the menstrual cycle and hormone support. Please consult your health care provider if you have any questions or concerns about your cycle.

Tracking the Menstrual Cycle

To understand what's normal for you, begin by writing down specific details about your cycle. I find that tracking this information for three months is a solid baseline for understating your cycle. Here are the important things to note with the usual diagnosis for each symptom in parenthesis:

> ## Endocrine Disrupters
>
> *These are chemicals that negatively affect the endocrine system. These chemicals appear everywhere—in pesticides, plastics, cosmetics, water sources, and the food we eat. Over time, exposure to endocrine disrupters causes problems in the body by affecting the production and natural flow of hormones. Problems include infertility, early puberty, attention deficit hyperactivity disorder (ADHD), metabolic disorder and obesity, and cancer.*

Last Menstrual Period (LMP)

The first day of the period is the first day of the menstrual cycle, or LMP. Note how many days the bleeding lasts and the quality of each day (i.e., bleed amount, color, clots, pain). Light spotting does not count as the first day, but it is important to note.

Period Flow

There is nuance to each day of the period. Is there any spotting or bleeding between cycles (due to Qi deficiency)? Are there gushes of blood, pauses in the flow, clots, or dark colors (due to Qi and Blood stagnation)? Is there a sticky, stringy consistency (a manifestation of dampness)? Does the flow seem heavier (excess) or lighter (deficiency) than usual? Track the heaviness of the flow by using menstrual cups or by noting the frequency of pad and tampon changes.

Pain

Is there any pain associated with your period? Pain in the lower abdomen (a result of Qi stagnation and/or cold)? Pain in the low back and hips (due to Kidney deficiency)? Is there down-bearing pressure in the vulva or thighs (related to Liver stagnation and/or dampness)? Is the quality of the pain stabbing (caused by Blood stagnation) or dull (due to Qi stagnation)? Does the pain start before the period (due to Qi or Blood stagnation) or with the period (a result of Qi and Blood deficiency)? Note the timing and number of days when you feel pain.

Emotions and Mental Health

Are there any changes in mood, behavior, or emotion with your cycle? Do you experience mood swings and irregular or volatile emotions (caused by Qi stagnation)? Do you experience depression, sadness, or anxiety (a sign of Qi and Blood deficiency)? Note the timing and number of days when you feel those emotions.

Premenstrual Syndrome/ Symptoms (PMS)

PMS can occur at any time of the cycle, but it is commonly associated with the luteal phase. Do you experience PMS with breast tenderness, hypochondriac pain, digestive upset, and mood swings (key signs of Liver Qi stagnation)? Is there insomnia, night sweats, heart palpitations, anxiety, restlessness, or feeling hot (related to Heart blood deficiency with heat)? Do you experience water retention, fatigue, heaviness, depression, numbness, and sweet cravings (manifestations of Spleen Qi with dampness)? Note the timing and number of days when you experience PMS.

Energetics of the Menstrual Cycle

Yin and Yang is a philosophy that describes all aspects of life, including the menstrual cycle. The first half of the menstrual cycle (the period and follicular phase) is considered the Yin part, and the second half (ovulation and the luteal phase) is the Yang part of the cycle. In Asian American herbalism, we look to Blood and Yin herbs to support healthy Yin during the first part the cycle. And we generally look to Qi and Yang herbs to bring balance during the second half of the cycle. However, the nature of Yin and Yang is never static. So, dividing the menstrual cycle into these two phases is simply a system of healing strategies for the practical use of herbal remedies in daily life and for herbal cycling.

Herbal cycling is the practice of choosing herbal medicine based on the energetics of the menstrual cycle and from tracking the menstrual cycle. I find this to be one of the most satisfying and rewarding herbal protocols as an herbalist. All the listed Traditional Chinese Medicine (TCM) formulas are for reference and can be looked up online.

The Yin

The Yin part of the cycle includes the period and the follicular phase. The beginning of the period is a time for pause, and herbal medicine is not typically taken during the first few days of the bleed. Herbal remedies begin on day three or four of the cycle when bleeding slows, and the follicular phase begins. This Yin part of the cycle is when healthy Blood and Qi are used to produce the uterine lining and the follicles that hold the ovum (egg). Yin fluids also increase cervical fluids and lubrication to the vagina leading up to ovulation. Issues observed during the period can be addressed with Blood tonic herbs that are appropriate for periods that are light, spotty, or absent, and for cramping or pains that begin with the bleed. Blood and Qi moving herbs are appropriate for periods that are heavy, irregular, clotted, sticky, dark, and that bring on stabbing pains and/or pain that starts before the bleed.

Treatment Principle: Nourish Yin and Blood
HERBS: Blood and Yin tonics
RECIPES FROM THIS BOOK: Moon Child Tea for General Menstrual Support (page 221); Lotus Decoction for Excess and Irregular Menstruation (page 219); Healing Wort Tea for Delayed and Light Periods (page 223)
HEALING PRACTICES: Eating nourishing foods and hydrating, moderate exercise, breath work, and baths
TCM FORMULA: Si Wu Tang (Blood deficiency and stagnation); Ba Zhen Tang (Qi and Blood deficiency); Liu Wei Di Huang Tang (Yin deficiency)

The Yang

The Yang part of the cycle includes ovulation and the luteal phase. Ovulation consists of the movement of the ovum (egg) as it is released from the ovary and the few days surrounding that. There are usually no specific herbal protocols for this phase. The luteal phase should be a time of harmonious movement as the egg is released and travels through the fallopian tubes to the uterus. However, this movement and flow can be interrupted by Qi stagnation, dampness, inflammation, or physical obstructions. Stagnation during this time leads to quintessential premenstrual syndrome (PMS). The symptoms include irregularity that affects the emotions (i.e., irritability and mood swings) and issues with pain, digestion, weight, and water retention. Healing herbs include invigorating herbs that address excesses, including Qi and Blood stagnation, dampness, heat, and cold.

Treatment Principle: Support Yang, Invigorate Qi

HERBS: Qi and Yang tonics, Qi invigorators

RECIPES FROM THIS BOOK: Moon Child Tea for General Menstrual Support (page 221); Citron Rose Tea (page 222) for PMS; Bonsai Herbal Tea (page 150) for PMS; Mandarin Black Tea (page 90) for damp stagnation; Daikon and Chrysanthemum Bath for Damp Stagnation in the Hips (page 226); Roasted Salt Pack for Abdominal Pain (page 227)

HEALING PRACTICES: Moxibustion, movement and exercise, meditation, and mind-body practices

TCM FORMULA: Xiao Yao Tang (Liver Qi stagnation and Blood deficiency); Jin Gui Shen Qi Wan (Yang deficiency)

Pain

When the Qi is not harmonious, there are almost always pain symptoms associated with the menstrual cycle. When and how this pain shows up tells us about the nature of imbalance within. Pain that occurs before the bleed but stops once the period starts is considered an excess pain rooted in the stagnation of Qi or Blood stagnation or coldness. Herbs that warm and move Blood and Qi are helpful. Warming and invigorating healing practices include moxibustion and gentle massage. Cramps and pain that occur once the period begins are rooted in deficiency—the body is so Qi deficient and Blood deficient that the loss of menstrual blood causes the body to contract. In these cases, healing herbs include Qi and Blood tonic herbs and herbs that calm and soothe the body.

Treatment Principle: Move Blood and Qi

HERBS: Blood tonics and invigorators

RECIPES FROM THIS BOOK: Moon Child Tea for General Menstrual Support (page 221); Lotus Decoction for Excess and Irregular Menstruation (page 219); Healing Wort Tea for Delayed and Light Periods (page 223); Roasted Salt Pack for Abdominal Pain (page 227); Fresh Ginger Compress for pain (page 190)

HEALING PRACTICES: Rest, gentle exercise, moxibustion, heat packs, honoring the desire to do less

TCM FORMULA: Si Wu Tang (Blood deficiency and stagnation)

Herbal Cycling – Herbs to Balance the Menstrual Cycle

There is a natural flow to the menstrual cycle, and healthy Qi facilitates a harmonious and easy monthly cycle. Herbal cycling is the practice of choosing herbal medicine based on the energetics of the menstrual cycle and tracking the menstrual cycle. This work is nuanced and enriching. All the listed Traditional Chinese Medicine (TCM) formulas are for reference and can be found on TCM websites.

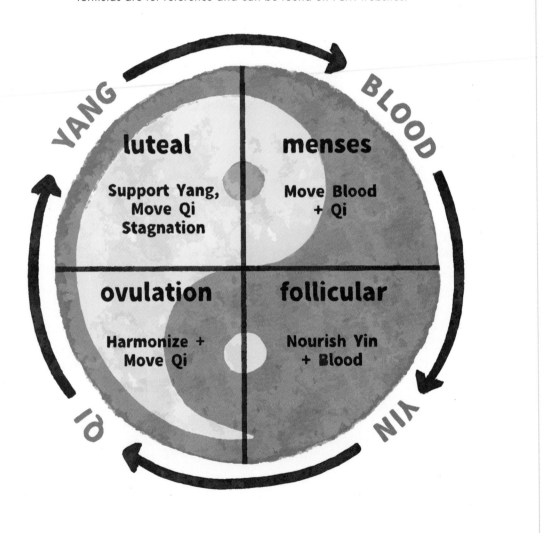

YANG

BLOOD

luteal

Support Yang, Move Qi Stagnation

menses

Move Blood + Qi

ovulation

Harmonize + Move Qi

follicular

Nourish Yin + Blood

QI

YIN

LOTUS DECOCTION FOR EXCESS AND IRREGULAR MENSTRUATION

Makes 4 cups (960 ml)

INGREDIENTS

1 ½ oz (40 g) dried lotus seeds

1 cup (12 g) dried black wood ear
    mushroom

10 dried jujube dates

2 dang gui slices, each about
    4 in (10 cm)

8 licorice slices, each about
    2 in (5 cm)

Certain situations call for strong herbal medicine and a heavy menstrual flow is one such case. This decoction includes healing seeds, roots, fruits, and mushrooms to heal ailments including heavy menstrual flow, unexpected starts and stops to the menses, and general irregularity of the cycle and emotions.

Black wood ear mushrooms and jujube dates strengthen Qi and Blood to address heavy or frequent bleeding. Lotus seeds have an astringent nature that prevents the leakage of body fluids by deeply drawing energies back into the core. Dang gui is a key herb for menstruation in Asian herbalism. It has a Yin-Yang balancing effect that moves Qi, strengthens Blood, and brings circulation to the abdomen. Licorice eases pain in the body and brings a subtle balance to the other herbs in the formula.

In a large pot, bring the dried lotus seeds, wood ear mushroom, jujube dates, dang gui, licorice, and 8 cups (2 L) of water to a boil. Turn the heat to low and simmer with the lid cracked for about 30 minutes, or until the liquid has reduced by half. Strain the herbs with a slotted spoon and discard. Reserve the tea and add fresh water if there are less than 4 cups (960 ml) of tea remaining. Store in glass jars in the refrigerator for up to 4 days. The medicinal dose is 1 cup (240 ml) twice per day for 1 week at a time. Warm before drinking and as with all tonic herbal formulas, stop taking during head colds or infections.

This formula must be taken regularly to effect real change (i.e., taking the medicinal dose for one week per month for 3 to 6 months). But the effort is well worth it, as the result is the preservation of precious vitality!

Contraindications: This tea is not recommended in cases of kidney disorders, hypertension, and congestive heart failure due to the licorice.

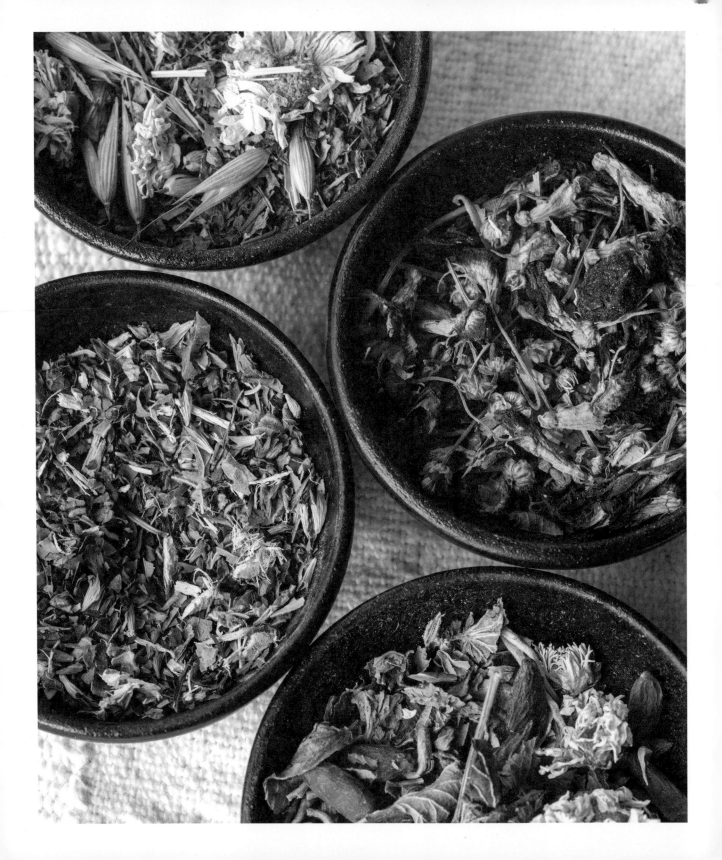

MOON CHILD TEA FOR GENERAL MENSTRUAL SUPPORT

Makes 3 ½ cups (200 g) loose-leaf tea

INGREDIENTS

1 cup (34 g) dried raspberry leaf

1 cup (120 g) dried mulberry fruit

½ cup (14 g) dried chamomile

½ cup (14 g) dried nettle

¼ cup (7 g) dried oat straw

¼ cup (6 g) dried alfalfa leaf

Moon Child is a tonic tea blend to support the uterus and mind-body balance. Raspberry leaf is a uterine tonic that supports the health of the uterus and the natural course of the menstrual cycle. Mulberry is a Yin tonic fruit that supports healthy Blood and body fluids and adds sweetness. Chamomile and oat straw are for stress and digestion. Alfalfa and nettle are nutrient-dense and add minerals to fortify the endocrine system. This blend can be taken freely during any part of the menstrual cycle.

Moon Child is also helpful for support during the last trimester of pregnancy, postpartum, and breastfeeding. The raspberry leaf prepares the uterus for birth and postpartum; chamomile and oats help with stress and digestion; and nettle and mulberries nourish Blood and body fluids, which is all key for breastfeeding and postpartum healing.

In an airtight container, combine the raspberry leaf, mulberry fruit, chamomile, nettle, oat straw, and alfalfa. Store in an airtight container away from heat, light, and moisture for up to 12 months.

To make a cup of tea, place 1 heaping tsp of the tea in a teapot and pour 1 cup (240 ml) of boiling water (200° F [95° C]) over the tea. Cover and steep for 15 minutes before straining. Drink immediately. The medicinal dose is 1 to 2 cups (240 to 480 ml) per day for 1 to 2 weeks, or as needed.

Contraindication: Omit nettles in cases of cardiac or renal failure.

CITRON ROSE TEA

Makes 2 cups (480 ml)

INGREDIENTS

¼ cup (15 g) diced fresh citron
    peel

1 knob of fresh ginger, peeled
    and cut in half

1 Tbsp dried rose petals

1 tsp honey or sugar for serving

This lovely blend is ideal for addressing hormone-related indigestion, pain, mood swings, and premenstrual syndrome (PMS). It gets right to the root cause of these discomforts: Liver Qi stagnation that drains the system and causes blockages. Citron is used in TCM to move Qi stagnation that shows up in the body as pain in the ribcage and mid-back, menstrual cramps, mood swings, and emotional strain (i.e., irritability, anger, rage, sadness, etc.). Fresh ginger also moves Qi and is particularly helpful for digestive issues, such as loose stools, nausea, gas, and bellyache. Rose and honey nourish the Qi and Blood dynamic and lend a Heart-centered softness to the mix.

In a small pot, bring the citron, ginger, and 2 cups (480 ml) of water to a boil. Turn the heat to low, cover, and simmer for 10 minutes. Add the rose and simmer 5 minutes more. Remove from the heat and strain. Add the honey, and stir until dissolved. Drink immediately and freely as often as you wish.

HEALING WORT TEA FOR DELAYED AND LIGHT PERIODS

Makes 2 cups (480 ml)

INGREDIENTS

1 Tbsp dried motherwort leaves

2 tsp dried mugwort leaves

½ cinnamon stick

1 tsp honey or sugar

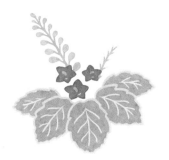

Herbal names that end with "wort" are the mark of a traditional healing plant. This herbal tea blend uses two well-known wort herbs: mugwort and motherwort. This tea was formulated to increase blood flow when periods become very light and spotty, delayed, or missed altogether.

Motherwort invigorates the Blood to address irregular menstruation, PMS, and pain. It is traditionally used to heal after times of long-term stress, depletion, or illness. Mugwort warms and invigorates organs in the abdomen to move out of cold stagnation and strengthen the Qi energy within. It relieves menstrual cramps that respond well to heat such as with a heating pad. The cinnamon stick adds flavor and plays on the warmth and invigorating nature of the wort herbs. Honey or sugar is used in traditional Chinese recipes to boost Qi and in this recipe, it also offsets the bitter taste of the herbs. Follow up with a cup of green tea once or twice a day when experiencing headaches associated with the cycle. For deep healing, moxibustion on the lower abdomen is also called for (see more on page 283).

In a teapot or large glass jar, combine the motherwort, mugwort, and cinnamon. Bring 2 cups (480 ml) water to a simmer (180° F [80°C]) and pour over herbs. Always take care when adding hot water to glass jars. It should never be boiling otherwise the jar can crack. Cover and steep for 10 minutes before straining. Add the honey and stir until dissolved. Drink immediately. The medicinal dose is ½ cup (125 ml) of tea every 30 minutes until menstrual cramps subside.

Follow up with a hot water bottle to warm the area or moxibustion treatment on the lower belly on acupuncture points Ren 4–6 (instructions on page 288).

Contraindication: This tea is not recommended during pregnancy or in cases of potential pregnancy because motherwort and cinnamon move Blood and stimulate the uterus.

YIN-YANG VITEX ELIXIR FOR HORMONE BALANCE

Makes 3 cups (720 ml)

INGREDIENTS

1 cup (120 g) dried vitex berries
   (Vitex agnus-castus)

4 dang gui slices, each about
   4 in (10 cm)

¼ cup (40 g) white peony root

¼ cup (20 g) licorice

2 cups (480 ml) 80 proof brandy

1 cup (240 ml) raw honey

Elixirs extract herbal medicine with a blend of alcohol and honey. This elixir recipe was formulated to balance hormones with elements of both traditional and modern herbalism. Dried vitex berry is a uterine tonic and the star of this recipe because of its capacity to heal hormone imbalance. It is helpful for menstrual pain, irregular cycles, emotional strain, PMS, and any issues that arise after taking the birth control pill or courses of hormonal contraception. And while vitex balances hormones for menstruating folks, it should not be taken after menopause. Dang gui and white peony root are both Blood tonics that have a synergistic effect on everything related to blood, including the menstrual cycle. Dang gui is warm and invigorating, whereas white peony root is cool and stabilizing. Together, they soothe and nourish. Licorice brings another layer of ease and pain relief to the body and harmonizes the other herbs in the formula.

In a 4 cup (960 ml) glass jar, combine the vitex berries, dang gui, white peony root, and licorice. Cover the herbs with brandy, filling the jar three-quarters of the way full. Add honey to the jar until the mixture is 1 in (2.5 cm) from the top of the jar. Cover with a plastic or non-reactive lid (or line metal lids with plastic wrap). Store away from heat, light, and moisture and gently shake the mixture every 1 to 3 days.

After 4 weeks, use cheesecloth or a fine-mesh sieve to strain the elixir; discard the herbs. Label the jar with the date and ingredients. The final elixir is stable at room temperature and can be kept for up to 3 years if stored away from heat, light, and moisture. You can tell if an elixir has spoiled by the change in smell or taste, and any visible signs of mold or fermentation. ↗

The medicinal dose is 1 tsp twice per day for the first 3 weeks. Continue to take 1 tsp per day for 3 to 6 months. Consistency, not perfection, is key for dosing this elixir. So, take it slowly over time until the desired effects are reached.

Note: Do not substitute Chinese vitex (man jing zi) in this recipe as that is a different species used for treating cold and flu due to wind-heat invasion.

Contraindications: This tea is not recommended in cases of kidney disorders, hypertension, and congestive heart failure due to the licorice. It is not recommended for postmenopausal women due to the vitex.

DAIKON AND CHRYSANTHEMUM BATH FOR DAMP STAGNATION IN THE HIPS

Yields 1 bath

INGREDIENTS

2 fresh daikon radishes with
leaves and stems

3 fresh chrysanthemum stems
with leaves, each about
12 in (30 cm)

1 cup (300 g) sea salt or Epsom
salt

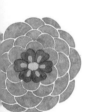

*Note: You may substitute turnip
greens for the chrysanthemum or
daikon. If using only one of the
greens listed in this recipe, double
the amount. To use dried greens
instead, substitute 1 to 2 cups of
dried greens and decrease the water
to 4 cups (960 ml).*

Dampness is a heavy, fluid stagnation caused by body fluids trapped in the body due to poor circulation and metabolism. It tends to settle down into the hips, creating issues for the uterus and menstrual cycle, including menstrual pain, vaginal discharge, prostate issues, cysts, fibroids, and urinary tract infections.

Daikon radish and chrysanthemum greens are used in many Asian cooking traditions. We use daikon leaves to increase circulation and remove damp stagnation in the lower abdomen for a healing bath. Chrysanthemum greens add an invigorating, Qi-moving energy. When making the bath tea, you will smell and sense the moving, green aromatics.

To prepare the greens, remove the leaves and stems from the daikon and reserve the daikon for another use. Gently wash the daikon and chrysanthemum greens under cool running water. Use scissors to cut the stems of all the greens into 3 in (7.5 cm) pieces.

Fill a large pot with 8 cups (2 L) of water and bring to a boil. Add the daikon and chrysanthemum greens, cover, and simmer for 15 minutes, or until the water turns dark yellow.

Meanwhile, draw a very warm bath. When the bath is ready, strain the herbs from the bath "tea" then add the bath tea, along with salt, to the bath water.

Soak for 20 minutes for a full therapeutic effect. Add more hot water as needed.

Hot compress method: Prepare the daikon and chrysanthemum tea as described in the daikon bath, but instead of pouring the tea into a bathtub, make a hot towel compress following the instruction on page 297. Place on the lower abdomen, on and above the pubic bone.

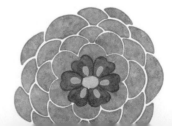

ROASTED SALT PACK FOR ABDOMINAL PAIN

Makes 1 reusable salt pack

INGREDIENTS

2 cups (600 g) coarse sea salt or
pink Himalayan salt

Roasted salt retains a penetrating heat that eases deep pains and soothes the body. Thus, a roasted salt pack is a natural heat therapy for pain that lies deep in the belly, hips, and low back. Salt is the taste of the energetic Kidney, and salt packs speak to healing aches and pains rooted in a Kidney deficiency. Kidney-deficient pain manifests as low back and hip pain, swelling and aches in the belly, menstrual cramps (especially those that come on with the period), chronic diarrhea, and painful gas. The salt pack's deep heat can also heal joint pain aggravated by cold, damp weather. It's important to use sea salt or pink Himalaya salt rather than table salt or Epsom salt, because they will not heat properly.

In a dry ceramic or stainless-steel pan, roast the salt over medium heat, stirring and shaking the pan frequently for 10 to 15 minutes, or until the salt becomes very hot. Carefully place the hot salt in a thick cotton dish towel or pillowcase. Tie up the salt pack with a piece of string and wrap it in a thick cotton hand towel. Place the salt pack directly on the area you wish to treat and hold with gentle pressure for 30 minutes, or until it cools. Save cooled salt to be roasted several more times until the salt turns grey and no longer retains heat. Repeat up to 3 times per week or as needed.

Note: When roasting the salt, do not use a cast-iron or aluminum pan; the material will adversely interact with the minerals in the salt. For the pack, do not use towels made of synthetic materials or socks as they will melt against the hot salt (most socks contain some synthetic stretch material).

SLEEP

Sleep is an enigma, and I find it one of the most challenging things to heal. Many people do not reach or fully maintain a restorative, restful state in sleep. Waking up frequently, dream-disturbed sleep, night sweats, jaw and teeth grinding, apnea, and light and noise disturbance all have a negative effect on sleep. Even with the information we glean from modern technology, the various sleep studies, and virtual apps, there is still some mystery around the mechanics of sleep. Herbs and healing practices can break the cycle of insomnia and improve how someone falls asleep, stays asleep, and wakes up feeling well rested and restored. Understanding not only the herbs but also the energetics of insomnia helps us create strategies and routines that draw the body into a restorative state that has a lasting effect on sleep and overall physical and mental wellness.

The Energetics of Sleep

There are energetic factors that commonly affect sleep quality and cause insomnia. Most often in the clinic, sleep difficulties are related to Blood deficiency (i.e., difficulty falling asleep), Yin deficiency (i.e., difficulty staying asleep), and heat (i.e., dream-disturbed sleep, sleeping hot, and night sweats). Sleep disturbed by Blood deficiency

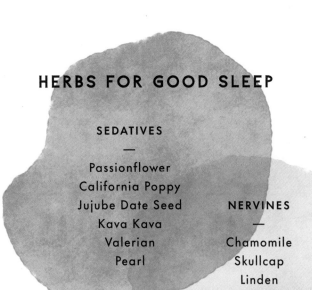

HERBS FOR GOOD SLEEP

SEDATIVES
—
Passionflower
California Poppy
Jujube Date Seed
Kava Kava
Valerian
Pearl

NERVINES
—
Chamomile
Skullcap
Linden
Lavender
Lemon Balm
Tulsi
Oat Straw and
Milky Oat Tops
Hops

BLOOD + YIN TONICS
—
Blueberry
Longan Fruit
Goji Berry
Marshmallow
White Wood Ear Mushroom
Reishi

Asian American Herbalism

generally manifests as resistance to or difficulty falling asleep. Low-grade cases of insomnia with resistance to sleep are not always identified as insomnia but significantly impact daily energy and fatigue.

Making improvements to long-standing insomnia is challenging and a dedicated course of herbal medicine is often needed to see results. To start, choose from the various recipes in this section and take one cup of tea twice per day for four days. Drink the tea slowly throughout the day, rather than in the evening, so that you do not have to wake up to go to the bathroom. After a few days of taking the tea consistently note any improvement to your sleep. Continue taking the tea for two to four days per week until sleep has improved. During this time you can switch freely between the various sleep tea recipes in this book. The general rule is that the longer the ailment has occurred, the longer the course of treatment required.

The Organ Clock

Stress and emotional strain are major factors in insomnia and sleep quality. When emotional factors are involved, I always consider the organ clock from traditional Chinese medicine (TCM). The organ clock is divided into two-hour segments related to each energetic organ.

According to the organ clock, the Large Intestine time (5:00 to 7:00 am) is the ideal time to wake up and have a bowel movement. The Earth element hours that follow are prime for eating the first meal of the day (Stomach) and work that requires concentration (Spleen). For deeply restorative sleep, it's important to go to bed by 9:00 pm and sleep undisturbed through 1:00 am. If you sleep during this energetic cycle (9:00 pm to 1:00 am), your system replenishes the well of energy that you draw from during the waking hours. This timeframe also brings healing to the body (Wood element) and mind (Fire element). Insomnia and waking during the Liver time (1:00 to 3:00 am) indicates issues associated with stress, anxiety, and overstimulation. As you might imagine, this is quite common because stress disturbs sleep! Another common time for insomnia is between the hours of the Lung (3:00 to 5:00 am), which is associated with grief and sadness. When grief and sorrow are not present, the insomnia may be caused by difficulty letting go of something or the need for emotional release.

The organ clock offers us so much information to draw from to understand not only issues with sleep but the natural, energetic cycles of each day. Taking cues on how to live in harmony with the energy of the day is in itself a healing practice. A person's specific condition determines which herbs are appropriate. However, one can simply take teas of nervines and relaxing herbs to prepare for sleep or take Liver herbs, such as chrysanthemum and mint, to unwind layers of stress when prone to waking during 1:00 to 3:00 am. Depending on the level of stress, some of the more heavy and sedative herbs can be incredibly powerful to support healing of patterns of fear, grief, and stress when waking during the Lung hours (3:00 to 5:00 am).

The Organ Clock

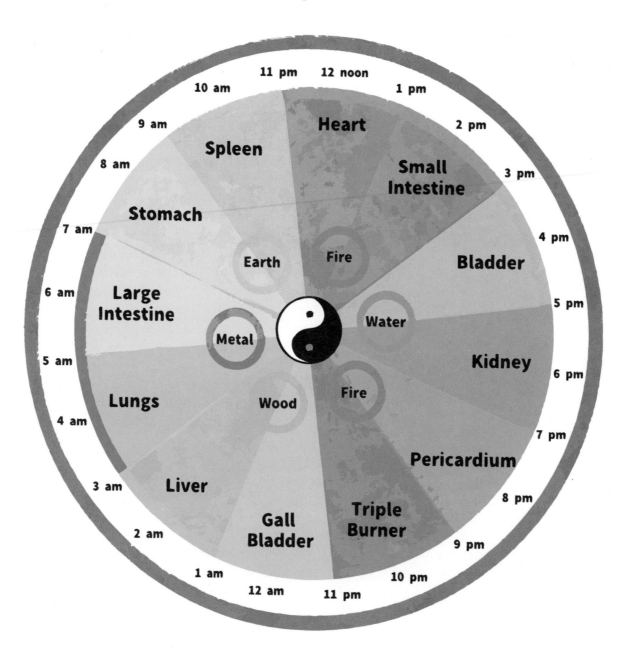

Asian American Herbalism

JUJUBE DATE SEED TEA FOR INSOMNIA WITH HEART BLOOD DEFICIENCY

Makes 4 cups (960 ml)

INGREDIENTS

2 Tbsp jujube date seeds, crushed in a mortar and pestle

10 pieces dried longan fruit

2 Tbsp codonopsis

5 licorice slices, each about 2 in (5 cm)

The depth and quality of one's sleep is always affected by the energetic Heart. Insomnia rooted in Heart Blood deficiency specifically includes difficulty falling asleep, feeling hot at night and tired during the day, restlessness, and poor memory. This herbal decoction is a mix of herbs traditionally used to nourish Heart Blood and improve the sleep-wake cycle. Jujube date seed and dried longan fruit are prized insomnia herbs for their ability to calm the spirit, reduce night sweats, and bring on restorative sleep. Codonopsis, on the other hand, balances the circadian rhythm (the natural sleep-wake cycle) by improving energy during the waking hours. Licorice supports the balanced energizing properties of the codonopsis.

In a large pot, bring the jujube date seed, longan fruit, codonopsis, licorice, and 8 cups (2 L) of water to a boil. Turn the heat to low and simmer with the lid cracked for about 30 minutes, or until the liquid has reduced by half. Strain the herbs with a slotted spoon and discard. Reserve the tea and add fresh water if there are less than 4 cups (960 ml) of tea remaining. Store in a glass jar in the refrigerator. Slowly drink over the course of 2 to 3 days. Warm each serving before drinking.

Contraindications: This tea is not recommended during pregnancy due to the jujube date seeds, which stimulate muscle, including the uterus. This tea is not recommended in cases of kidney disorders, hypertension, and congestive heart failure due to the licorice.

Fresh Longan Fruit Tea

When available, fresh longan fruit can be prepared as a tea to benefit the Heart, Blood, and Spleen Qi to heal sleep patterns and increase overall vitality. To prepare, place 10 pieces of fresh longan fruit in a double boiler and steam for 15 minutes. Place in a teapot with 2 cups (480 ml) of boiling water (200° F [95° C]). Cover and steep for 10 minutes before straining. Drink up to 2 cups (480 ml) per day. As with any medicinal fruits, use with caution in cases of indigestion because they can increase bowel movements.

REISHI DECOCTION FOR YIN DEFICIENCY INSOMNIA WITH NIGHT SWEATS

Makes 4 cups (960 ml)

INGREDIENTS

10 dried astragalus slices, each
about 2 in (5 cm)

1 Tbsp dried marshmallow root

1 Tbsp schisandra berries

5 in (12 cm) slice dried reishi
mushroom

Insomnia due to Yin deficiency with heat requires strong medicine, such as this decoction made with reishi mushroom. The key symptom of Yin-deficient insomnia is a heat that feels like it is radiating from deep within and night sweats. Marshmallow root is a Yin tonic that simultaneously supports Yin fluids and cools heat arising from Yin deficiency. Reishi mushroom benefits the Heart, which is the house of the spirit, and is key for deep, restorative sleep. Ongoing night sweats can become a vicious cycle that depletes Yin fluids through the loss of body fluids (sweat). Thus, the astragalus and schisandra work together to specifically protect Yin fluids by preventing (astringing) excessive sweating. To further address night sweating, take Wild Sage Foot Baths (page 233) as needed.

In a large pot, bring the astragalus, marshmallow, schisandra, reishi mushroom and 8 cups (2 L) of water to a boil. Turn the heat to low and simmer with the lid cracked for about 30 minutes, or until the liquid has reduced by half. Strain the herbs with a slotted spoon and discard. Reserve the tea and add fresh water if there are less than 4 cups (960 ml) of tea remaining. Store in glass jars in the refrigerator for up to 4 days. The medicinal dose is 1 cup (240 ml) twice per day until positive changes to your sleep are noticed. Warm each serving before drinking and as with all tonic herbal formulas, stop taking them during head colds or infections.

Note: This formula is for night sweats due to Yin deficiency. The tongue will appear red, raw, dry, peeled, or have a patchy coat. Cases with significant damp heat (the tongue will have a thick yellow coat) need to be addressed with more nuanced herbs under the guidance of a trained herbalist.

WILD SAGE FOOT BATH

Yields 1 foot bath

INGREDIENTS

4 cups (90 g) fresh sage leaves
and stems

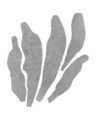

Wild California sage (*Artemisia californica*) is native to the United States and grows along the Pacific coast, from Oregon to Mexico. Any fresh sage can be used for a foot bath. Even dried culinary sage can be used, although much less is needed. Sage is renowned for its ability to protectively hold in fluids. This applies to both spontaneous daytime and nighttime sweating. Night sweats are a symptom of Yin deficiency insomnia. And while sage doesn't treat the root cause of insomnia, stopping the sweats helps preserve precious Yin fluids. Sage is also useful for decreasing milk flow when weaning and thus should not be used as medicine when actively breastfeeding.

To prepare the sage, use scissors to cut the stems into 2 in (5 cm) pieces.

In a large pot, bring the sage stems and leaves and 4 cups (960 ml) of water to a simmer. Remove from the heat, and steep for 30 minutes while preparing a very warm foot bath in a large basin or bucket to soak the feet and ankles comfortably.

When the bath is ready, strain the herbs and discard. Reserve the bath "tea" and add the tea to the soaking basin. Sit in a comfortable chair and soak your feet for 20 minutes for a full therapeutic effect.

Keep a hot water kettle on the stove to reheat the foot bath as needed.

Note: To use dried sage instead, substitute 1 cup (20 g) of dried sage and decrease the water to 2 cups (480 ml).

SPIRITED AWAY TEA

Makes 2 ¾ cups (200 g)
loose-leaf tea

INGREDIENTS

1 cup (170 g) unsweetened dried
   blueberries
½ cup (14 g) dried chamomile
½ cup (10 g) dried lemon balm
¼ cup (3 g) dried blue pea
   flower
¼ cup (6 g) dried lemon verbena
¼ cup (7 g) dried linden leaf and
   flower

This tea is visual medicine that calms the body and mind. I formulated this blend with my daughter, Zoë, as a fun, flavorful sleepy time tea. Once steeped, the blue pea flowers release a vibrant blue color that speaks to one's inner child and reflects my daughter's colorful spirit.

This gentle sleep tea is led by soothing chamomile, which eases nervous energy in the body and mind. It is especially good for nervous energy affecting the stomach. Linden is a nervine that is especially good for insomnia with an edge, including tension, anxiety, and restlessness. The combination of lemon balm and lemon verbena work together to move Qi and balance this soothing and emotionally supportive medicine. And blueberry is a Blood tonic that grounds this formula with sweetness and nourishing medicine. This tea is lovely with a spoonful of honey to bring out all the flavors.

In an airtight container, combine the blueberries, chamomile, lemon balm, blue pea flower, lemon verbena, and linden. Store away from heat, light, and moisture for up to 12 months.

To make a cup of tea, place 1 heaping tsp of herbal tea in a teapot and pour 1 cup (240 ml) of boiling water (200° F [95° C]) over the tea. Cover and steep for 15 minutes before straining. Drink immediately. Drink freely before bed or anytime you please.

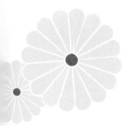

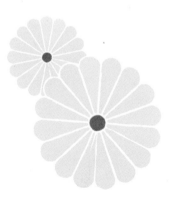

GOOD NIGHT MOON TEA — A LUNAR INFUSION

Makes 2 ½ cups (160 g)
loose-leaf tea

INGREDIENTS

1 cup (120 g) dried mulberries

½ cup (14 g) dried oat straw
and/or milky oat tops

½ cup (10 g) dried rose petals

¼ cup (5 g) dried California
poppy flowers

¼ cup (7 g) dried skullcap

¼ cup (6 g) dried passionflower
leaves

*Note: To substitute fresh poppy flowers
in the recipe, add 6 fresh flower heads
per cup of tea. Fresh mulberries can also
be used in this recipe. Make the Fresh
Mulberry Tea (page 111) and steep the
Good Night Moon Tea (without dried
mulberries) for 10 minutes in the warm
mulberry tea. Strain the herbs and drink
freely. Store in the refrigerator for up to
3 days.*

This is an herbal blend useful for chronic insomnia, including difficulty falling or staying asleep and sleeplessness due to tension. While it can be made as a simple tea, it is a meaningful blend to make as a lunar infusion. Lunar infusions are infused under the light of the moon.

Mulberries lead this blend with their sweet, nourishing energy. They benefit insomnia and memory by strengthening Yin and cooling agitating heat. Passionflower leaves are sleepy time herbs that are particularly useful for when stress and emotional strain manifest in the body, such as with headaches, bellyaches, and heartaches. Skullcap and California poppy are sedative herbs that sedate the body and draw the mind into a restful state. Rose speaks to the spiritual aspects of sleep by touching the Heart's energy. And milky oat tops and oat straw heal the nerves and buffer the stress response, which is central to any relaxation.

In an airtight container, combine the mulberries, oat straw and/or tops, rose, poppy, skullcap, and passionflower. Store away from heat, light, and moisture for up to 12 months.

To make a single cup of tea, place 1 heaping tsp of the tea in a teapot and pour 1 cup (240 ml) of boiling water (200° F [95° C]) over the tea. Cover and steep for 15 minutes before straining. Drink immediately.

To make a lunar infusion: Place ¼ cup (16 g) of the tea in a jar, add 4 cups (960 ml) of cool water, cover, and place outside in the light of the moon. Set an intention for healing and envision your most peaceful night's sleep. The next morning, strain the herbs and discard. Reserve the infusion and casually sip throughout the day. Store in the refrigerator for up to 3 days.

LUCID DREAMS MUGWORT BATH

Yields 1 bath

INGREDIENTS

5 cups (100 g) fresh mugwort
   leaves and stems
2 cups (400 g) Epsom salt

Mugwort baths bring to my mind the herbal steam rooms of Korean spas. The herb's deep, comforting heat has been used for generations in Korea and across Asia to relieve physical pains and exhaustion and increase circulation. Adding Epsom salt to this recipe increases its effect for healing the nervous system. The mythology around mugwort is that it brings forward lucid dreams, which are moments of waking consciousness during sleep. It also deepens intuition and attunement with the energies within. Its magic can be brought forth internally as tea, in the air as smoke or smudge, and in the water as a bath. Mugwort healing occurs on all levels—the physical, emotional, and spiritual planes.

To prepare the mugwort, use scissors to cut the stems into 2 in (5 cm) pieces. In a large pot, bring the mugwort stems, leaves, and 8 cups (2 L) of water to a simmer. Remove from the heat, cover, and steep for 15 minutes while drawing a very warm bath.

When the bath is ready, strain the herbs from the bath "tea" then add the tea, along with the Epsom salt, to the bath water. Soak for 20 minutes for a full therapeutic effect.

Note: To substitute dried mugwort instead, add 3 cups (180 g) of dried mugwort.

Down to Earth Guided Meditation

We know that meditation is beneficial for sleep and brings a busy, distracted mind to a place of stillness. However, I've found that the idea of meditating can be intimidating for many folks. Guided meditations are wonderful because they allow you to release control and remove the pressure to do things the "right way." To try this yourself, prepare by recording the meditation and playing it back to yourself, or have a friend read it aloud to you. I've written the mediation as I would say it aloud, with pauses between each line. When ready, find a comfortable place to rest and sleep once the guided meditation has been recited. Remove distractions and noises and create a space where you can fully tap into the moment and release the stress and tension of the day.

Meditation:

→ Find a comfortable reclined position and feel your body fully supported.

→ Following your natural breath, take a moment to come into the space, into the moment.

→ And with each breath, with each exhalation, start to soften and release the body.

→ Soften the belly, the fingers, and the toes.

→ Release the chest and throat, the jaw, tongue, and eyes.

→ Take a moment to notice any areas that may feel tight, stuck, painful, or numb. Send a breath to any such area. Breathe directly into that space. (Pause for 10 seconds.)

→ Now bring your awareness to the very top of your head.

→ Visualize a soft light; the color is gold or silver.

→ And that light moves down over the face and scalp. Washing over and gently hugging the brain.

→ From there, the light draws downward, following the course of the spine. Glowing brightly at heart center. And all the way down, glowing in the soft of the belly and hips.

→ The light reaches each fingertip. And each toe. See it clearly.

→ The energy within is so strong and vital that it not only fills you but also radiates from you, forming a soft, energetic boundary around your entire body. A protection.

→ With this in place, begin to let go. Allowing thoughts, sensations, even little movements to pass right through you.

→ As you settle in, breath by breath. Again and again.

FACE AND COMPLEXION

How we care for our skin affects our health on every level. And while the mainstream beauty industry sells quick fixes and cover-ups, holistic beauty practices cultivate inner and outer beauty. Taking the time from our hurried, overburdened lifestyles to care for ourselves is an act of healing. And doing so with joy and alignment is a self-nurturing act. Healthy skin and a glowing face communicate wellness. We lead with our eyes and talk with our mouths in face-to-face interactions. The face is how we communicate with the world around us. Thus, the most profound effect of modern Asian beauty treatments, including jade rolling, acupuncture, facial massage, and gua sha, is the release of emotional holding from the face. This includes authentic emotion, such as a heartfelt smile when seeing a friend. It's also about how we hold emotion in our faces as a defense mechanism, such as when feeling insecure in a new situation or interacting with a threatening person. Emotional holding patterns are even brought to the surface at night with teeth grinding and jaw clenching. True wellness includes an awareness of these holding patterns and finding ways to release them.

Making and using clean and natural herbal skin care products, such as cleansing grains and oils, is important for health, because the skin absorbs everything. Making clean skincare products at home gives you the power to choose ingredients and the knowledge that what you are putting on your skin is safe and effective. Many commercial products contain endocrine disrupters and other harmful ingredients, such as parabens, phthalates, and BPA, so it is important that you check the safety of the ingredients in products you buy.

Energetic Facial Map

The skin and face are a microcosm of the rest of the body. Different areas on the face reflect the health of the Zangfu organs. For example, the forehead represents the Liver, and the presence of Liver Qi stagnation is held in the brow. Skin quality also reflects the health of Qi, Blood, and body fluids. Dull and dry skin indicates Qi and Blood deficiency. Oily and blemished skin reflects dampness and an imbalance of Spleen Qi. Thus, energetic face mapping gives us a window into our internal health and wellness.

Forehead

The forehead is ruled by the Liver and Gallbladder. The health of these organs is related to good physical movement, digestion, and the smooth flow of Qi and Blood. Skin issues on the forehead, such as acne, dryness, wrinkles, furrows, tension, and asymmetry, indicate a deeper issue with the Liver and Gallbladder. Stress and internal stagnation are almost always at play in these cases.

The forehead also has a high concentration of oil glands and is susceptible to acne. Stress and poor sleep quality can further worsen acne on the forehead because they stagnate Liver Qi and weaken the immune system. Deep horizontal lines across the forehead indicate an overactive nervous system and poor digestion manifesting as irritable bowel syndrome (IBS) or uncomfortable gas and bowel movements.

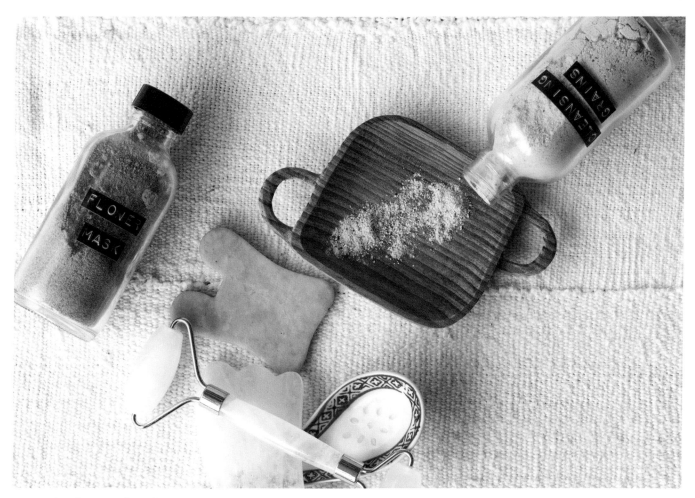

Facial grains and gua sha

People with frustration and anger are likely to have deep furrows between their eyebrows. If the body is overburdened with toxins due to stress, emotions, food, and the environment, it also shows up in this area. More lines on the left side of the brow indicate repressed emotions, especially anger and issues with how you relate to the Yang aspects of your personality (i.e., action, ambition, adventure). The right side of the brow holds pent-up emotions due to worry and overthinking. In my clinic, I've found that this indicates issues in relating to the Yin aspects of your personality (i.e., rest, creativity, personal expression).

Support Liver Qi and the Gallbladder with Yin activities, including meditation, rest, relaxation, play, and breath work to balance the nervous system. Drink more water and incorporate bitter flavors, such as turmeric, dandelion, and leafy greens, into the diet. Facial massage is a wonderful way to reduce the tension in your forehead and overall face, which will enhance your beauty (for more on facial massage, see page 252).

Sides of the Face and Temples

The sides of the face and temples reflect the health of the Kidney, Urinary Bladder, and adrenals. The Kidney is sensitive to chronic fear and overreactive stress response. Medications, chronic infections, inflammation, and excessive behavior (i.e., alcohol, smoking, poor diet) also weaken these energetic organs. Wrinkles, lines, dark spots, and acne in this area indicate internal imbalance. Puffiness, swollen lower eyelids, and dark circles also represent impaired Kidney energy.

Support the Kidney by reducing stress with healing practices, including meditation, acupuncture, yoga, qigong, and tai chi. Staying hydrated with healthy fluids (i.e., spring water, raw coconut water, herbal tea) is also key, as the Kidney rules the water element. Take mineral- and nutrient-dense foods and herbs, such as goji berry, nettle, he shou wu, and seaweed. Avoid sugar, processed foods, and excess caffeine, as they weaken the Kidney.

Cheeks

The cheeks are linked to the Stomach, Spleen, and Lung. There is good vitality in the complexion when the Stomach, Spleen, and Lung are healthy. Red inflammation on the cheeks near the nose indicates Stomach heat, and is often a sign of a food sensitivity to dairy or gluten. Patchiness or discoloration on the cheeks can indicate poor metabolism and low absorption of nutrients such as folic acid and iron. Acne on the cheeks is also caused by dirty cellphones, pillowcases, or a tendency to touch your face. The Lung will carry dampness in the form of phlegm and mucus when the Stomach is unhealthy. With this dynamic, people will start coughing up phlegm, especially in the morning. If there is acne, redness, dry skin, and irritation on your cheeks, they are likely caused and aggravated by diet. For healing, check out Medicine Meal (page 269).

Chin and Jawline

The chin and jawline represent the health of the Large Intestine and Stomach. Your chin is where hormonal imbalances will make themselves known, which means you're more likely to break out around your menstrual cycle. Studies have proven that chin and jawline acne is often caused by an excess of androgens and hormones that overstimulate oil glands. Often, with surges of hormones in the luteal phase, hormone imbalance is related to diet and overall gut health, especially if you're eating high-carb foods or dairy with added hormones. Another sign of imbalance is a swollen or puffy jawline with flabby skin. This is due to inflammation and aggravated by dampness.

Reducing stress as much as possible, getting adequate sleep, and getting regular exercise will help heal skin issues and blemishes on the jawline. For the health of the Kidney, cut back on sugars, white bread, processed foods, and dairy. My favorite healing treatment for a more profound balance of Kidney Yin and Yang is moxibustion on the lower abdomen and back (see page 283 for more on moxibustion). Moxibustion helps the water metabolism and brings down inflammation to reduce a puffy jawline.

MIMOSA FLOWER TEA FOR A CHEERFUL SPIRIT

Makes 1 cup (240 ml)

INGREDIENTS

1 to 2 Tbsp dried mimosa flower

The mimosa flower is called he huan hua in Mandarin Chinese, which means "collective happiness flower." This happiness flower calms the mind by moving stagnant Liver Qi and harmonizing energy within the body and mind. Mimosa is a beautiful medicine for healing depression or anxiety that causes a feeling of oppression in the chest, pain, irritability, restlessness, forgetfulness, and insomnia. Like most flower medicine, its effect is mild and gentle and should be taken over time for the full benefit.

Place the mimosa in a teapot and add 1 cup (240 ml) of boiling water (200° F [95° C]). Cover and steep for 10 minutes before straining. Drink immediately.

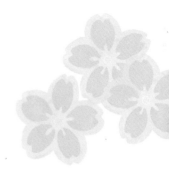

MIDORI PEARL JASMINE GREEN TEA

Makes 3 oz (85 g) loose-leaf
tea

INGREDIENTS

3 oz (85 g) loose Jasmine pearl
   green tea
½ tsp freshwater pearl
   powdered extract

This magical, floral cup of green tea is infused with jasmine flowers and dusted with pearl powder. In traditional Chinese medicine, Pearl powder is a beauty tonic and medicinal to calm the mind. Green tea draws excess heat and tension from the face and mind. And jasmine flowers harmonize Qi to prevent stagnation and have a gentle warming quality that balances the cooling nature of the green tea. This tea is named in honor of my beautiful sister, Tara Midori. Midori means "green."

I make this blend with a hand-rolled green tea pearl as a play on words with the pearl powder, but it can be made with any loose-leaf jasmine green tea.

In an airtight container, gently combine the green tea with the pearl powder extract. Store away from heat, light, and moisture for up to 12 months.

To make a cup of tea, place 1 tsp of the tea in a teapot and pour 1 cup (240 ml) of barely simmering water (170° F [75° C]) over the tea. Cover and steep for 1 to 2 minutes before straining. Drink immediately. If desired, re-steep by pouring fresh, simmering water over the tea for a second cup.

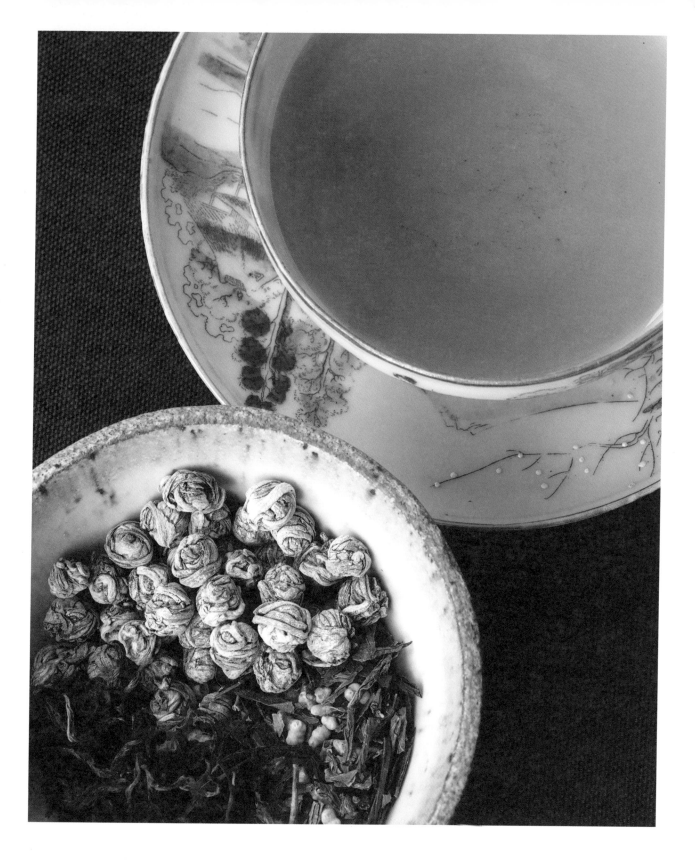

ROSY COMPLEXION TEA

Makes 6 cups (1.4 L)

INGREDIENTS

8 dried jujube dates
¼ cup (45 g) pearl barley
8 dried chrysanthemum flowers
2 Tbsp dried rose petals
Honey or maple syrup, for
  serving

A healthy, rosy complexion reflects the wellness of the energetic Heart. When the Heart is overwhelmed from stress and emotional strain, it shows up on the face as redness and irritation. Rose is a classic herb for healing the Heart and harmonizing Qi. Chrysanthemum also harmonizes Qi and cools heat that can present as inflammation. In folk traditions, jujube dates are considered a beauty tonic because they are excellent for tonifying Qi and Blood. And pearl barley clears dampness so fresh Qi can rise to the face.

In a small pot, bring the jujube dates, pearl barley, and 6 cups (1.4 L) of water to a boil. Turn the heat to low and simmer for about 10 minutes, or until the dates are very soft. Remove from the heat then add the chrysanthemum and rose, cover, and steep for 10 minutes before straining. Slowly drink 1 to 3 cups (240 to 720 ml) over the course of a day, adding honey or maple syrup to sweeten. Store in a glass jar in the refrigerator for up to 3 days.

TEA LEAVES CLEANSING GRAINS AND MASK

Makes 2 cups (240 g)

INGREDIENTS

¼ cup (3 g) dried
    chrysanthemum
¾ cup (75 g) green tea powder
¼ cup (35 g) rice powder
1 cup (130 g) green or white
    kaolin clay
Rose water or hydrosol
    (optional)

Green tea and chrysanthemum make for a cooling and astringent blend for oily skin. Green tea powder and rice powder should be purchased premade when possible (see Resources on page 312). You can make green tea powder by grinding green tea leaves in a blender. Do not use matcha powder; it is too fine for making cleansing grains.

In a blender, pulse the chrysanthemum into a fine powder. Remove any large or rough pieces; the mixture should be grainy yet soft, because the flowers will always have some grit. Take care not to breathe in the fine dust. Transfer to an airtight container then add the green tea powder, rice powder, and clay and mix to combine. Store away from heat, light, and moisture for up to 12 months.

To cleanse, place 1 Tbsp of the mixture in the palm of your hand or in a small bowl. Mix in just enough water, rose water, or hydrosol to make a soft paste. Gently massage the cleansing grains paste onto your face using the lightest pressure of your fingertips. Rinse off with warm water. To make a mask, leave the facial grains on the skin until dry and gently wash off with warm water and a soft towel.

Topical Recipes – Cleansing Grains Three Ways

Cleansing grains are an excellent way to clean and exfoliate the skin using herbs and natural materials. They work well for many skin types, especially if you're sensitive to the chemicals and preservatives in commercial cleansers. Gentle exfoliation removes dead skin cells, increases circulation, and brings fresh Qi and Blood to the face for a fresh glow. They can be used daily on many skin types and are great for removing sunscreen and light makeup.

THE FLOWERS CLEANSING GRAINS AND MASK

Makes about 2 cups (200 g)
for 24 masks

INGREDIENTS

½ cup (40 g) old-fashioned
   rolled oats

2 Tbsp dried rose petals

2 Tbsp dried hibiscus flowers

1 cup (130 g) pink or white
   kaolin clay

2 Tbsp rice powder

1 tsp freshwater pearl powder
   extract

Rose water or a hydrosol
   (optional)

This natural mask combines oats and flowers to brighten and soften the skin. After you make the grain mixture you will mix that with a little bit of water or, preferably, rose water or a hydrosol. Hydrosols are herbal waters that are a byproduct from making essential oils, and they can be purchased at most health food stores and herb shops. Powders such as chamomile and rice powder should be purchased premade when possible (see Resources on page 312). You may use other dried flowers such as chrysanthemum, violet, lavender, calendula, and jasmine. When grinding whole herbs and flowers, remove any large chunks and stems that do not break down into a fine powder. An electric coffee grinder that is only used for herbal preparations will also work in place of a blender.

In a blender, pulse the oats, rose, and hibiscus into a fine powder. Remove any rough or large pieces; the mixture should be grainy yet soft, because the flowers and oats will always have a gritty texture. Take care not to breathe in the fine dust. Transfer to an airtight container then add the kaolin clay, rice powder, and pearl powder and mix to combine. Store away from heat, light, and moisture for up to 12 months.

To cleanse, place 1 Tbsp of the mixture in the palm of your hand or in a small bowl. Mix in just enough water, rose water, or hydrosol to make a soft paste. Gently massage the cleansing grains paste onto your face using the lightest pressure of your fingertips. Rinse off with warm water. To make a mask, leave the facial grains on the skin until dry and gently wash off with warm water and a soft towel.

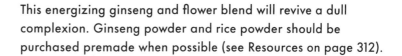

RICE GRAINS ENERGIZING GINSENG MASK AND CLEANSING GRAINS

Makes 2 ½ cups (280 g)

INGREDIENTS

¼ cup (4 g) dried calendula

2 Tbsp dried chamomile flowers

1 ½ cups (195 g) white kaolin clay

½ cup (70 g) rice powder

2 Tbsp ginseng powder

2 Tbsp poppy seeds

Rose water or hydrosol (optional)

This energizing ginseng and flower blend will revive a dull complexion. Ginseng powder and rice powder should be purchased premade when possible (see Resources on page 312).

In a blender, pulse the calendula and chamomile into a fine powder. Remove any large or rough pieces; the mixture should be grainy yet soft, because the flowers will always have some grit. Take care not to breathe in the fine dust. Transfer to an airtight container then add the kaolin clay, rice powder, ginseng powder, and poppy seeds and mix to combine. Store away from heat, light, and moisture for up to 12 months.

To cleanse, place 1 Tbsp of the mixture in the palm of your hand or in a small bowl. Mix in just enough water, rose water, or hydrosol to make a soft paste. Gently massage the cleansing grains paste onto your face using the lightest pressure of your fingertips. Rinse off with warm water. To make a mask, leave the facial grains on the skin until dry and gently wash off with warm water and a soft towel.

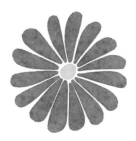

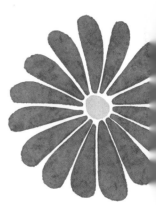

CHRYSANTHEMUM TSUBAKI FACIAL OIL

Makes 8 fl oz (240 ml)

INGREDIENTS

⅔ cup (160 ml) tsubaki camellia oil

3 Tbsp jojoba oil, preferably clear

2 Tbsp meadowfoam seed oil

2 Tbsp rose hip seed oil

½ tsp vitamin E oil

8 drops blue chamomile essential oil

8 drops helichrysum essential oil

Rose water, a hydrosol, or water, to prep skin before applying oil

Chrysanthemum Tsubaki Facial Oil was created to use in facial acupuncture treatments at my clinic. I fell in love with this subtle oil and now use it every morning after misting clean skin with rose water or a hydrosol spray. The tsubaki camellia oil is slightly dry, so it absorbs quickly into the skin. Jojoba and rose hip seed oil nourish and hydrate the skin. The meadowfoam seed oil has a luxurious feel yet is shelf stable, absorbs well, and doesn't have a strong odor. Blue chamomile and helichrysum essential oils are classics for skin integrity and give this blend a fresh scent. Add rose geranium essential oil for a more floral aroma. It is vital to use organic oils because the skin absorbs *everything*.

In a large glass jar, combine the tsubaki camellia oil, jojoba oil, meadowfoam seed oil, rose hip seed oil, vitamin E oil, blue chamomile essential oil, and helichrysum essential oil. Use a chopstick to stir the oils together and fully incorporate them. Cover and leave to rest so that the oils thoroughly combine. Store in an 8 fl oz (240 ml) glass jar with a dropper for ease of use. The oil will last up to 12 months if stored away from heat, light, and moisture.

To use, prep clean skin by misting with water, rose water, or a hydrosol. Rub 20 drops of the oil between your hands and gently pat into the skin.

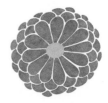

TAMANU FACIAL OIL

Makes 3 fl oz (90 ml)

INGREDIENTS

2 Tbsp clear or yellow jojoba oil

1 Tbsp plus 1 tsp tamanu nut oil

1 Tbsp plus 1 tsp avocado oil

2 tsp argan oil

½ tsp vitamin E oil

8 drops lavender essential oil

8 drops blue chamomile
   essential oil

Tamanu Facial Oil is a hydrating oil for dry and delicate skin. I formulated this oil for facial massage, jade rolling, and gua sha and find it luxurious and hydrating. Tamanu nut oil replenishes the skin and encourages skin regeneration, while avocado oil absorbs deeply to address dryness and discoloration. Argan oil has a smooth texture that brightens and revitalizes skin texture. And jojoba oil is similar to skin sebum, absorbing quickly and adding a protective barrier that prevents dehydrated skin. This blend has an earthy, nutty scent that works well with lavender essential oil, which is calming and acts as a natural preservative.

In a large glass jar, combine the jojoba oil, tamanu nut oil, avocado oil, argan oil, vitamin E oil, lavender essential oil, and blue chamomile essential oil. Use a chopstick to stir the oil together and fully incorporate them. Cover and leave to rest so that the oils thoroughly combine. Store in a 4 fl oz (120 ml) glass jar with a dropper for ease of use. The oil will last up to 12 months if stored away from heat, light, and moisture.

To use, prep clean skin by misting with water, rose water, or a hydrosol. Rub 20 drops of the oil between your hands and gently pat into the skin.

ICHI NI SAN THREE-PURPOSE OIL

Makes 7 fl oz (210 ml)

INGREDIENTS

⅓ cup (80 ml) tsubaki camellia oil

⅓ cup (80 ml) Calendula Sun Oil (page 176)

2 Tbsp jojoba oil, clear or yellow

1 Tbsp plus 1 tsp apricot seed oil

½ tsp vitamin E oil

15 drops hinoki cypress essential oil

This three-purpose oil can be used as a body oil, hair oil, or oil cleanser. Ichi Ni San means "one-two-three" in Japanese. Tsubaki oil is a dry oil that readily absorbs into the skin and hair. Apricot oil absorbs quite quickly and is rich in omega fatty acids to tone and hydrate. The Calendula Sun Oil (page 176), an excellent skin healer, is infused with calendula flowers. If you do not have this infused calendula oil on hand, you can substitute plain safflower oil or more of the apricot seed oil. Jojoba oil contains a natural anti-inflammatory called myristic acid that helps to reduce wrinkles, stretch marks, and acne scars and balance the skin's natural oils.

In a large glass jar, combine the tsubaki camellia oil, Calendula Sun Oil, jojoba oil, apricot seed oil, vitamin E oil, and hinoki cypress essential oil. Use a chopstick to stir the oils together and fully incorporate them. Cover and leave to rest so that the oils thoroughly combine. Store in 4 fl oz (120 ml) glass jars with a dropper for ease of use. The oil will last up to 12 months if stored away from heat, light, and moisture.

To use as a body oil, simply rub it into the skin. It works particularly well on slightly damp skin, such as after a shower. As hair oil, rub a few drops between your hands and apply them to the ends of the hair. As an oil cleanser, apply to a dry face and gently massage it with the lightest pressure of your fingertips. Wet a soft towel with very warm water, ring it out, and gently blot and wipe away the oil.

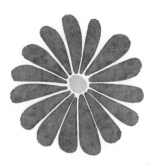

Asian American Herbalism

FLOWER POWER BEAUTY STEAM

Makes 1 steam

INGREDIENTS

1 cup (60 g) dried elderflower

1 cup (30 g) fresh or dried mixed
flowers (i.e., rose, lavender,
chamomile, etc.)

Steams are a time-tested way to hydrate delicate facial skin and bring fresh Qi to the face. Elderflower is a release-the-exterior herb that draws energy to the surface of the skin. Although it has a dispersing effect, it is also moistening and has an astringent quality that prevents skin irritation and dryness. Elderflower steams also help reduce congestion and mucus in the sinuses to address sinusitis, allergies, and headache. While this steam can be made with elderflowers alone, adding other garden flowers that you may have on hand is lovely. My favorite facial care flowers are rose, lavender, chamomile, calendula, and chrysanthemum.

Fill a large pot with 8 to 10 cups (2 to 2.4 L) of water. Bring to a boil then remove from the heat, add the elderflowers and mixed flowers, cover, and steep for 10 to 15 minutes. Place a bath towel under a large bowl on a table in front of a comfortable chair. Carefully pour the steaming tea and flowers into the bowl. Wrap another bath towel over your head and shoulders and hold tight under the chin. Sit on the chair and drape the towel that is over your head around the steaming pot to create a tent to trap the steam. Steam for 5 to 15 minutes. The heat of the steam should feel comfortably warm so you can breathe freely. If the steam is too hot or overwhelming, open the towel and allow the steam to cool until it is a comfortable temperature.

Facial Massage – Jade Rolling and Gua Sha

For many years I specialized in facial acupuncture treatments, which always included facial massage, jade rolling, and facial cups. Facial gua sha and jade rolling are akin to lymphatic massage and energetic healing. They are lovely and effective modalities, but it is essential to call them what they are—a modern take on traditional healing practices. Ten years ago, almost no one who came through my clinic had ever heard of gua sha, let alone facial gua sha. However, facial gua sha has recently become very popular in mainstream culture. When facial gua sha first started to gain popularity, I was excited to see increased interest in Asian healing practices. However, how it has been presented in the mainstream is an overwhelming example of cultural appropriation. Presenting gua sha as a superficial, new-age beauty treatment is not only wrong but hurtful to the traditional culture and medicine.

Moreover, there is seldom any talk about the painful history in America of Asian immigrants being persecuted for using such techniques. In the 1970s and 1980s, gua sha markings on children were misunderstood by schoolteachers and law enforcement as child abuse. This is why gua sha can be a challenging subject. I share these practices here for home use because they are a big part of my work as an acupuncturist and East Asian medicine practitioner. And I practice with the belief that we need more, not less, access to healing therapies. For more in-depth information and the traditional uses of gua sha, see page 284.

What Does Gua Sha and Facial Massage Do?

- Releases emotional holding from the face for more symmetry and balance.
- Smoothes fine lines by relaxing tight facial muscles.
- Increases circulation of Blood and Qi to the skin and tissues.
- Improves blood circulation and stimulates cells to produce natural collagen and elastin.
- Moves out stagnant body fluids and lymph to reduce puffiness and swelling.
- Clears out inflammation and redness and strengthens the vascular integrity of the face.

Because of its invigorating properties, do not gua sha the face until 8 weeks after fillers, Botox, or chemical or surgical treatments on the face.

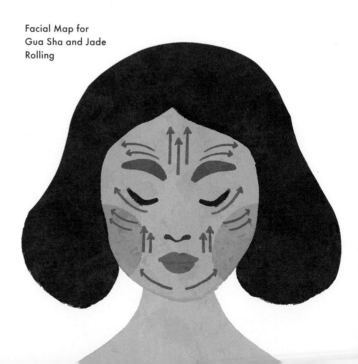

Facial Map for Gua Sha and Jade Rolling

Facial Massage – The Treatment

→ Start with clean skin. Moisten the skin with a hydrosol or plain water. Apply facial oil to the face, neck, and upper chest. The skin should be slick to allow the gua sha tool to glide gently across the skin.

→ You will need a jade roller or gua sha tool, which are readily available online (see Resources on page 312).

→ Use very light pressure! Never pull on the skin or massage deeply. Facial gua sha should never leave markings on the skin.

→ The motions should be upward and outward, starting from the midline of the face and body. Perform each motion 3 to 5 times.

→ Start at the center of the chest at the sternum and sweep the tool along the upper chest at the collarbones and to the shoulders.

→ Next, bring the tool to the back of the head at the base of the neck and sweep down the neck to the tops of the shoulders.

→ For the front of the neck, carefully hold the skin taught so that the sweeping motion doesn't drag the delicate skin. Sweep up from the collarbones to the base of the jaw and chin.

→ From the front of the chin, sweep along the jawline to just under the ear. Pay attention to any tension in the chewing muscle (the masseter) at the corner of the jaw. It will be sore and tense if you are prone to jaw clenching and teeth grinding at night.

→ Work on the cheeks in three sections, moving in long, slightly curved upward motions from the midline of the face to the ear. Start at the corner of the lip up to the ear. Then from the nose to just below the cheekbone and the ear. And finally, from the nose to just above the cheekbone and the ear.

→ Apply constant, even pressure under each eye, being careful not to pull the lower eyelid.

→ At each temple, apply very light pressure and move the tool in a clockwise circle for nine rotations. Draw the tool down from the temple, over the jaw, and down the neck to the collar bones. Sweep the tool across the collarbone, as you did in the first step, to encourage lymphatic drainage.

→ To work the forehead, start between the eyebrows by combing out the furrows with a zigzag motion.

→ Starting at the inner eyebrow (orbital bone), sweep across the eyebrow to the temple. Then work upwards from the eyebrow to the hairline in five sweeps.

→ If you don't mind getting your hair oily, continue to sweep the tool past the hairline and across the scalp. You can use more pressure on the scalp, like a gentle massage.

→ Finish by working back down the face in the reverse order you started. Still working from the midline toward the ear, move the tool in a single sweep across the forehead, the cheeks, the jaw, the neck, and ending at the chest.

→ Afterward, you will notice a refreshed flush of energy on your face. With practice, this treatment takes just a few minutes. It should never cause pain and should never leave markings on the face.

→ Repeat this treatment every three days or as desired.

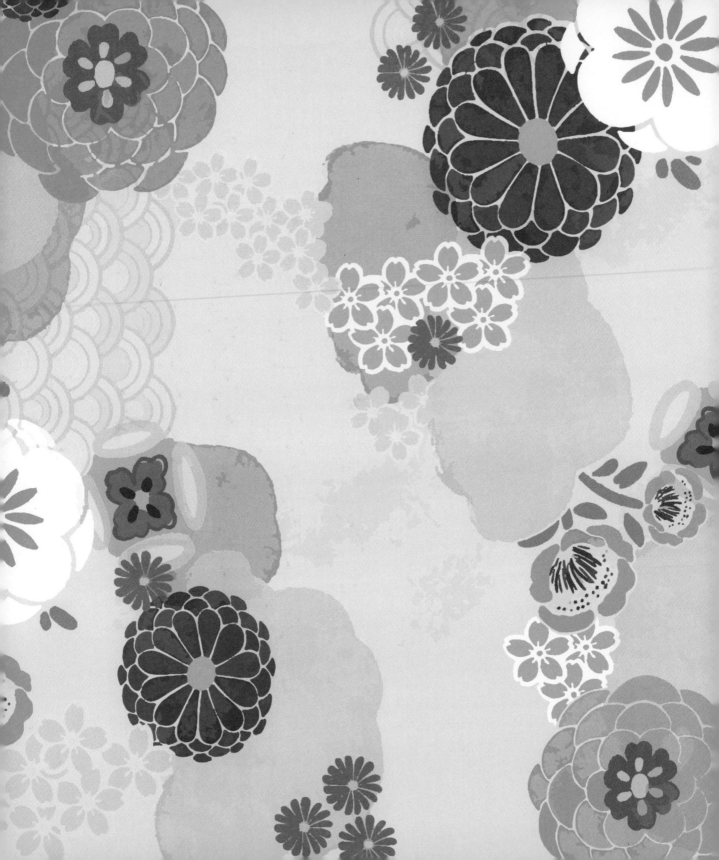

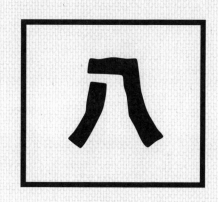

CHAPTER EIGHT

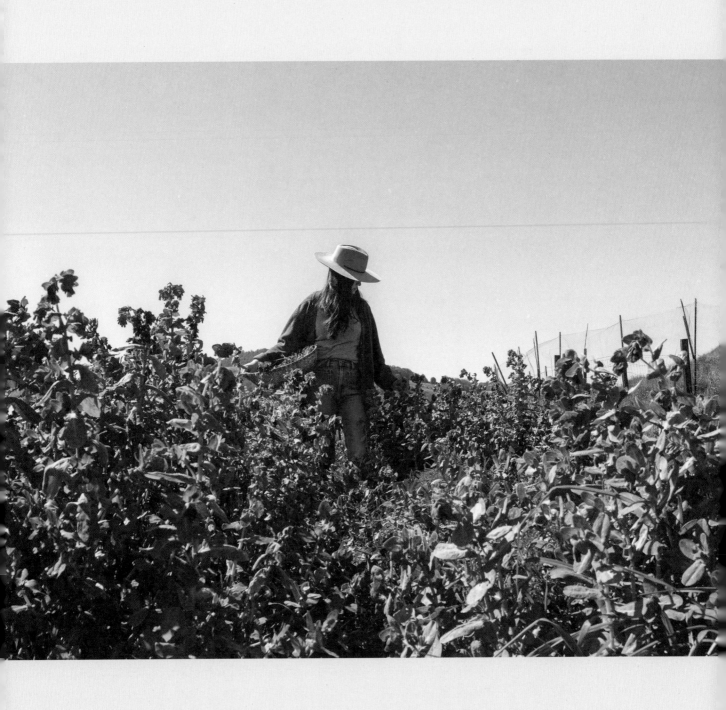

LIVING IN HARMONY AND MAINTAINING HEALTH

———

Our mind and body are a reflection of the world around us. Even with all our modern-day conveniences—lights, cell phones, alarms, heaters, and air conditioning—we are still hardwired to the day and night. The sun and the moon. The harmony and flow of the seasons. East Asian philosophy offers a clear and poetic perspective on how to live in accordance with the seasons.

SEASONAL WELLNESS

A common misconception about the flow of the seasons is that the equinox and solstice are the beginning of each season. According to the lunar calendar these points are the peak of each season rather than the beginning. In this way, the spring begins with the second full moon of the year, sometime in late January to early February. That is why spring festivals including Chinese Lunar New Year coincide with this timing.

Following the natural rhythms of each season gives us clues on how to live in harmony with nature. Living in accordance with the seasons protects your deep reserve of Qi and sets the tone for the year to come.

Spring

The true nature of the spring, from late January to early May, is uneven, modest, and tender. As the heaviness of winter lifts, spring energy helps us to thaw hard layers and holding patterns. The sun shines a little brighter and encourages us to get outside, move, and grow. However, with change comes instability, and this season can bring with it restlessness or irritability that is hard to place. The edgy nature of spring can increase Liver Qi stagnation and irregularity, which show up as mood swings, irritability, having trouble unwinding from the day's activities, and difficulty letting things go. Yet, with age and wisdom, we see that transitional times hold considerable potential for conscious growth. This season asks us to reconsider tired, played out habits.

As we move away from the rich stews and roots vegetables of winter, spring foods are light and crisp in nature. And as the season progresses, we have access to more fresh greens and vegetables, including kale, chard, bok choy, dandelion, and chrysanthemum greens. Quick and light cooking preparations, such as steaming and stir fry, are appropriate for the season. A moderate amount of raw foods is also healthy. Seasonal foods tend to be sour, cool, and spicy: asparagus, radish, peas, fava beans, nettles, spring onions, lemons, mandarins, kumquats, grapefruit, and mushrooms. The sour taste of lemon water, fermented pickles, and vinegar is healing for the energetic Liver, the organ of spring.

Spring is often considered a good time for detoxification, and a balanced diet supports the body's natural capacity to cleanse the body from the inside out. I do not recommend harsh detoxification techniques, such as fasting, enemas, or minimal, restrictive diets, because they invite imbalance by depleting the Spleen Qi and draining Blood and body fluids. A healthier way is to incorporate healing foods and herbs that help the liver process toxins. Fermented foods and cooling herbs, including miso, mung bean, mushroom, and seaweeds help the body to clear out physical toxins, such as heavy metals, and reduce the effects of radiation exposure when eaten daily for three to six months. Another important piece is to limit or eliminate processed foods, fried food, alcohol, smoking, irregular eating habits, and disordered eating, all of which slows the Qi and leads to a buildup of dampness and stagnation.

SPRING

Yang within Yin
Vision
Tendons
Liver
Gallbladder
Wood Element
Wind
Flexibility
Irregularity
Friction
Patience
Discernment

CREAMY NETTLE SOUP

Serves 4

INGREDIENTS

2 Tbsp olive oil or avocado oil

2 leeks (white parts only), thinly
   sliced

2 zucchini, chopped

1 ½ cups (27 g) fresh nettle
   leaves, stems removed (or
   ¾ cup [21 g] dried nettle)

6 cups (1.4 L) homemade
   chicken stock or canned broth

3 Tbsp grass-fed unsalted
   butter, such as Kerrygold,
   melted

Sea salt and pepper

Crème fraîche or sour cream, for
   serving

I fondly remember hosting seasonal wellness workshops with a team of dear friends at Tara Firma Farms in Petaluma, California. Carrie Kane is a nutritionist who always brought a depth of knowledge to share with the community and a delicious seasonal dish. Her Creamy Nettle Soup is unforgettable. It is a perfect balance of light and fresh, with a rich, satisfying flavor. Nettles are a mineral-rich and nutrient-dense herb that grow freely during the spring rainy season. Be sure to wear gloves to process them, because the hairs on the leaves will sting the skin until cooked. Dandelion greens and other dark leafy greens can be substituted. The recipe calls for grass-fed butter, which is special to spring, as it's when the cows can be sent out to pasture to graze on the fast-growing green grasses.

In a large soup pot, heat the oil over medium heat. Add the leeks and zucchini and sauté for a few minutes, or until soft. Stir in the nettles and stock then cover and simmer for 15 minutes.

After 15 minutes, add the melted butter and use an immersion blender to blend into a creamy soup consistency. (If using a regular blender, blend in small batches and let the steam out carefully.) Season with salt and pepper. Divide into bowls, top with a dollop of crème fraîche or sour cream, and serve immediately.

Contraindication: This recipe is not recommended in cases of cardiac or renal failure due to the nettles.

DANDELION VINEGAR

Makes 1 ½ cups (360 ml)

INGREDIENTS

1 cup (55 g) fresh dandelion leaves (or 2 Tbsp dried dandelion)

½ cup (15 g) fresh nettle leaves, stems removed (or 1 Tbsp dried nettle)

2 cups (480 ml) unrefined apple cider vinegar

Dandelion vinegar is a quintessential springtime recipe with an invigorating mix of sour and bitter tastes. While you can use any vinegar, unrefined apple cider vinegar has beneficial bacteria that add to the health benefits. The acid of vinegar is excellent for extracting medicine from mineral-rich and nutrient-dense herbs, such as dandelion and nettle. When sourcing dandelions for medicine, it is best to find the greens at your local market or CSA farm; dandelions with yellow blooms and puffballs are not the correct variety.

Prepare any fresh leaves by rinsing off any dirt, drying thoroughly (excess water will spoil the final product), and chopping into ½ in (12 mm) pieces.

In a 2 cup (480 ml) jar, combine the dandelion and nettle. Pour the vinegar over the herbs, filling the jar three-quarters of the way full. There should be a 2 in (5 cm) space between the herbs and the top of the jar. Reserve any leftover vinegar to top off the mixture as the herbs absorb the liquid during the first week of tincturing. Cover with a plastic or non-reactive lid (or line a metal lid with parchment or plastic wrap). Label the jar with the date and the ingredients. Store away from heat, light, and moisture for three months (or up to eight months if refrigerated) and gently shake the mixture every 1 to 3 days.

After 2 to 4 weeks, use a cheesecloth or fine-mesh sieve to strain the herbs and discard. Reserve the vinegar and store in a clean glass jar away from heat, light, and moisture. Take ½ to 1 tsp before meals to stimulate the digestive system. Mix with sparkling water for a digestive drink. Sprinkle on sautéed greens and salads.

Contraindication: Omit nettles in cases of cardiac or renal failure.

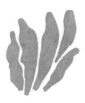

Early Summer

In Eastern tradition, summer includes two distinct seasons. Early Summer, from early May to early August, is what we usually consider the summer. It is the most Yang time of year, with daylight, activity, and expansion at a peak. Summer foods lend themselves to a lighter, simpler diet that calms the Heart and focuses the mind. Sautéing, steaming, light pickling, and raw preparations allow us to minimize our efforts and our use of the oven. Stimulating foods (i.e., coffee, chocolate, sugar, alcohol), hot spices, rich foods, iced food and drink, irregular eating habits, and disordered eating overstimulate the mind and lead to anxiety and restlessness. Unhealthy eating habits can cause health issues year-round, however, we are more vulnerable to the negative effects during the summer season. Seasonal foods tend to be bitter, cool, and spicy: kale, chard, collard greens, mustard greens, arugula, cucumber, mushroom, celery, lettuce, dill, basil, green onion, sprouts, tomato, garlic, ginger, raspberry, strawberry, sunflower seed, almond, pistachio, amaranth, quinoa, red lentil, whole grain wheat, rice, and oats.

Each season is represented in natural phenomena. The body parts that correspond to the summer are the Heart, blood vessels, Spleen, and muscles. The Heart and blood vessels correspond with the early summer season. This includes the physical heart and the energetic Heart, which governs the mind, emotions, sleep, and spirit. Imbalances of the Heart's energy manifest as anxiety, insomnia, heart flutters or palpitations, depression, mental fogginess, poor memory, and focus. The blood vessels are affected when the Heart's energy is out of balance, which can cause easy bruising, blood pressure issues, and poor blood circulation and Qi energy.

EARLY SUMMER

Yang
Blood Vessels
Circulation
Heart
Small Intestine
Fire Element
Fire
Heat
Expansive
Joy
Growth
Emotions

ROSE HONEY

Makes 1½ cups (360 ml)

INGREDIENTS

2 cups (160 g) fresh rose petals
and rosebuds (or 1 cup [20 g]
dried rose petals)

2 cups (480 ml) honey

Working with flowers and making sweet medicines like this one speak to the joy of herbalism. Roses are the flower of the Heart and thus the ideal flower to use in this summer recipe. There is a lot of grace with a honey infusion, so we measure with the heart here. Keep it simple and work with fresh petals and buds from your own garden or a neighbor's garden. Otherwise, dried rose petals can be ordered online (see Resources on page 312).

Prepare fresh roses by shaking off any dirt or bugs.

Fill a 2 cup (480 ml) glass jar with roses and pour honey over the flowers until the jar is almost full. There should be a 1 in (2.5 cm) space between the honey and the top of the jar. Use a chopstick to poke and stir the mixture to fully incorporate the ingredients. Reserve the extra honey to top off the mixture as the herbs absorb the honey during the first week of the infusion. Cover with a plastic or non-reactive lid (or line a metal lid with parchment or plastic wrap). Label the jar with the date and the ingredients. Store away from heat, light, and moisture for 4 to 6 weeks.

When ready to use, you can leave the flowers in the jar or strain them out. To strain, heat the honey jar in a double boiler until it liquefies. Pour the honey mixture through a cheesecloth or fine-mesh sieve and discard the flowers. Store in a clean glass jar at room temperature. The natural enzymes in the honey will allow it to keep for many years. Use to your heart's content.

Late Summer

Late summer is a time of transition. This fifth season includes the weeks leading up to the fall equinox and, to some extent, the seasonal transitions that occur during other times of the year. Transitional periods like this leave us quite vulnerable—the body is more susceptible to illness, and the mind is more prone to unnecessary, circular thinking. Seasonal transitions, however, are also the time of year when there is the greatest potential to tap into the deep well of balance within. Self-care and family care are particularly fruitful during this time, because the strides we make during this period are reflected in the following months.

Think of this as an opportunity to recalibrate and balance the mind, body, and spirit. Prepare simple meals, eat moderately, and limit or omit refined sugar and sweeteners. Sweet is the taste of this season, but it is not the sweetness of refined sugar. Consider the natural sweetness of foods, such as rice, potatoes, fruit, and honey. Other seasonally appropriate foods include egg, sweet potato, pea, apricot, green bean, melon, cherry, date, apple, currant, fig, mulberry, carrot, squash, onion, oats, barley, millet, chickpeas.

The Spleen and muscles are represented in the late summer season. According to Eastern philosophy, the Spleen is key to digestion, and this view is radically different from the Western concept of the spleen. When our Spleen is healthy, digestion functions properly, and the muscles are strong and supple. When the Spleen is weak, symptoms include muscle weakness, bloating, fatigue after eating, loose stools, diarrhea, heavy limbs, water retention, blood sugar imbalance, and unclear thinking. The Spleen thrives on routine and regularity, which speaks to the key habits for late summertime. And this intuitively makes sense as we know that our bodies take in nutrients from food most efficiently when we eat regularly and take time to focus, chill out, and enjoy simple meals.

LATE SUMMER

Yang
Muscles
Digestion
Spleen
Stomach
Earth Element
Damp
Sweetness
Transition
Focus
Overthinking
Vulnerability

BARLEY WATER

Serves 4

INGREDIENTS

The peel of 1 fresh tangerine (or
   2 tsp dried tangerine peel)
½ cup (90 g) pearl barley
Honey, for serving

Barley is traditionally used as both a food and a medicinal. It's rich in vitamins and minerals that nourish the nervous system. As a food and drink, barley drains Damp from the body and is useful for easing arthritis, inflammation, digestive upset, and water retention. Tangerine peel and citrus invigorate Qi and clear damp. Fresh and freshly dried tangerine peel is a wonderful remedy for pesky coughs and coughing up clear phlegm. It's ideal for mild coughs due to phlegm and dampness obstructing the Lung. Often people with this condition will cough up phlegm in the morning upon waking.

Wash the fresh tangerine peel well and tear it into 1 in (2.5 cm) pieces. Rinse the pearl barley and discard the water.

In a medium pot, bring the pearl barley, dried tangerine peel (if using), and 8 cups (2 L) of water to a boil. Turn the heat to low and simmer for about 30 minutes or until the liquid has reduced by half. Remove from the heat and skim any foam that collects on the top. Add the fresh tangerine peel (if using), cover, and steep for 10 minutes before using a cheesecloth-lined colander or fine-mesh sieve to strain. Discard the spent barley and tangerine peel. Reserve the barley water. Sweeten with honey and drink 2 to 4 cups (480 to 960 ml) per day. You may notice an increase in urination as the body purges the excess dampness.

Note: Use one whole dried tangerine peel for more profuse or stubborn phlegm.

Autumn

The transition from summer to autumn, in mid-September to early November, is often quite abrupt, and people tend to have difficulty adjusting. Energetically, it is a time of deep transition and letting go. You may find yourself preoccupied with getting clear on what isn't serving you well and, in the process, letting go of patterns and people that hinder your well-being. This may open you up to grieving and sadness as you process genuine loss. This work is not easy but when done in a way that feels safe and supported, transitional times allow for a fresh perspective. By releasing old holding patterns, you give yourself permission to occupy space and live more authentically. This will enable you to receive input more readily from the outside world, process and keep what feels right, and release the rest.

In Chinese medicine, the energetic patterns of autumn are ruled by the Lung and Large Intestine. These organs take nourishment from the outside world and when functioning correctly, determine what is useful and what must go. Because of the direct relationship between the internal body and the outside world, the body is more susceptible to getting sick during this season. Easily catching every cold or flu, chronic sinus infections, congestion, as well as dried, chapped, and other skin issues often occur. You may also notice that you're unintentionally absorbing other people's energy and issues more easily. Support your immunity and energetic boundaries by drinking more warm drinks and eating more cooked food, as well as spicy foods, including garlic, black pepper, and ginger.

When the Lung and Large Intestine are irritated by stress, overstimulation, or environmental toxins, their natural response is to secrete excessive mucus, which impairs breath and digestion. You can gently guide your energy inward by slowing down and allowing yourself some grace. Yoga and breath work strengthen the Lung. Enjoying regular, peaceful meals benefits the Large Intestine. Eating seasonally and taking herbs to balance the system helps to regulate phlegm and mucus during this time of year and into the rest of the year.

AUTUMN

Yin within Yang

Skin

Immune System

Lung

Large Intestine

Metal Element

Wind

Dry

Contraction

Discernment

Elimination

Boundaries

MUSHROOM – RICE WINE VINEGAR

Makes 1 ½ cups (360 ml)

INGREDIENTS

2 cups (200 g) fresh wild
   mushrooms, such as shiitake,
   maitake, or lion's mane

1½ cups (360 ml) unsweetened
   rice wine vinegar

The essence and flavor of herbs can be preserved quite nicely by vinegar. For mushroom vinegar, I use a high-quality unsweetened rice wine vinegar. This recipe lends itself to making yummy, seasoned rice for homemade sushi and onigiri. Mushroom growers are becoming more common with a wide variety of offerings at farmers' markets and natural food stores. My favorites are shiitake, maitake, and lion's mane, however, any single variety or combination of mushrooms will do.

Prepare the mushrooms by removing any dirt with a dry paper towel and chopping into ½ in (12 mm) pieces.

Put the mushrooms in a 2 cup (480 ml) glass jar and pour the vinegar over the herbs until the jar is three-quarters of the way full. There should be a 2 in (5 cm) space between the mixture and the top of the jar. Reserve the leftover vinegar to top off the mixture as the mushrooms absorb the liquid during the first week of the infusion. Cover with a plastic or non-reactive lid (or line a metal lid with parchment or plastic wrap). Label the jar with the date and ingredients. Store away from heat, light, and moisture and gently shake the mixture every 1 to 3 days.

After 2 to 4 weeks, use a cheesecloth-lined colander or fine-mesh sieve to strain the herbs and discard. Reserve the vinegar and store in a clean glass jar away from heat, light, and moisture for three months (or up to eight months if refrigerated). Use to season rice for onigiri or rice bowls. Sprinkle on sautéed greens and salads.

Winter

During winter, from early November to early February, the sun sets early and rises late. Cold weather and long nights draw our energies inward. It is naturally a time of year to retreat into our homes, cultivate warmth, and pause to restore and replenish our deep energy reserves. It's a time to consider how to purposefully turn our focus inward to become more restful during the winter. What demands can you let go of to reclaim more time for yourself? What are activities that recharge and excite you?

Winter is the season of the Kidney, which encompasses the deepest energies of the body, including our inner fire—our creative spark, drive, willpower, and vitality. Kidney energy oversees lifelong growth, aging, bone health, hormones, sexuality, and reproduction. When Kidney energy and inner fire are weak, there are symptoms including low back and knee pain, exhaustion, anxiety, insomnia, night sweats, memory issues, infertility, frequent urination, low libido, and water retention.

Kidney fire naturally declines with age and is accelerated by overwork, overstimulation, chronic stress, disease, sleep disturbances, drug use, chemical exposure, excessive sex, and poor diet. Drinking coffee to push through tiredness, working late, strenuous exercise, and the holiday hustle all deplete our reserves when we need them the most. Exhaustion at this time is more harmful than any other season, even though the consequences may not be felt until later in the year, when the energy you expect to have isn't there. Fortunately, there are herbs and remedies to prevent or slow the pace of this natural decline.

To replenish the Kidney energy, you need rest and not just for a day or a long weekend. This kind of restorative practice takes a dedicated effort. Prioritize time for solitude. Take time to reflect, dream, share stories, meditate, journal, and nap. Dress warmly to maintain body heat and keep your lower back and waistline warm because this is where the deep vitality fires of the Kidney lie. Use moxibustion over your lower abdomen, low back, and hips. Roast your buns near an open bonfire. Reconsider what it takes to fill your cup.

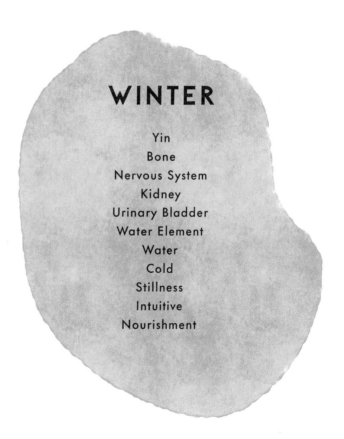

WINTER

Yin
Bone
Nervous System
Kidney
Urinary Bladder
Water Element
Water
Cold
Stillness
Intuitive
Nourishment

MANY MUSHROOMS SOUP

Serves 4

INGREDIENTS

1 cup (100 g) fresh maitake
mushrooms

1 cup (100 g) fresh oyster
mushrooms

1 cup (100 g) fresh shiitake
mushrooms

3 Tbsp grass-fed unsalted
butter, such as Kerrygold,
or olive oil

2 Tbsp wakame seaweed

2 tsp chopped garlic

2 tsp fresh ginger, peeled and
grated

3 baby bok choy, thinly sliced
(or 1 bunch of chard, stems
removed)

3 green onions, finely chopped

4 cups (960 ml) vegetable broth
or chicken stock

¼ cup (70 g) miso paste,
preferably yellow

½ tsp sea salt

Pinch of cayenne pepper
(optional)

Juice of 1 lime

Mushrooms are celebrated in both traditional and modern healing traditions for their ability to support life. They are important every season, but there is a special resonance with winter. Mushrooms thrive in darkness. They consume dying plant matter in nature, which reflects their ability to eat death within, as we see with their antitumor and anticancer properties.

This recipe is courtesy of my friend, Carrie Kane, a nutritionist and mother of four, which means she knows how to cook for a crowd! When she made this soup for an autumn-winter seasonal wellness workshop, it was indeed a crowd-pleaser.

Prepare the mushrooms by removing any dirt with a dry paper towel and chopping into ½ in (12 mm) pieces.

In a heavy large pot, melt the butter over medium heat. Add the mushrooms and sauté for 10 minutes, or until they release and reabsorb their juices. Add the wakame, garlic, ginger, bok choy, and green onions and sauté for 3 to 5 minutes, or until everything has softened. Add the stock and bring to a simmer. Continue simmering over medium-low heat for 10 minutes then remove from heat.

Meanwhile, in a small bowl, dissolve the miso paste, salt, and cayenne pepper (if using) in 1 cup (240 ml) of the warm soup. Add this back to the soup and taste for seasoning. Finish with a squeeze of lime juice. Serve immediately.

MEDICINE MEAL—
EATING FOR WELLNESS AND VITALITY

An awareness of what we eat and how we eat it is an essential part of Asian American herbalism. Many of the herbs in this book are found in daily meals—green and black tea, rice, honey, barley, ginger, umeboshi, thyme, seaweeds, burdock root, and mushrooms. My perspective always goes back to the Japanese yakuzen culture of making food that is both delicious and medicinal. Yakuzen means "medicine meal" and I learned this concept from my friend and tea ceremony teacher, Sachiko Knappman. Growing up in Japan, Sachiko learned from her mother and grandmother how to prepare foods according to the seasons and to maintain wellness.

Modern food systems differ significantly from the ancient ways. Many foods we eat today are out of balance with nature due to being highly processed, grown with chemicals, harvested out of season, and imported from all over the globe. The long-term combination of all these factors is an insidious cause of illness, which makes an awareness of the quality of food in our diet more important than ever.

The simplest way to improve your diet is to incorporate seasonal foods that are available where you live. Farmers' markets, family-owned CSAs, and your garden are sure ways to know the bounty of summer strawberries and winter citrus, but it's not always easy to know what is in season because of our year-round access to foods such as bananas and cucumbers.

Illness can also result from eating in the wrong way. Conditions that interfere with good digestion are eating at irregular times, eating too quickly, overeating, skipping meals, eating while working, and eating while under stress and emotional strain. Even high-quality, seasonal foods can aggravate internal imbalances for some. For example, bananas and dairy can generate dampness for some folks. Melon, cucumbers, and tofu can be too cooling for others.

The way we eat also affects energetic imbalances:

- Qi deficiency leads to low appetite or a lack of desire to eat.
- Restricted and disordered eating leads to Qi deficiency with dampness.
- People who have a voracious appetite have a heat imbalance.
- People who are vegetarian or vegan tend to be Blood and Yin deficient.
- People who overindulge in meats, processed foods, or alcohol have damp and phlegm issues.

How to Eat for Wellness

Digestion is simply the process of transforming food and drink into Qi. In East Asian theory, this process is ruled by the Spleen and Stomach, which break down food so that the resulting Qi can be distributed to the rest of the body for energy and wellness. Poor digestion and irregular elimination are signs that the Spleen and Stomach need care through a healing diet. Rejuvenating the Spleen and Stomach is a slow and steady process, so start slow and be gentle with yourself. The traditional healing diet, known as Qing Dan, is made up of warm, clear, pure, light, and bland foods. Warm, cooked meals are easier to digest, so think of grains, leafy greens, whole fruits and vegetables, legumes, sprouts, herbs, tea, and water. Processed foods are avoided, as they are difficult to digest and significantly increase inflammation. Here are some basic guidelines:

- Eat regular, frequent, small meals.
- Eat earlier in the day (before 8 pm).
- Relax and focus on eating.
- Drink a small cup of room temperature water, stock, or herbal tea with each meal.
- Incorporate small portions of animal proteins (1 serving = 4 oz / 100 g).
- Avoid eating exclusively raw and chilled meals, including iced drinks.
- Avoid processed foods with white flour, sugar, hydrogenated oils, fillers, and preservatives.
- Avoid eating out frequently, especially fried, greasy, and oily foods.

Dampness, Water Retention, and Weight

When discussing herbs to address weight gain and water retention, I walk a fine line. We live in a society with a deeply ingrained cultural prejudice that assigns morality and strength of character to how skinny, firm, or taut we can make our bodies. There are toxic cultural standards around the ability to control and maintain external appearances. So, you will not find a diet or regimen to follow in this book. Instead, I wish to offer and share herbs that support becoming strong energetically in a way that allows the system to discern what to hold onto and release. And how to let go of the uncomfortable, heavy, tight, itchy, oppressive layers of holding that not only affect the physical body but can also reflect mental and spiritual stagnation.

SIGNS FOR DAMPNESS

MIND
—

unclear thinking
poor memory
fogginess
poor discernment
compulsiveness
circular thinking
dulled senses
confusion
depression
exhaustion

BODY
—

feeling heavy
water retention
edema of low body
swollen, heavy, or stiff joints
abdominal fullness
gas, nausea
urinary discomfort
loose stools
oozing rashes
mucus or discharge
swollen tongue body,
with a thick coat

Asian American Herbalism

Dampness

Dampness is one of the leading causes of disease in modern times. Dampness feels heavy like a fog that settles over and clouds the mind. It usually arises from a place of Qi deficiency, burnout, and low-grade stress that over time creates an environment where the body becomes stuck in unhealthy holding patterns. These holding patterns feel like carrying the weight of the world and reflect the weight of stagnant fluids that should be eliminated from the body. Dampness is also created by taking in an excess of damp-forming substances, food, and drink (i.e., antibiotics, alcohol, and processed foods).

Symptoms of dampness include digestive upsets, a general feeling of heaviness in the body and limbs, a dull ache of the muscles, joint pain, heaviness and swelling of the joints, arthritis, chronic urinary tract infections (UTIs), coughing up phlegm, acne, water retention, and weight gain. There can also be difficulty with discernment, dulled senses, poor memory, and in severe cases, mania. Discernment is the ability to know what is useful and what is not. Energetically, this applies to our thoughts and keeps unhealthy, circular, obsessive thought patterns at bay. Discernment also affects what we hold in the physical body—releasing wastes by elimination and sweat rather than holding on to it as water retention and uncomfortable excess weight. In all these cases, herbs that transform damp are key, such as pearl barley, cleavers, plantain, and bee balm. Example recipes are Calm and Clear Pee Tea (page 211), First Aid Oil (page 178), Barley Water (page 264), and Barley and Greens Congee (page 279).

HERBS FOR DAMPNESS

Cleavers
Plantain
Red Clover
Elecampane
Bee Balm
Nettle
Blessed Thistle

Pearl Barley
Tangerine Peel
Oolong Tea
Poria
Atracylodes
Astragalus

WAKAME MISO SOUP

Serves 4

INGREDIENTS

2 Tbsp dried wakame seaweed

4 cups (960 ml) Kombu Shiitake
   Dashi (page 273)

¼ cup (70 g) red or yellow miso
   paste

4 oz (115 g) tofu, cut into small
   cubes

Soy sauce, for seasoning

2 green onions, thinly sliced

Wakame miso soup combines ingredients from the land (i.e., mushrooms and soy) and sea (i.e., kombu and bonito). It is a simple, comforting, grounding meal for any time of day. The recipe is adapted from Sonoko Sakai's *Japanese Home Cooking: Simple Meals, Authentic Flavors.*

To prepare the wakame, rehydrate in 2 cups (480 ml) of water for 15 minutes. Drain and cut into ½ in (12 mm) pieces.

In a medium pot, bring the dashi to a boil over medium heat then reduce the heat to low and simmer while you prepare the miso.

In a small bowl, dissolve the miso in ½ cup (120 ml) of the warm dashi. Add this back to the soup with the tofu and prepared wakame. Turn off the heat once the tofu is heated through, about 1 minute. Taste for seasoning and add some soy sauce if needed. Divide the soup among 4 bowls, sprinkle with the green onions, and serve immediately.

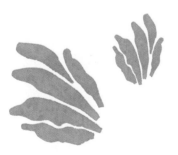

Asian American Herbalism

KOMBU SHIITAKE DASHI

Makes 4 cups (960 ml)

INGREDIENTS

1 piece kombu seaweed, about
    2 × 5 in (5 × 12 cm)
3 dried shiitake mushrooms
3 cups (20g) bonito flakes

Dashi is a Japanese stock base used for many recipes, including miso soup. It can be made with a variety of ingredients, and I grew up with homemade dashi made of kombu, shiitake mushrooms, and katsuobushi (bonito flakes from dried tuna). Grandma Masako would use it to make miso and noodle soups with shiitake and tofu. Kombu and mushrooms impart a Yin-nourishing medicine to this everyday staple. The recipe is adapted from Sonoko Sakai's *Japanese Home Cooking: Simple Meals, Authentic Flavors.*

In a medium pot, combine the kombu, shiitake mushrooms, and 5 cups (1.2 L) of filtered water. Warm over low heat until bubbles form around the kombu. Remove the kombu right before the water reaches a boil. Once the water comes to a boil, remove it from the heat. Add the bonito flakes and infuse for 2 minutes. Using a cheesecloth-lined colander or fine-mesh sieve, strain the dashi. Allow the mixture to filter slowly and do not press out the bonito flakes, or it will make the dashi cloudy. Use immediately or refrigerate for up to 4 days.

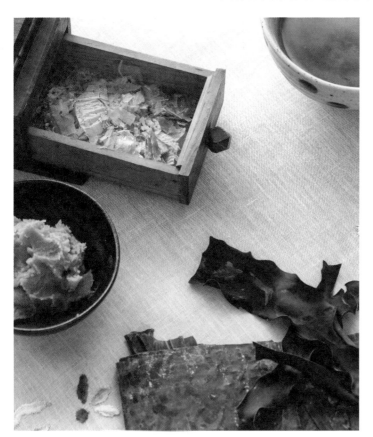

MEDICINAL HERB STOCK

Makes 4 quarts (3.8 L)

INGREDIENTS

4 quarts (3.8 L) chicken stock or
 vegetable broth
The Qi Herbs (page 88), Blood-
 Nourishing Herbs (page 100),
 or Yama Herbs for Yin and
 Yang (page 117).

Adding herbs to stocks is a cornerstone of home cooking. Asian American herbalism plays on this kitchen medicine by adding tonic herbs with specific benefits. Tonic herbs are safe to take regularly and in moderation when infused into daily food and drink.
There are three recipes in this book to choose from: The Qi Herbs (page 88), Blood-Nourishing Herbs (page 100), and Yama Herbs for Yin and Yang (page 117). Medicinal herb stocks can be a stand-alone meal or used in various everyday recipes, including soups and porridges. When making rice, legumes, or grains, use the stock to replace half of the cooking water. For a quick probiotic tonic drink, add a pinch of salt, a crushed garlic clove, and a splash of sauerkraut juice to a cup of warmed medicinal herb stock.

In a large stockpot, bring the stock and herb blend to a boil. Reduce the heat to low and simmer for 45 minutes. There is no need to reduce the liquid. Using a cheesecloth-lined colander or a fine-mesh sieve, strain the stock and use as you normally would. Store in the refrigerator for up to 5 days or in the freezer for up to 3 months.

MAMA FAYE'S TINOLANG MANOK

Serves 4

INGREDIENTS

2 Tbsp vegetable oil

1 medium onion, sliced

3 garlic cloves, chopped

1 knob of fresh ginger, peeled
and cut into thin strips

½ whole chicken, quartered

2 Tbsp fish sauce

1 chayote squash or unripe
papaya, peeled and cut into
wedges

2 cups (300 g) fresh moringa
leaves (malunggay)

Steamed white rice, for serving

Healing foods come directly from our people, cultures, and families. Sapho Flor helped research the cultural foodways of the Asian diaspora for this book and, in the process, shared this recipe from their mama, Faye Docuyanan Teologo. Tinolang Manok is a Filipino dish that elegantly incorporates the healing foods of its home country. Moringa (malunggay), ginger, and garlic infuse this meal with nutrient-dense herbs to invigorate Qi, support the immune system, and reduce inflammation. The chicken adds protein and depth of flavor to the dish and energetically nourishes Blood and Qi. Sapho wrote this recipe with specific measurements, but Mama Faye measures the ingredients from the heart.

In a large soup pot, warm the oil over medium heat. Add the onion, garlic, and ginger and sauté for a few minutes, or until soft. Add the chicken and cook, turning as needed, until browned. Add the fish sauce and 3 cups (720 ml) of water and bring to a boil. Turn the heat to low and simmer for 40 minutes, skimming any foam that rises to the top of the soup. Add the chayote or papaya and cook for 5 minutes more. In the last 2 minutes of cooking, add the moringa leaves. Season with salt and pepper and serve with steamed rice.

Porridge

Porridge is a healing meal that is easy to digest and is often taken when recovering from illness. Grains strengthen Qi, and rice is the most common grain used for Asian porridges. However, barley, millet, oats, and wheat are also used. Medical herbs, foods, and teas are infused into porridges for flavor and to increase the healing properties.

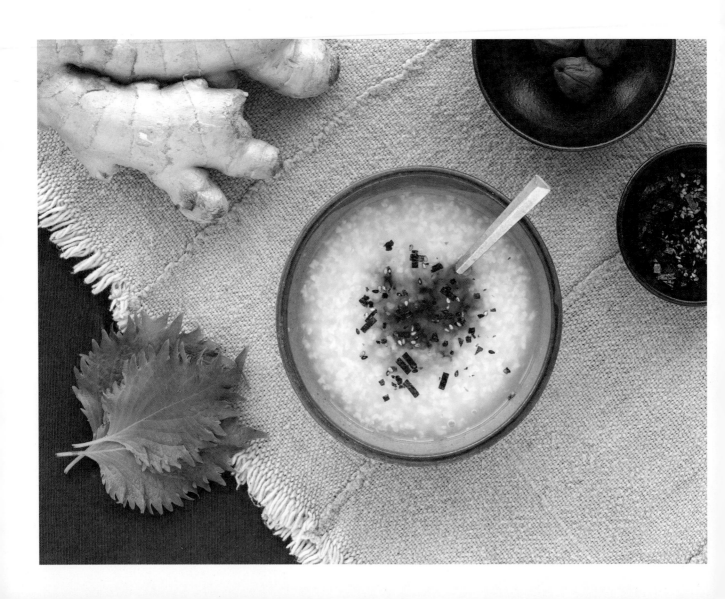

OKAYU - JAPANESE RICE PORRIDGE

Serves 4

INGREDIENTS

1 cup (200 g) uncooked
   medium-grain white rice

½ tsp salt

—

Toppings:

2 green onions, finely chopped

Soy sauce

Shiso Gomashio (page 280)

Egg, soft hard boiled and cut in
   half

Umeboshi plum

Sesame oil

Chile crunch or chile oil

In Japan, okayu is a healing food eaten when sick or recovering from illness. It is a light and restorative meal and my go-to dish when I feel overly full from eating too many rich, heavy foods. Like a thick congee, this recipe follows a five:one rice-to-water ratio. For more flavor, dashi or chicken stock can be used to cook the porridge.

Rinse the rice in water 3 to 5 times until the water runs clear. Transfer the rice to a large soup pot, add 5 cups (1.2 L) of water and bring to boil. Turn the heat to low and simmer, stirring occasionally to prevent scorching, for 30 minutes. Remove from the heat, cover, and let steam for 10 minutes. The rice should be soft and thick. Mix in the salt and serve in individual bowls garnished with the toppings of your choice.

The names of rice porridge:

Congee or Jook – **China**
Kola Kanda – **Sri Lanka**
Okayu – **Japan**
Babor – **Cambodia**
Juk – **Korea**
Khao Piak Sen – **Laos**
Bubur Ayum – **Indonesia**
Lugaw – **Philippines**
Chok – **Thailand**
Chao Ga – **Vietnam**
Akki Ganji, Khichdi – **Southern Asia**

MEDICINAL CONGEE RICE PORRIDGE

Serves 6 to 8

INGREDIENTS

The Qi Herbs (page 88), Blood-Nourishing Herbs (page 100), or Yama Herbs for Yin and Yang (page 117)

1 cup (200 g) uncooked medium white rice

Soy sauce, for serving (optional)

Green onions, thinly sliced for serving (optional)

Gomashio, for serving (optional)

Rice porridge is a dish of many names across the Asian diaspora. Congee is a simple rice porridge made by slowly cooking water and rice using an eight:one ratio. Medicinal congee takes just a few extra steps to be infused with traditional Asian roots and healing herbs. My preferred method for making a medicinal congee is to replace half of the cooking water with an herbal decoction made from tonic herbs. A shortcut is to add a muslin bag filled with a batch of tonic herbs to the pot while the congee cooks. For the tonic herb recipes, see The Qi Herbs (page 88), Blood-Nourishing Herbs (page 100), or Yama Herbs for Yin and Yang (page 117).

In a small pot, bring the herbs and 3 cups (720 ml) of water to a boil. Reduce heat and continue simmering for 45 minutes, or until reduced to 2 cups (480 ml) of tea. Use a cheesecloth-lined colander or fine-mesh sieve to strain the herbs and discard. Transfer the medicinal tea to a large pot, add the rice and 6 cups (1.4 L) of water and bring to a boil. Turn the heat down to low, cover, and gently simmer, stirring occasionally to prevent scorching, for 1 hour. Serve with soy sauce, green onions, gomashio, or toppings of choice. Store leftovers in an airtight container in the refrigerator for up to 3 days. Reheat congee over low heat on the stovetop, stirring in additional liquid as needed.

The medicinal dose is 1 cup (200 ml) of congee twice per day for 3 days.

Note: If using a slow cooker to make Medicinal Congee Rice Porridge, cook overnight or for at least 8 hours.

BARLEY AND GREENS CONGEE

Serves 6 to 8

INGREDIENTS

Blood-Nourishing Herbs
(page 100)

½ cup (90 g) pearl barley

½ cup (100 g) uncooked
medium grain white rice

1 cup (20 g) roughly chopped
fresh spinach

1 cup (15 g) roughly chopped
kale, chard, or other greens

6 cups (1.4 L) chicken stock
(optional)

1 Tbsp unsalted butter

1 tsp sea salt

1 tsp pine nuts

1 tsp black sesame seeds

Barley congee is about balancing healthy bodily fluids, including Blood. The barley and greens strengthen the body in a way that slows hair loss, resolves constipation, and reduces bloating. It is a wonderful healing meal to make when you need deep hydration and a reset for the digestive system. This recipe was adapted from *Book of Jook: Chinese Medicinal Porridges* by Bob Flaws.

In a large soup pot, bring the Blood-Nourishing Herbs, pearl barley, rice, spinach, greens, and 6 cups (1.4 L) of water or chicken stock to a boil. Turn the heat to low, cover, and simmer, stirring occasionally to prevent scorching, for 45 minutes to 1 hour. Stir in the butter and salt. Serve warm topped with pine nuts and black sesame seeds. Store leftovers in an airtight container in the refrigerator for up to 5 days. Reheat congee over low heat on the stovetop, stirring in additional liquid as needed.

The medicinal dose is one to two bowls per day for three days.

Note: If using a slow cooker to make Barley and Greens Congee, cook overnight or for at least eight hours.

SHISO GOMASHIO

Makes 1 ¼ cups (170 g)

INGREDIENTS

1 Tbsp dried shiso leaves

1 cup (140 g) white or black
    sesame seeds

2 Tbsp fine sea salt

1 Tbsp dulse seaweed powder

Gomashio is a Japanese condiment that is translated in English as "sesame salt." My great-grandma Hana simply called her blends "goma." This blend combines the classic sesame seed and salt mixture with herbs to benefit digestion and balance Yin and Yang energies. Dulse powder adds a nice umami flavor and increases the Yin-nourishing properties. Shiso leaves benefit the belly (Spleen and Stomach) to ease indigestion, gas, and nausea. Green or red shiso can be used in this recipe, although it is easier to find green shiso at your local Asian market.

In a dry cast-iron or heavy skillet, roast the dried shiso leaves over medium heat, stirring constantly with a wooden spoon, for less than 1 minute, or until the leaves just start to crisp. Remove from the pan and set aside to cool. Add the sesame seeds to the hot pan and toast, stirring constantly to prevent burning, for about one to three minutes, or until just starting to turn fragrant. Remove from the heat and set aside to cool.

Using a suribachi or mortar and pestle, grind the toasted shiso leaves to a coarse powder. Transfer the shiso to an airtight container then use the suribachi to grind the sesame seeds and salt into a uniform powder. Add the sesame seed-salt mixture and the dulse seaweed powder to the shiso. Store away from heat, light, and moisture. Sprinkle on rice, grains, salads, and other dishes as a condiment.

Note: If working with fresh shiso leaves, leave them on the stalk and tie them into small ½ in (12 mm) bundles. Hang to dry with the stems pointing up, out of direct sunlight, and with good air circulation for a few days and up to 1 week. The leaves are ready when they crumble when pinched. Remove leaves from the stems.

Contraindication: This recipe is not recommended in cases of diabetes due to shiso's effect on regulating blood sugar.

Asian American Herbalism

KKAENIP KIMCHI

Serves 6

INGREDIENTS

32 fresh green shiso leaves

¾ cup (180 ml) soy sauce

1 small white or yellow onion, sliced

1 green onion, thinly sliced

1 to 2 garlic cloves, grated

1 Tbsp gochugaru (Korean red chile flakes)

1 Tbsp brown sugar

1 Tbsp sesame oil

1 Tbsp sesame seeds

Kkaenip Kimchi is a quick spicy pickle made with shiso leaves (kkaennip) and gochugaru (Korean red chile flakes). This recipe is from Nina Jung, an acupuncturist and herbalist friend in the San Francisco Bay Area. It is traditionally made in Korea during the summer and autumn, when shiso grows in abundance. Quick pickles contain enzymes that benefit digestion. Shiso and chile flakes also increase appetite and digestive fire!

Prepare the shiso leaves by rinsing them in water. Gently shake the water from the leaves and dry in a colander while preparing the sauce.

In a small bowl, combine the soy sauce, onion, green onion, garlic, gochugaru, brown sugar, sesame oil, and sesame seeds and mix well to combine.

Put 3 shiso leaves in the bottom of a large, shallow airtight glass container and spread 1 spoonful of sauce on the leaves. Repeat this process of layering for the rest of the shiso leaves and sauce. Cover and refrigerate for 1 day to marinate the shiso leaves. Serve with steamed rice. Store in the refrigerator for up to 1 week.

Contraindication: This recipe is not recommended in cases of diabetes due to shiso's effect on regulating blood sugar.

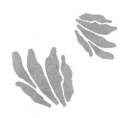

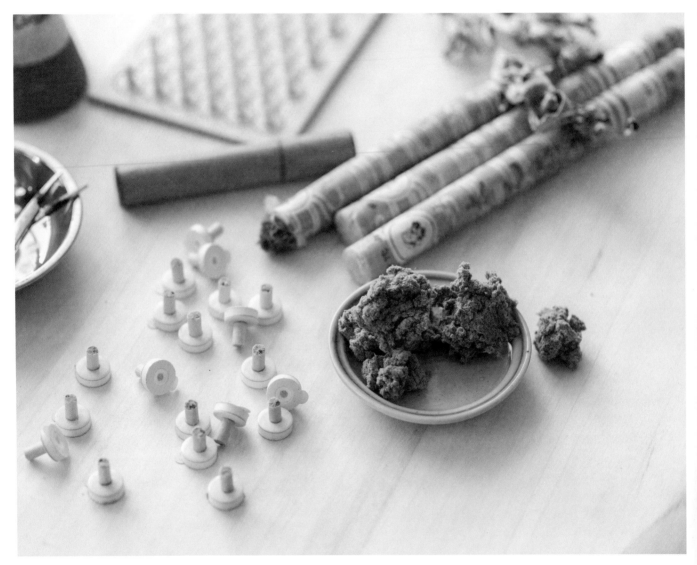

Moxibustion – Stick Moxa and Direct Moxa on the Skin

HEALING PRACTICES

Asian medicine in the United States is often reduced to the practice of acupuncture. However, folk traditions, including moxibustion, gua sha, massage, and acupressure, predate acupuncture by many generations. Home remedies tend to be the most accessible, common sense medicine, such as heat therapy and gentle massage. Moxibustion is a heat therapy that uses mugwort to warm areas of the body and various acupuncture points. Gua sha is a scraping massage that increases healthy circulation and removes stagnation, pathogens, and toxins from the body. Acupressure and acupuncture are the application of pressure (massage) and needles on specific points to heal a wide array of illnesses. The following is a guide to the most common things I teach patients in my clinic for home care. It is meant to empower you to take these practices into your own hands to heal at home and on your own terms.

Moxibustion

Moxibustion is the use of moxa herbs to warm acupuncture points for therapeutic benefit. It provides a deep penetrating heat that is healing and comforting. Its use predates written history and is thought to have paved the way for mapping out the acupuncture channels as we know and use them today. Moxa is made from mugwort leaves that are crushed and pounded into soft fiber, that looks and feels like herbal cotton. Modern moxa comes in many forms, from sticks to little stick-on patches. Moxa can be purchased from your local acupuncturist, Asian herb shops, and online (see Resources on page 312).

Benefits of Moxibustion

- Increases energy
- Increases circulation and the smooth flow of Qi and Blood
- Strengthens Qi and raises Yang
- Resolves dampness
- Benefits digestion
- Eases nerve and muscle pain
- Reduces back and abdominal pain
- Strengthens the immune system to prevent disease
- Calms the nervous system and reduces stress
- Enhances sexual function and fertility
- Balances hormones and promotes a healthy menstrual cycle

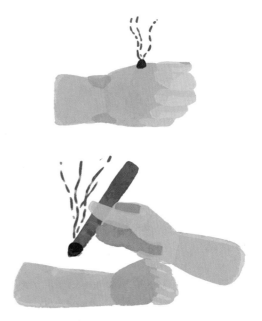

How To Give a Moxibustion Treatment

→ Rest in an area with ventilation that is free from drafts. Peel the outer paper wrapper off the moxa stick. Do not remove the thin, inner tissue paper. Always use fire safety precautions when working with moxa.

→ Light the moxa stick with a lighter and blow on the end until there is an orange ember covering the end of the stick. As ash forms on the stick, roll off excess ash into an ashtray until the lit end of the stick has a slight cone shape. It will radiate a pleasant warmth.

→ Hold the lit end of the stick over the area to be treated, just 1 in (2.5 cm) away from the skin. The moxa stick is moved slowly over the area being treated in a circular or pecking motion without ever coming into direct contact with the skin. Move the stick in small clockwise circles (about 1 in [2.5 cm] in diameter) until the area becomes warm and slightly pink. Continue by doing moxa on the other areas until treatment is complete.

→ Ash that forms on the end of the stick is brushed or tapped off in an ashtray or jar so that the ash does not fall off and burn the skin. Never touch the lighted end of a moxa stick even if it no longer appears to be glowing. Relight if there is no longer any heat coming from the stick. When finished, snuff out the stick, with the lit end pointing down, in an ashtray or jar with sand. The stick can be relit and used for repeated treatments.

Caution and Contraindications:

- Do not moxa skin that is red or inflamed.
- Do not moxa the face, head, neck, or groin.
- Do not moxa the abdomen and low back during pregnancy.
- Do not moxa on skin that is numb or has nerve damage.

Common Points for Wellness and Longevity:

- Spleen 6 for stress and hormone balance
- Stomach 36 for energy, circulation, and digestion
- Kidney 3 to increase vitality, energy, and sexual function
- Ren 4 – Ren 6 for abdominal discomfort, digestion, and fertility
- Du 4 for back pain, vitality, and energy
- See the following section on acupressure and acupuncture (page 287) for detailed locations.

Gua Sha

Gua Sha is a scraping massage used in homes in China and across the Asian diaspora since before written history. It is traditionally done along the back of the neck to prevent head colds, but it is also a folk remedy to address various aches and pains. Popularized through traditional Chinese medicine, this type of folk medicine has been practiced by families and healers in every culture. It is also known as cao gio in Vietnam, kerokan in Indonesia, and coining and scraping in the U.S. What I'm sharing is in the vein of home care—it is what has been passed down by the aunties. For specific treatments, see Gua Sha to Ward Off a Early-Stage Head Colds (page 162), How to Gua Sha a Painful Joint (page 197), and Facial Massage:

Jade Rolling and Gua Sha (page 252). Working with a skilled practitioner may look different than the advice I outline here for the home herbalist.

Gua means "to scrape" in Mandarin Chinese, and sha is the word that describes the marks that come to the skin's surface. Sha is a pathogen—the same as wind, heat, or damp—that becomes stuck in the body and is expressed on the skin through gua sha. Sha indicates stagnation and represents a blockage in the flow of Qi and Blood.

Gua Sha is done with a smooth, solid tool, such as a porcelain soup spoon, a jade or stone tool, a thin river rock, or a large smooth coin. Oil is first applied to the skin to help the tool glide smoothly. The tool is then drawn down the skin in a single direction for thirty to sixty seconds. The scraping pressure is the same as you would desire in a strong massage. A red or brown flush (sha) usually comes up to the surface of the skin if there is a stagnation present. The sha is not a bruise and should not cause intense pain or burning. The colors that come up with treatment depend on what is being held just below the surface of the skin in the connective tissue, fascia, and muscles. Rosy, unmarked skin generally indicates good health. Light pink and pale colors are a sign of depletion or weakness. Red color with heat is a sign of inflammation and stagnation. If the area becomes dark red or purple, there is deep stagnation, toxins, or a deep injury. Gua sha increases circulation and brings immune cells to the area for healing.

When color (sha) develops on the surface of the skin during a treatment, you can stop scraping the area once the color has fully expressed (stops becoming darker). Gua sha should be repeated on affected areas three to four times or until the issue being treated has resolved. Wait three to five days between treatments for the skin to heal and the sha to dissipate. With continued use, the presence of sha will disappear and healthy color and sensation will return to the area.

Gua Sha Cautions and Contraindications:

- Sha and markings on the skin only occurs with body gua sha. Facial gua sha should never mark the skin.
- Do not gua sha over an acute injury (less than two days from the source of the injury), new bruising, abrasions, or open wounds.
- Do not gua sha pimples or moles because it can stimulate growth.
- Avoid sunburns, rashes, irritated or inflamed skin.
- Avoid very soft skin and areas with many glands, including the neck, groin, armpits, and breasts.
- Do not gua sha on people with blood conditions, migraines, high blood pressure, or during pregnancy.

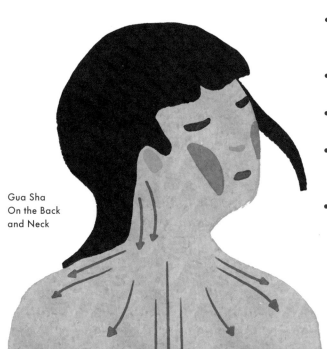

Gua Sha
On the Back
and Neck

ACUPRESSURE AND ACUPUNCTURE

Acupressure and acupuncture are healing techniques that balance Qi's flow in the energy meridians. There are more than three hundred points along the fourteen main energy meridians, also known as acupuncture channels, and they all have specific healing properties. These practices were developed over thousands of years and are still effective for relieving symptoms of illness (i.e., pain) and addressing the root causes of disease (i.e., stagnation and inflammation). Acupressure is a massage technique that applies finger pressure to points along the energy meridians. Acupuncture is the practice of inserting sterile, hair-fine needles at these points. Moxibustion is also done on these points for therapeutic benefit. Modern studies have given us some scientific insight into how this all works. Some studies measured the electrical currents in the fascia to illustrate how Qi flows just below the skin's surface. Other studies observed the presence of specialized neurons in the body that correspond to specific acupuncture points' location and function. However, we do not need studies to prove or verify how the medicine works. They simply add to our sophisticated, complex understating of this body of work.

Acupressure Basics

Start simple. Select the points you wish to work with and note your reasons and desired effect. I find that once annoying issues and ailments are resolved with acupressure, it is easy to forget how bothersome they once were or if they even existed at all!

Press and massage the acupressure point on both sides of the body using your thumb. Hold the pressure or make a slow clockwise movement on the point while taking six long inhalations and exhalations.

There is a cumulative effect. Repeat acupressure on your selected points every 20 minutes for acute issues, such as headaches or nausea, until symptoms resolve. For chronic issues, including insomnia and stress, incorporate acupressure massage into your wellness routines or practices as needed. Home care is important, and I also recommend trying out acupressure and acupuncture treatments from skilled practitioners to feel the flow of energy that occurs when receiving a healing session.

A wide variety of everyday ailments can be addressed with basic knowledge of the healing properties of commonly used points. The following are the greatest hits of acupressure points that I recommend in my clinical practice for home care.

Acupressure Points to Know

Liver 3 (LV 3)

LOCATION: On top of the foot, where the bone of the big toe meets the second toe, about 1 inch (2.5 cm) back from the web between these two toes. Often tender or sore with strong pressure, but this means you're hitting the right spot!

- Apply acupressure or moxibustion.
- Increases circulation and moves holding patterns.
- Reduces pain in the body.
- A key point on the Liver channel to move Liver Qi stagnation.

Pericardium (PC 6)

LOCATION: On the inside of the wrist, between the two tendons running down the midline of the forearm. Three fingers' widths from the wrist.

- Apply acupressure.
- Moves Qi in the chest and upper torso to ease nausea, motion sickness, and pain in the chest.
- A strong influence on the Heart, mind, and spirit.
- Calming for anxiety, restorative sleep, and general stress.

Kidney 3 (KD 3)

LOCATION: On the inner ankle, between the inner ankle bone and Achilles tendon.

- Apply acupressure or moxibustion.
- Commonly used for low back pain, hip instability, and weak knees.
- Restores deep energy and vitality.
- Graceful aging point.
- A notable influence on the Kidney, Yin, and Yang.

Large Intestine (LI 4)

LOCATION: On the hand, between the web of the thumb and first finger. Often tender or sore with strong pressure.

- Apply acupressure.
- Decreases pain and tenderness in the body.
- Particularly good for treating the head and face, such as with headache, head cold, flu, and congestion.
- Influences the flow of Qi in the entire body, particularly in the torso (San Jiao).

Spleen 6 (SP 6)

LOCATION: On the inner calf above the ankle, four finger widths above the inner ankle bone (medial malleolus). Often tender or sore with strong pressure.

- Apply acupressure or moxibustion.
- A common use for hormonal imbalance with PMS, irregular and painful periods.
- Influences the flow of Qi and Blood.
- Moves stagnation for stress and pain.
- A nourishing, Yin quality to this point.
- A crossing point with the Kidney and Liver meridians.

Stomach 36 (ST 36)

LOCATION: On the lateral (outer) side of the shin bone, four finger widths below the bottom of the knee cap.

- Apply acupressure or moxibustion.
- Improves energy and circulation.
- Strong impact on Qi and Blood.
- A grounding point that draws Qi down from the head and to the gut.
- Eases pain and muscle cramps.
- Regulates digestion, metabolism, and appetite.

Conception Vessel 4–6 (Ren 4–6)
LOCATION: On the lower abdomen, the line connecting the belly button to the top of the pubic bone. These three points are 3 to 5 finger widths below the belly button.

- Apply moxibustion.
- Influences the back and organs of the lower abdomen.
- For issues with digestion, urination, the menstrual cycle, hormone balance, and fertility.
- Restores Kidney Yin and Yang.
- Enhances vitality.
- Eases pain due to stagnation and deficiency.
- Increases circulation.

Governing Vessel 4 (Du 4)
LOCATION: On the low back, along the spine, and three finger widths above the top of the hips.

- Apply moxibustion.
- For infertility, impotence, incontinence, or any bladder or reproductive organs issues.
- Has the same indications as the Conception Vessel points, but with more influence on the back body, hips, and spine.

HERBAL PREPARATIONS

Herbal preparations are all about finding the most effective and tasty ways to take your herbs. In this way, there is always a balance between convenience, preservation or shelf life, and the final experience. Water-based medicine is the dearest to my heart because it is the way I learned from my teachers and family. These are humble and universal preparations, including teas, infusions, stocks, soups, and decoctions. Elixirs, syrups, and honey are medicines that are sweet to the taste and have a relatively stable shelf life ranging from one month to many years. Tinctures and powder extracts have even greater long-term preservation and have many uses in the clinic and the kitchen. And then there are external preparations for use on the skin, such as infused oils, salves, liniments, compresses, baths, steams, and compresses. Herbal preparations are an important and foundational skill set for the home herbalist.

Internal Preparations

Herbal Tea Infusions
Infusions are simply herbs that have been infused or steeped in water. There are many spins on this technique, including using hot water, cool water, or the energy of the moon and sun.

Warm Infusion
The method for making a classic cup of herbal tea is an ideal preparation to extract medicine from leafy herbs, flowers, and delicate plant material. To make a cup of tea, pour 1 cup (240 ml) of boiling water (200° F [95° C]) over over 1 heaping

teaspoon of herbs, cover, and steep for five to ten minutes. Strain and drink immediately. Tea may be stored in the refrigerator for up to three days. There are many examples of warm infusions in this text, such as Bonsai (page 150), which is one of my all-time favorites and one I made with my Grandpa Hiroshi in mind.

Cold Infusion

The method for making tea with cool water is the most effective way to extract medicine from hydrating, mucilaginous (slippery) herbs, such as marshmallow root, chamomile, rose, and slippery elm bark. I also prefer this method for fresh aromatic herbs, including mint and lemon balm. To make a batch of tea, fill a pitcher or large glass jar with 4 cups (960 ml) of cool water. Stir in ¼ cup of dried herbs or 1 cup of fresh herbs. Cover and steep at room temperature (less than 70° F [21º C]) for at least four hours and up to overnight. In temperatures greater than 70° F [21º C], steep in the refrigerator so the cold infusion doesn't ferment. Strain and drink slowly over the course of a day or two. Store in the refrigerator for up to three days. Examples are the Marshmallow and Rose Cold Infusion (page 110) and the Fresh Lemon Balm Water (page 136).

Tea (Ocha)

All non-herbal tea leaves come from the same plant, *Camellia sinensis*, and are processed in different ways to create various aromas, tastes, and appearances. The right flavors are bright, fresh, and soft. Tea leaves must be steeped for a short time, and with water that is just the right temperature. Tea develops a bitter or unpleasant flavor when steeped for too long or in water that is too hot. Good quality tea can be steeped up to five times as the flavor evolves and becomes more subtle with each steep. In this way, we honor the tea plant and the labor of the many hands that create a single cup of ocha.

Black Tea

Black tea undergoes an oxidation-fermentation process that changes the tea leaves to shades of brown and black. This creates a tea that is slightly easier to digest than green tea. Good quality black tea smells sweet without any artificial or perfumed scent. To make a cup of tea, pour 1 cup (240 ml) of simmering to boiling water (180 to 200° F [80 to 95º C]) over 1 tsp of tea. Cover and steep for three to five minutes before straining. Drink immediately. Re-steep as you please. For an example of an herbal black tea recipe, see Floral Black Tea Latte (page 101).

Green Tea

Green tea is a less oxidized tea because it is quickly removed from heat exposure upon harvest. This preserves the vibrant green color and flavor of the tea leaves. Good quality green tea is green, whole, and has a bright scent. To make a cup of tea, pour 1 cup (240 ml) of barley simmering water (170 to 180° F [75 to 80° C]) over 1 tsp of tea. Cover and steep for one to two minutes before straining. Drink immediately. Re-steep as you please. For an example of an herbal green tea recipe, see Hana Bancha Green Tea (page 127) or Midori Pearl Jasmine Green Tea (page 242).

Decoctions

Decoctions are the best preparation for making teas from roots, bark, seeds, and hard materials. The double-boil method is how I was taught to make traditional Chinese medicine formulas. However, I often simplify things with a single-boil method in my clinical practice. This is also the method to make the base for syrups.

Single-Boil Method

This method is suitable for everyday medicine and common ailments, including cold and flu, digestion, and stress reduction. To make a batch of tea, add herbs and 12 cups (2.8 L) of water to a large pot and bring to a boil. Turn the heat to medium and simmer with the lid cracked until the liquid has reduced by half (about 30 minutes). Strain the herbs with a slotted spoon and reserve the tea. Add fresh water if there are less than 6 cups (1.4 L) of tea remaining. Store in glass jars in the refrigerator for up to 4 days. Warm each serving of tea before drinking. This is also

the method for adding herbs to soups, such as The Qi Herbs (page 88).

Notes: After straining the herbs from the decoction, they may be used again to make one more batch of tea. Store the herbs in the freezer for future use.

Double-Boil Method

This method is key for extracting the most medicine from tonic herbs, like ginseng and pearl. It is the preferred method for making deeply restorative tonic teas like Jujube Date Seed Tea for Insomnia (page 231). To make a batch of tea, add herbs and 8 cups (2 L) of water to a large pot and bring to a boil. Turn the heat to medium and simmer with the lid cracked until the liquid has reduced by half (about 30 minutes). Strain the herbs with a slotted spoon and reserve them for a second pot of tea. Reserve the tea by pouring it into a large pitcher or glass jar. Repeat this process with the same herbs by putting them back in the pot with a fresh 8 cups (2 L) of water. Bring to a boil and simmer to reduce by half again. Strain out the herbs and discard them. Mix the second batch of tea into the first batch of tea. You may add fresh water if there are less than 8 cups (2 L) of tea remaining. Store in the refrigerator for up to 4 days. Take 1 cup (240 ml) twice per day. Warm each serving of tea before drinking.

Syrups and Elixirs

These are medicines that go down nice and easy. Syrups are made from herbal decoctions that are sweetened and thickened with honey. Like cordials and herbal liqueurs, elixirs are steeped over time in a blend of alcohol and honey. The sweetness helps mask the medicine's intense, sometimes bitter herbal flavors. Moreover, the sweet taste of honey is a Qi tonic that has a nourishing and hydrating effect. It's the reason that a spoonful of honey is given to ease a sore throat. For folks who do not use honey, maple syrup, agave, and glycerin are common substitutes.

To make a syrup, add 2 oz (55 g) of dried herbs and 4 cups (960 ml) of water to a pot and bring to a simmer. Stir and simmer, uncovered, until the liquid has reduced by half (about 30 minutes). Once the liquid is reduced to about 2 cups (480 ml), remove from the heat and add any aromatic herbs, such as vanilla or fresh tangerine peel. Cover and steep for 5 to 10 minutes before straining through a cheesecloth-lined colander or fine-mesh sieve. Discard the spent herbs. Once the liquid cools to lukewarm, stir in 1 cup (240 ml) of honey. Do not cook the honey, as high temperatures will damage its beneficial enzymes. Store in the refrigerator for several months. Syrups may be canned in glass jars for long-term storage. Herbal syrups for reference are Elderberry Syrup (page 163) and Loquat Cough Syrup (page 172).

I find that proper syrups are too sweet, but to make a thick syrup, increase the honey so that it is equal to the liquid (i.e., 2 cups [480 ml] liquid to 2 cups [480 ml] honey). Adding 2 Tbsp of brandy or vodka to the final product will extend the life of the syrup and add an invigorating quality to the medicine. The more honey and liquor added, the longer it will keep.

Tinctures

A tincture is an herbal medicine that steeps over time in a solvent, such as alcohol, vinegar, or vegetable glycerin. Tinctures are strong, concentrated medicine, as well as very shelf-stable and long-lasting. They can keep for nearly a decade when stored away from heat, light, or moisture.

To make a tincture, place dried herbs in a 4 cup (960 ml) glass jar and pour a solvent over the herbs until the jar is three-quarters of the way full (leaving 2 inches [5 cm] between the mixture and the top of the jar). Reserve any leftover liquid to top off the mixture during the first week of tincturing when the herbs absorb the liquids that they are steeping in. Tightly cover the jar with a plastic or non-reactive lid (or line metal lids with parchment or plastic wrap). Label the jar with the date and ingredients. Store away from heat, light, and moisture and gently shake the mixture every one to three days.

After four to six weeks, strain the herbs out with cheesecloth or a fine-mesh sieve and discard. Store in a clean glass jar away from heat, light, and moisture. Tinctures will easily keep for five years if stored properly. You can tell if your preparation has spoiled by changes in smell or taste, or signs of visible mold or fermentation. Mix with warm water, sparkling water, or juice to dilute. Tinctures for reference are Burdock Root Bitters (page 202) and Mushroom-Rice Wine Vinegar (page 266).

Powders and Powder Extracts

Herbal powders and powder extracts are two very different things—powders are raw, and powder extracts have been cooked. Herbal powders are herbs that have simply been ground into a uniform powder. These were used in ancient and traditional herbal recipes to make it easy to use preparations. They are also used in topical preparations such as Tea Leaves Cleansing Grains and Mask (page 245). I don't often recommend raw herbal powders be taken internally, because many herbs are not easy to digest and benefit from being extracted in water or other solvents.

Powder extracts are modern-day herbal medicines that are super convenient and famously used in Kampo Japanese herbalism. They are liquid herbal decoctions that have been dehydrated to a solid form and powdered with binders such as potato starch. To make tea, they are rehydrated with hot water, and I often compare them to the herbal equivalent of dehydrated coffee. Powder extracts are easy to use and my go-to for coffee drinkers because they blend well into lattes.

Topical Preparations

Infused Oils

Infused oils are carrier oils infused with fresh or dried herbs. They are rubbed into the skin to benefit the skin, but they also go deeper as the healing properties are absorbed into the body.

For beginners, using dried herbs to make infused oils is easier, because the water content of fresh herbs can lead to mold and spoilage. To prepare fresh herbs, let them wilt in the sun for a day then use scissors to cut them into small pieces. For dried herbs, pulse them in a blender ten to twenty times until broken into smaller pieces.

Solar-Infused Oil

The sun is a time tested and a well-loved way to infuse healing oils. It takes much longer than heating the oils on a stove, but there is something undeniable gained by the warm glow of the summer sun. An example is Calendula Sun Oil (page 178).

Carrier Oils

While you can use various carrier oils, my favorite oil for infusing herbs is safflower. Safflower oil is light, inexpensive, similar to the skin's natural oils, and works for all skin types. Plus, safflowers are used in Asian herbal traditions to invigorate Blood and move stagnation.

Best carrier oils:
safflower oil, olive oil, fractionated coconut oil, and sunflower oil

Oils to blend with infused oils:
tamanu nut oil, tsubaki camellia seed oil, jojoba oil, rose hip seed oil, avocado oil, and vitamin E oil

Essential oils to prevent spoilage:
tea tree essential oil, rosemary essential oil, lavender essential oil, and lemon essential oil

---

To make a sun oil, pour the herbs into a 2 cup (480 ml) glass jar and cover the flowers with oil (about 1¼ cups [300 ml]). There should be 1 to 2 in (2.5 to 5 cm) of oil covering the top of the herbs, so they do not spoil. Save the remaining oil to top off the herbal mixture when the herbs absorb the oil. Cover tightly and place the jar in a sunny window or a warm spot to infuse for two to four weeks. Gently shake the mixture every few days to mix and prevent mold from growing on top of the oil mixture. Strain the oil with a cheesecloth or fine-mesh sieve and squeeze all

Solar infused oils rarely go rancid during the sunny infusion time; however, once strained, they will go rancid if near heat or sunlight.

Common Herbs for Infused Oils

Calendula: Antiseptic and renowned healing properties; beneficial for cuts, scrapes, dry skin, rashes, skin irritations, and generally healthy skin

Comfrey: For deep and superficial injuries, including cuts, burns, bruises, sprains, strains, and broken bones (for external use only)

Arnica: Anti-inflammatory for acute trauma—bruises, sprains, strains, swelling, and pain (for external use only, not for open skin)

Plantain: A fresh poultice is the best cure for a bee sting, bug bites, cuts, scrapes, and minor infections

the oil out of the flowers with your hands or the back of a wooden spoon. Allow the water in the mixture to settle to the bottom of the jar. Take care not to pour off any water that settles at the bottom of the jar, as it will spoil the finished oil. Pour the finished oil into clean, dry glass jars and label with the date, ingredients, and "for external use only." Store away from heat, light, and moisture for up to one year.

Stove Top Infused Oil

This method can quickly make an infused oil within hours by heating it on a stove or in a crockpot. An example is Mugwort Warming Massage Oil (page 192). To make an infused oil, place the herbs in a double boiler and cover with the safflower oil (or carrier oil of choice). Slowly heat the oil for 30 to 60 minutes over very low heat. Do not simmer or overheat the oil—it will turn the oil rancid and fry the herbs. If tiny bubbles begin to appear, remove the oil from the heat. You'll know when it's done because it will take on the scent or the color of the herbs. Once it's cool enough to strain, press the oil out of the herbs through a cheesecloth-lined colander or fine-mesh sieve. Allow the oil to cool to room temperature then pour the oil into clean, dry glass jars or metal tins and label with the date, ingredients, and "for external use only." Take care not to pour in any water or plant materials

that may have settled to the bottom of the oil. Store away from heat, light, and moisture for up to one year.

Salves

A salve is a topical preparation of oil and beeswax applied to the skin for hydration and healing. Adding a hardening agent like beeswax to an infused oil helps hold it on the skin so that the medicinal properties can fully absorb. While I use beeswax in my salves, there are other hardening agent options, including shea butter, cocoa butter, various waxes, and animal fats. A salve is usually made with a one to eight ratio of wax to oil. This looks like 1 oz (30 g) wax to 8 oz (240 ml) oil.

Examples of salves are First Aid Salve (page 179) and Wow Gao (page 194).

To make a salve, place 8 oz (240 ml) of oil and 1 ounce (30 g) of beeswax in a pot and carefully warm over low heat. Stir often until the beeswax has fully melted into the oil. Check the consistency by using the spoon test (see sidebar below). Remove from the heat and add 10 drops of essential oil as a natural antiseptic and preservative. Immediately pour the mixture into clean, dry glass or metal containers. Once cool and hardened, secure with a lid, label with the date, ingredients, and "for external use only." Store away from heat, light, and moisture for up to one year.

The Spoon Test

To test the consistency of a salve before it hardens, dip a metal spoon into the mixture while it's still warm then cool in the refrigerator or freezer for a few minutes to solidify. The consistency is right when the mixture is solid yet easy to scoop and rub into to the skin with a fingertip. At this point, you can make the final product firmer by adding more hardening agents such as beeswax or softer by adding more oil. Reheat the oil mixture gently to incorporate it fully.

Liniments

Liniments are alcohol-based topical preparations made the same way as a tincture. They heal deep injury by absorbing through the skin and drawing the herbal medicine down to the connective tissue and muscle. In martial arts traditions, liniments support healing after training for bruises, strains, and injuries to joints and muscles. Unlike salves and oils, liniments dry quickly and should be lightly massaged into the injured area for fifteen minutes multiple times daily. An example is Kick-Ass Liniment (page 195).

To make a liniment, place dried herbs in a 4 cup (960 ml) glass jar and pour rubbing alcohol over the herbs until the jar is three-quarters of the way full (leaving 2 in [5 cm] between the mixture and the top of the jar). Add additional alcohol to top off the mixture during the first week of tincturing when the herbs absorb the liquids. Tightly cover the jar with a plastic or non-reactive lid (or line metal lids with plastic wrap). Label the jar with the date, ingredients, and "for external use only." Store away from heat, light, and moisture and gently shake the mixture every one to three days.

After four weeks, strain the herbs out with cheesecloth or a fine-mesh sieve and discard. Store in a clean glass jar away from heat, light, and moisture for up to six years. You can tell if an alcohol-based preparation has spoiled by changes in smell or taste, or signs of visible mold or fermentation.

Baths and Soaks

Baths are a time-honored ritual across many cultures. They are also an excellent way to take in herbal medicine. Energetically, baths and soaks reconnect us to the natural world of water that is in us and all around us. There are many lessons to learn from a bath. It is a dedicated time to be held, supported, and lifted up in our busy lives. It is the grace to allow things to wash over us. It is the embodiment of going with the flow.

Herbal Baths

When I was growing up, baths were an everyday event. As a child, I often woke up to the sound of my Grandpa Hiroshi filling the tub. This practice is still strong in my home with the addition of various herbs and healing elements. Asian bathing culture isn't just about getting clean; it's for healing. When drawing an herbal bath, it is best to make a strong herbal bath "tea" rather than putting the herbs directly in the bath water, which is a messy and unpleasant experience. However, other healing add-ins, such as salt and coconut milk powder, can and should be dissolved directly into the bath water. Examples of herbal baths are Milky Oat Bath (page 154), Mugwort and Nuka Bath for Smooth Skin (page 175), Lucid Dreams Mugwort Bath (page 236), and Daikon and Chrysanthemum Bath (page 226).

To make a bath tea, place 3 cups (150 g) of fresh herbs into a large pot with 6 cups (1.4 L) water. Simmer gently for fifteen minutes and remove from the heat. Steep for 15 minutes more while running a very warm bath. When the bath is ready, strain the herbs, and add the bath tea and any other additions to the bath water. Soak for twenty minutes for a full therapeutic effect. To use dried herbs instead of fresh, substitute 1 cup (20 g) of dried herbs for the 3 cups (150 g) of fresh.

To make herbal bath salts, in a blender, pulse 1 cup (20 g) of dried herbs and 1 cup (260 g) of sea salt into a coarse powder. Gently mix in another 3 cups (900 g) of salt. Add a cup of any other additional dry ingredients at this time (see Bath Add-Ins for ideas). Store away from heat, light, and moisture for up to one year. To use, add a handful of herbal bath salts to a warm bath.

Epsom Salt Baths

These baths are quite popular for easing body aches and pains. Epsom salt is not a salt at all; it is a magnesium crystal. Magnesium is a mineral necessary for proper nervous system function. It plays a part in nerve impulse and muscle contraction, including for the heartbeat, brain function, bodily sensations, physical recovery, and the ability to relax. There are many magnesium supplements out there. However, magnesium is easily absorbed through the skin (transdermal absorption). Epsom salt baths and soaks are my preferred method of magnesium supplementation, because it feels good and doesn't have the laxative side effect of some supplements.

Foot Bath

Foot baths are a grounding, peaceful therapy that brings folks out of their heads by drawing stagnant energy from the mind, face, and neck back down to the gut. The energetic healing here involves getting more in touch with instincts and a sense of "trusting the gut." Examples of foot baths are the Heart-Centered Shio Foot Soak (page 140) and Wild Sage Foot Bath (page 233).

To prepare a foot bath, place herbs and 4 cups (960 ml) of water in a large pot. Bring to a simmer, remove from the heat, cover, and steep for thirty minutes while preparing a very warm foot bath in a soaking basin. When the bath is ready, strain the herbs, saving the tea. Add the tea to the soaking basin with Epsom salts and essential oils (if using). Sit in a comfortable chair and soak your feet for twenty minutes for a full therapeutic effect. Keep a hot water kettle on the stove to reheat the foot bath as needed.

Steams

Just like heat, steam rises. Thus, herbal steams are ideal for ailments affecting the head, sinuses, and eyes. The moisture in steams is also great for hydrating delicate lung tissue to help the body cough up stubborn phlegm from the airways. Two options for steams are a hot pot or a cool-mist humidifier. An example is Thyme Steam for Cough and Congestion (page 170).

Cool-Mist Humidifier

It can be hard to handle the intensity of a hot steam pot when you're ill. I started using a cool-mist humidifier at the recommendation of my kids' pediatrician for nighttime croup and coughing. Adding essential oils to the humidifier gives off a healing mist throughout the night that is effective for coughs that are worse at bedtime or when lying down.

Prepare by filling a cool-mist humidifier with cold water and adding 1 to 5 drops of essential oil (i.e., thyme, oregano, eucalyptus, lavender). Adjust the amount of essential oil so that the scent is strong but not bothersome. Diffuse near the bedside while napping or overnight. Repeat one to two times per day for up to five days or until symptoms are relieved.

Hot Pot Steam

A hot pot is the traditional way to steam. It is used for healing everyday ailments or as a hydrating beauty treatment. You will need one large bath towel for this method. Fill a large pot with 8 cups (2 L) of water and herbs of choice. Bring to a boil, remove from the heat, and steep for fifteen minutes. Place a large basin on the floor in front of a comfortable chair. Carefully pour the hot liquid into a soaking basin; do not scald or burn the skin. Wrap a bath towel over your head and shoulders and hold tight under the chin. Sit on the chair and drape the towel from over your head around the steaming basin to create a tent to trap the steam. The steam and heat should feel comfortably warm so that you can breathe freely. Steam for five to fifteen minutes. If the steam is too hot or overwhelming, open up the towel and allow the steam to vent until it feels comfortable. You may wish to close your eyes when using strong aromatic herbs or essential oils.

Compress

A compress is a moist, heat therapy used externally on the skin. It promotes circulation to heal aches, injuries, skin irritations, congestion, and inflammation. The simplest compress is a hot wet towel—the image that comes to mind is a damp rag on the forehead of a feverish child. A poultice is an herbal compress made from gently cooked or macerated herbs and water. And a plaster compress is made in the same way as a poultice but mixed with a binding agent and held in place by a fabric bandage.

Compresses are slow, old-school medicine. To be effective, they need to be applied with care and consistency. For acute ailments, they should be applied for fifteen to thirty minutes at a time and repeated every few hours until symptoms resolve. Discontinue use if any skin irritation or adverse reaction occurs.

Hot Towel Compress

A hot towel compress is a humble, comforting treatment. It can be made by simply soaking a cloth with hot tap water or dipping it in a pot of hot water. To make a compress, you will need two washcloths and hot water. For the tap water method, run tap water until hot. Hold a small cotton towel by the ends and soak in the hot water. For the hot pot method, heat 4 cups (960 ml) water until very hot to the touch but not boiling. If using herbs to increase healing properties, steep them in the very hot water for fifteen minutes at this time. Remove from the heat. Hold the towel by a corner and dip it into a hot pot of water.

When the towel is cool enough to handle, fold it into thirds and wring out excess water. Place on the body area you wish to treat and cover with a dry towel to retain heat. Gently hold it in place until it cools (a few minutes) and then rewarm

---

Herbs for Compresses:

Cure-alls: chamomile,
red clover, burdock root

Skin: plantain, gotu kola, lavender,
mulberry,
green tea, violet

Pain: comfrey, fresh ginger,
red clover, hyssop, mugwort, turmeric

Congestion: lotus node,
lily root, chrysanthemum greens,
daikon greens, onion,
mustard seed

---

and reapply for about fifteen minutes or until the skin becomes warm and rosy. This may be done daily or as needed until the pain or ailment subsides.

Poultice

Poultices are compresses made from gently cooked herbs. To make one, chop a few handfuls of fresh or dried herbs into small bits. Place in a pot with enough water to just cover and bring to a boil. Remove from the heat, cover, and steep until just cool enough to handle. Gently wring out small handfuls of the herbs, so they do not drip and lay them over the body area in need. Make a ½ inch (12 mm) thick poultice of herbs on the skin and secure it with a cotton wash cloth or fabric bandage to hold it in place. Let sit for fifteen to thirty minutes and reapply three times per day until symptoms resolve. A spit poultice is made by chewing herbs before putting them on the skin. Take care to only do this with edible herbs, such as plantain, which is a traditional spit poultice for bee stings and bug bites!

Plasters

A plaster is a compress made from an herbal paste or simple dough. Herbal plasters are sophisticated poultices that are ideal to use with herbs that are too loose or chunky to sit cleanly on the skin. Chinese medicine pain patches are examples of modern-day plasters. For each plaster, you will need pieces of cotton fabric or flannel (about 3 × 5 inches [7.5 × 12 cm]) that can be purchased new or cut from old clothes and rags.

Prepare the fresh herbs by chopping them finely or grating them with a metal grater. Place in a pot with enough water to cover and bring to a boil. Continue boiling until the herbs are soft. Remove from the heat and mash into a paste. Add just enough arrowroot powder or flour to thicken the mash into a soft dough, with a consistency similar to thick mashed potatoes or very soft modeling clay. Spread a ¼ in (6 mm) layer of the dough on a piece of cotton fabric and apply with the herb side against the skin. Allow to cool and dry on the skin for twenty to sixty minutes. Repeat daily until symptoms resolve or for up to one week.

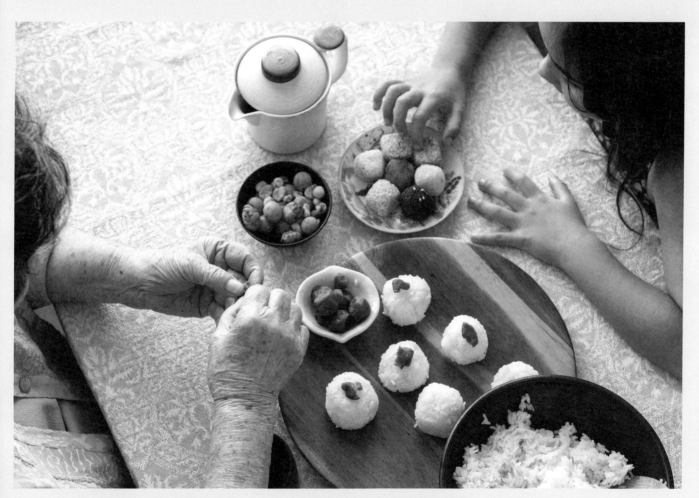

Grandma Masako and Zoë Wilkins making umeboshi rice balls, Petaluma, California, 2022

SINGLE HERB PROFILES

The following is a guide to the herbs used in this book.
The purpose is to simply increase understanding and confidence in
practicing herbal medicine at home.

Herb Profile Key

Herb name: Each herb is first listed by its common name in English. It is followed by the pinyin name in parenthesis if it is also identified that way in the United States. Pinyin is a Romanized system of Mandarin Chinese that uses English letters rather than Chinese characters. The botanical name is then listed in italics—this is the Latin or scientific name identifying the plant species.

Taste: The flavors of an herb determine some of its energetic healing effects on the body. The five tastes—bitter, sweet, sour, salty, and pungent/spicy—are explained on page 53.

Temperature: The thermal nature of an herb is an energetic healing property that affects the temperature of the body. The temperatures—hot, warm, neutral, cool, and cold—are explained on page 55.

Zangfu organs: Each herb has a special correspondence to at least one Zangfu organ. This is an energetic organ and is not the same as the physical anatomical organs. See page 63 for more on the Zangfu organs.

How it works: This section describes the way that the herb effects change in the body, its therapeutic actions, and its energetic healing properties.

Dose: The listed dosages are for dried herbs to be made as a decoction. Dosages are given as a range, with an average size adult (about 150 lb [70 kg]) in mind. See page 31 for more on dosing and how to adjust based on the individual.

American Ginseng

(Xi Yang Shen)

Panax quinquefolius

Taste: Sweet, bitter

Temperature: Cold

Zangfu organs: Kidney, Heart, Lung

How it works: Tonifies Qi; tonifies Yin; benefits energy and vitality; cools heat; generates body fluids.

Dose: 3 to 6 g

Notes: Use in moderation for stagnation or significant heat symptoms.

Arnica

Arnica montana

Taste: Pungent/spicy

Temperature: Very warm

Zangfu organs: Heart, Pericardium, Liver

How it works: Invigorates and moves Blood; heals bruises and trauma; relieves pain; warming; anti-inflammatory.

Notes: Apply infused oil liberally for skin conditions and injury. Topical and external applications only, as it is slightly toxic if ingested.

Ashwagandha

Withania somnifera

Taste: Sweet, bitter, pungent/spicy

Temperature: Warm

Zangfu organs: Lung, Heart, Spleen

How it works: Tonifies Yang and Jing (essence); benefits the immune system; tonifies Wei Qi; calms the spirit; adaptogenic; anti-inflammatory.

Dose: 0.5 to 3 g

Notes: Contraindicated in pregnancy. Considered safe unless taken in high doses, which can cause nausea, vomiting, and diarrhea.

Astragalus

(Huang Qi)

Astragali Radix

Taste: Sweet

Temperature: Warm

Zangfu organs: Spleen, Lung

How it works: Tonifies Qi; lifts Yang and Qi; benefits Wei Qi and the energetic boundary; increases circulation of body fluids; heals skin; diuretic; adaptogenic.

Dose: 10 to 15 g

Notes: Use in moderation for cases of stagnation or significant heat symptoms.

Bee Balm

Monarda herba

Taste: Pungent/spicy, bitter

Temperature: Warm

Zangfu organs: Spleen, Stomach, Urinary Bladder

How it works: Aromatic; transforms damp; releases the exterior (wind-cold); eases nausea; diaphoretic; anti-inflammatory.

Dose: 3 to 10 g

Black Sesame Seed

(Hei Zhi Ma)

Sesamum indicum

Taste: Sweet

Temperature: Neutral

Zangfu organs: Liver, Kidney

How it works: Tonifies Yin and Jing (essence); nourishes Blood; benefits digestion and constipation.

Dose: 3 to 30 g

Blessed Thistle

Centaurea benedicta

Taste: Bitter, pungent/spicy

Temperature: Cool

Zangfu organs: Liver, Gallbladder, Spleen

How it works: Clears heat; dries damp; moves Qi stagnation; antibacterial, diuretic.

Dose: 3 to 6 g

Notes: Use with caution with Yang-deficiency cold.

Blueberry

Vaccinium

Taste: Sweet

Temperature: Neutral

Zangfu organs: Kidney, Liver

How it works: Tonifies Blood; nourishes the Liver; benefits the eyes.

Dose: 6 to 30 g

Boat Seed

(Pang Da Hai)

Sterculia lychnophora

Taste: Sweet

Temperature: Cold

Zangfu organs: Lung, Large Intestine

How it works: Resolves phlegm; cools heat; stops cough; nourishes Lung Yin.

Dose: 3 to 5 seeds

Burdock Root

(Niu Bang Gen)

Arctium lappa

Taste: Bitter, slightly pungent/spicy

Temperature: Cool

Zangfu organs: Liver, Kidney, Urinary Bladder, Stomach

How it works: Cools heat; drains damp; invigorates and moves Qi; nourishes Qi and Yin; heals skin; diuretic.

Dose: 6 to 15 g

Notes: It is also known as "gobo"

in Japanese. Due to its drying nature, use moderately with Yin deficiency dryness.

Calendula

Calendula officinalis
Taste: Pungent/spicy, bitter
Temperature: Cool
Zangfu organs: Liver, Lung
How it works: Invigorates and moves Blood; cools heat; stops pain; heals skin and bruises; anti-inflammatory; benefits digestion.
Dose 2 to 6 g. Apply infused oil liberally for skin conditions and injury.
Notes: Contraindicated in pregnancy because of its Blood moving properties.

California Poppy

Eschscholzia californica
Taste: Pungent/spicy, bitter
Temperature: Cold
Zangfu organs: Liver, Gallbladder, Heart
How it works: Calms the spirit; cools heat; invigorates Qi; relieves Qi and Blood stagnation; relieves pain; sedative.
Dose: 4 to 12 g

Cardamom

(Bai Dou Kou)
Amomum kravanh (round or brown cardamom); *Angelica archangelica* (green cardamom)
Taste: Pungent/spicy
Temperature: Warm
Zangfu organs: Lung, Spleen, Stomach
How it works: Transforms dampness; invigorates and moves Qi; warms the middle jiao (abdomen); relieves nausea; aromatic.
Dose: 3 to 6 g
Notes: Round or brown cardamom is typically used in traditional Chinese medicine, and green cardamom is a common culinary spice in South Asian cuisine. These are different varieties, yet their energetic properties are interchangeable. Green cardamom is used in the recipe in this book.

Chamomile

Matricaria recutita
Taste: Bitter, sweet, pungent/spicy
Temperature: Cool
Zangfu organs: Liver, Heart, Stomach
How it works: Calms the spirit; benefits the Heart; cools heat; resolves Liver Qi stagnation; benefits digestion; releases the exterior; antispasmodic; nervine; sedative.
Dose: 3 to 12 g

Chinese Yam

(Shan Yao)
Rhizoma dioscoreae
Taste: Sweet
Temperature: Neutral
Zangfu organs: Kidney, Lung, Spleen
How it works: Tonifies Spleen Qi; tonifies Kidney Yin.
Dose: 10 to 30 g
Notes: Use in moderation for cases of heat or stagnation.

Chrysanthemum

(Ju Hua)
Chrysanthemum morifolium
Taste: Sweet, bitter
Temperature: Cool
Zangfu organs: Lung, Liver
How it works: Regulates Qi; moves Liver Qi stagnation; releases the exterior (wind-heat); cools heat; calms the mind; reduces stress; benefits the eyes.
Dose: 4.5 to 15 g
Notes: Use in moderation with significant Qi deficiency. May cause allergies in people who are sensitive to ragweed.

Cinnamon Bark

(Rou Gui)
Cinnamomum cassia
Taste: Pungent/spicy, sweet
Temperature: Hot
Zangfu organs: Heart, Kidney, Liver, Spleen
How it works: Tonifies and warms Kidney Yang; deeply warming; addresses water retention; relieves pain; increases circulation.
Dose: 2 to 5 g
Notes: Contraindicated in pregnancy. Use with caution if experiencing heat symptoms including Yin-deficiency fire and bleeding conditions.

Cinnamon Twig

(Ghi Zhi)
Cinnamomum cassia
Taste: Pungent/spicy, sweet
Temperature: Warm
Zangfu organs: Heart, Lung, Urinary Bladder
How it works: Releases exterior wind (wind-cold); tonifies Yang;

stops pain; invigorates Qi; circulates body fluids.

Dose: 3 to 9 g

Notes: Contraindicated in pregnancy. A large overdose can cause a burning sensation in the eyes, cough, thirst, dry mouth, or dizziness.

Citron

(Fo Shou)

Fructus Citri Sarcodactylis

Taste: Pungent/spicy, bitter

Temperature: Warm

Zangfu organs: Liver, Lung, Stomach, Spleen

How it works: Regulates Qi; resolves Liver Qi stagnation; eases pain; benefits digestion; resolves phlegm.

Dose: 3 to 10 g

Cleavers

Galium aparine

Taste: Bitter, salty

Temperature: Cold

Zangfu organs: Kidney, Urinary Bladder, Spleen, Lung

How it works: Drains damp; cools heat; clears toxins; softens hardness; transforms phlegm; diuretic.

Dose: 5 to 15 g

Notes: Due to its draining, diuretic energy, use with caution in Yin deficiency.

Codonopsis

(Dang Shen)

Codonopsis pilosula

Taste: Sweet

Temperature: Neutral

Zangfu organs: Spleen, Lung

How it works: Tonifies Qi; increases energy and strength; nourishes Blood and body fluids; calms the mind; benefits the Lung; stops cough.

Dose: 6 to 10 g

Comfrey

Symphytum officinalis

Taste: Bitter, sweet

Temperature: Cool

Zangfu organs: Stomach, Lung, Liver, Kidney

How it works: Clears damp-heat; Cools Blood.

How it works: Cools heat; disperses swelling; nourishes Yin; heals skin; anti-inflammatory.

Dose: 5 to 15 g

Notes: Apply infused oil liberally for skin conditions and injury. Topical and external applications only due to liver toxic pyrrolizidine alkaloids.

Cordyceps

(Dong Chong Xin Cao)

Cordyceps sinensis

Taste: Sweet

Temperature: Warm

Zangfu organs: Lung, Kidney

How it works: Tonifies Yang and Jing (essence); benefits the Lung; reduces phlegm.

Dose: 5 to 10 g

Notes: Side effects of overuse include headache, irritability, restlessness, swelling, and nose bleeds.

Damiana

Turnera diffus

Taste: Pungent/spicy, sweet

Temperature: Warm

Zangfu organs: Kidney, Spleen, Heart

How it works: Tonifies Yang; benefits Kidney and Heart; antidepressant; aphrodisiac.

Dose: 3 to 6 g

Dandelion

(Pu Gong Ying)

Taraxacum officinale

Taste: Bitter

Temperature: Cool

Zangfu organs: Liver, Stomach, Urinary Bladder

How it works: Cools heat; drains damp; moves Liver Qi stagnation; eases pain; diuretic.

Dose: 3 to 9 g

Notes: Use in moderation with Yang deficiency cold.

Dang Gui

(Chinese Angelica Root)

Angelica sinensis

Taste: Sweet, pungent/spicy

Temperature: Warm

Zangfu organs: Heart, Liver, Spleen

How it works: Tonifies, invigorates, and moves Blood; relieves pain; increases energy; improves circulation; heals skin.

Dose: 5 to 15 g

Notes: Dang gui, also translated as dong quai, is listed in this book under its Chinese pinyin name to distinguish it from Western angelica root (*Angelica archangelica*) which is an entirely different herb. Use caution with Yin-deficiency heat and severe Spleen Qi deficiency. It will cause nosebleeds if taken in excess. Western species of angelica root (*Angelica archangelica*) are also used to address Liver Qi stagnation, pain, and menstrual disorders. They are used similarly to dang gui, but they move Qi more strongly than Blood.

Echinacea

Echinacea purpura
Taste: Pungent/spicy, bitter
Temperature: Cool
Zangfu organs: Lung, Liver, Urinary Bladder
How it works: Cools heat; clears toxins; dispels wind; transforms phlegm; stops bleeding; anti-inflammatory.
Dose: 3 to 9 g
Notes: Only use cultivated herbs because of overharvesting and wildcrafting.

Elder, Elderflower, Elderberry

(Jie Gu Mu)
Sambucus nigra
Taste: Pungent/spicy, bitter
Temperature: Cool
Zangfu organs: Lung, Urinary Bladder, Liver
How it works: Releases exterior wind (wind-heat); dries damp; clears heat toxins; expresses rashes; anti-inflammatory; diaphoretic; antibacterial; antiviral.
Dose: 1 to 6 g
Notes: Use black elderberries only, as red elderberries (S. Racemosa) are toxic. Only take teas and cooked preparations of the flowers and berries (never raw).

Elecampane

Inula helenium
Taste: Bitter, pungent/spicy
Temperature: Warm
Zangfu organs: Spleen, Stomach, Lung
How it works: Reduces and transforms dampness; tonify Spleen Qi; resolves phlegm; benefits digestion.

Dose: 3 to 9 g
Notes: Use with caution in Yin deficiency.

Eleuthero, Siberian Ginseng

(Ci Wu Jia)
Eleutherococcus senticosus
Taste: Pungent/spicy, bitter
Temperature: Warm
Zangfu organs: Spleen, Kidney, Heart
How it works: Tonifies Qi and Yin; benefits energy, sleep, and mental clarity; regenerates white blood cells after chemotherapy and radiation; adaptogenic.
Dose: 10 to 30 g
Notes: Not a true ginseng but similar in nature to ginseng (ren shen).

Eucommia Bark

(Du Zhong)
Eucommia ulmoides
Taste: Sweet
Temperature: Warm
Zangfu organs: Kidney, Liver
How it works: Tonifies Yang and Jing (essence); relieves joint pain; benefits the bones; reproductive tonic.
Dose: 10 to 15 g

Frankincense

(Ru Xiang)
Boswellia carterii
Taste: Pungent/spicy, bitter
Temperature: Warm
Zangfu organs: Heart, Liver, Spleen
How it works: Invigorates and moves Blood; heals skin; moves and invigorates Blood and Qi; heals skin; reduces swelling; relieves pain.
Dose: 3 to 10 g

Notes: Contraindicated for internal use during pregnancy. It is essential to source ethically harvested frankincense.

Galangal

(Hong Dou Kou)
Alpinia Galanga
Taste: Pungent/spicy
Temperature: Warm
Zangfu organs: Spleen, Lung
How it works: Dries and transforms damp; stimulates appetite; benefits digestion.
Dose: 3 to 6 g
Notes: Use in moderation for Yin-deficiency heat.

Gentian

(Long Dan Cao)
Genetiana lutea
Taste: Bitter
Temperature: Cold
Zangfu organs: Liver, Gallbladder, Stomach
How it works: Clears heat; transforms damp; benefits digestion; heals skin.
Dose: 3 to 6 g
Notes: Use in moderation with Spleen Qi deficiency.

Ginger, Dried

(Gan Jiang)
Zingiber officinale
Taste: Pungent/spicy
Temperature: Hot
Zangfu organs: Heart, Lung, Spleen, Stomach
How it works: Warms the middle jiao (abdomen); dissolves phlegm; dispels cold; transforms damp; relieves pain.

Dose: 3 to 10 g
Notes: Use caution during pregnancy and with any heat symptoms.

Ginger, Fresh

(Sheng Jiang)
Zingiber officinale
Taste: Pungent/spicy
Temperature: Warm
Zangfu organs: Lung, Spleen, Stomach
How it works: Releases exterior wind (wind-cold); invigorates and moves Qi; harmonizes the middle jiao (abdomen).
Dose: 3 to 9 g
Notes: Use in moderation for Qi deficiency, Yin-deficiency heat, and hypertension.

Ginkgo Biloba Leaf

(Yin Xing Ye)
Ginkgo biloba
Taste: Sweet, bitter
Temperature: Neutral
Zangfu organs: Kidney, Lung
How it works: Astringent; invigorates Qi and Blood; stops pain; enhances memory and vitality.
Dose: 3 to 6 g
Notes: Do not take with blood thinners, including ibuprofen, aspirin, and fish oil supplements.

Ginseng

(Ren Shen)
Panax ginseng
Taste: Sweet, slightly bitter
Temperature: Warm
Zangfu organs: Lung, Spleen
How it works: Tonifies Qi; boosts Wei Qi; benefits the immune system; nourishes Blood and body fluids; calms the spirit.

Dose: 5 to 10 g
Notes: Use in moderation for cases of stagnation or significant heat symptoms.

Goji Berry

(Gou Qi Zi)
Lycium barbarum
Taste: Sweet
Temperature: Neutral
Zangfu organs: Liver, Kidney, Lung
How it works: Tonifies Qi, Blood, and Yin; benefits the eyes; nourishes the Lung.
Dose: 5 to 15 g
Notes: Use with caution during pregnancy as it may stimulate the uterus.

Gotu Kola

(Ji Xue Cao)
Centella asiatica
Taste: Sweet, slightly bitter
Temperature: Cool
Zangfu organs: Kidney
How it works: Tonifies Yin and Jing (essence); clears heat; improves memory; heals skin; anti-inflammatory.
Dose: 10 to 15 g
Notes: Can cause sleepiness. Rare side effects on the skin include burning sensations and redness.

Green Tea

(Lu Cha)
Camellia sinensis
Taste: Bitter
Temperature: Cold
Zangfu organs: Stomach
How it works: Cools heat; clears the mind; clears dampness; harmonizes the Stomach.

Dose: 3 to 12 g
Notes: Use in moderation with Spleen Qi deficiency with diarrhea.

Hawthorn, Chinese

(Shan Zha)
Crataegus cuneata
Taste: Sweet, sour
Temperature: Warm
Zangfu organs: Liver, Spleen, Stomach
How it works: Benefits digestion; relieves food stagnation; resolves Qi and Blood stagnation.
Dose: 10 to 15 g

Hawthorn, Western

Crataegus monogyna
Taste: Sweet, slightly bitter
Temperature: Warm
Zangfu organs: Heart, Pericardium
How it works: Tonifies Qi and Blood; invigorates and moves Blood; calms the spirit; benefits the Heart, mind, and sleep.
Dose: 3 to 9 g
Notes: Can increase the effects of pharmaceutical heart medicine.

He Shou Wu

(Foti)
Polygonum multiflorum
Taste: Sweet, bitter
Temperature: Warm
Zangfu organs: Kidney, Liver
How it works: Tonifies Blood and Jing; benefits the hair; enhances vitality; astringent.
Dose: 1 to 9 g
Notes: Should only be taken for two weeks at a time and not exceed the recommended dose on the product because of hepatotoxicity. Do not store or prepare in metal

containers. While it is possible to use raw he shou wu, the product you will find in stores is pre-processed with black beans to prevent a laxative effect.

Hemp Seed

(Huo Ma Ren)

Cannabis sativa

Taste: Sweet

Temperature: Neutral

Zangfu organs: Spleen, Stomach, Large Intestine

How it works: Benefits digestion; relieves dry constipation; moistens dryness; benefits the hair.

Dose: 10 to 15 g (crush before cooking)

Honeysuckle

(Jin Yin Hua)

Lonicera japonica

Taste: Sweet

Temperature: Cold

Zangfu organs: Lung, Stomach, Large Intestine

How it works: Clears heat toxins; moves Qi stagnation; releases the exterior (wind-heat); stops pain; diaphoretic.

Dose: 10 to 20 g

Notes: Use with caution with Yang deficiency and cold symptoms.

Jujube Date

(Da Zao, Hong Zao)

Ziziphus jujuba

Taste: Sweet

Temperature: Warm

Zangfu organs: Spleen, Stomach

How it works: Tonifies Qi and Blood; calms the spirit; improves vitality, energy, physical stamina, and beauty.

Dose: 3 to 12 fruits or 10 to 30 g

Notes: Use in moderation with existing dampness and heat.

Jujube Date Seed

(Suan Zao Ren)

Ziziphys jujuba

Taste: Sweet, sour

Temperature: Neutral

Zangfu organs: Heart, Liver, Spleen, Gallbladder

How it works: Calms the spirit; nourishes the Heart; stops sweating due to Qi and Yin deficiency.

Dose: 9 to 15 g (crush before decocting)

Notes: Contraindicated in pregnancy because it stimulates the muscles, including the uterus.

Korean Mint

(Huo Xiang)

Herba Agastache

Taste: Pungent/spicy, aromatic

Temperature: Slightly warm

Zangfu organs: Spleen, Stomach, Lung

How it works: Dispels Damp; harmonizes the Spleen and Stomach; alleviates nausea and vomiting; releases-the-exterior.

Dose: 5 to 10 g

Notes: In English, it is also known as purple or giant hyssop. It shares a name in Chinese pinyin with patchouli (guang huo xiang), and they can be used interchangeably.

Lemon Balm

Melissa officinalis

Taste: Pungent/spicy, bitter, slightly sweet

Temperature: Cool

Zangfu organs: Stomach, Liver, Heart

How it works: Calms the spirit; tonifies Blood; invigorates Qi; cools Liver heat; releases the exterior (wind-heat); stops pain; anti-inflammatory, diaphoretic.

Dose: 1 to 6 g

Licorice, Chinese

(Gan Cao)

Glycyrrhizae uralensis

Taste: Sweet

Temperature: Neutral

Zangfu organs: Spleen, Stomach, Lung, Heart

How it works: Tonifies Qi; relieves pain; clears toxins and phlegm; harmonizes Qi; relieves pain; stops cough; adaptogenic.

Dose: 3 to 10 g

Notes: Licorice is one of the most common herbs used in Traditional Chinese Medicine. For the recipes in this book, it can be used interchangeably with Western licorice (*Glycyrrhiza glabra*). Honey-fried licorice (zhi gan cao) is sweet, warm, and is a stronger Qi tonic than raw licorice. Contraindicated in large doses for kidney disorders, hypertension, and congestive heart failure. Large doses can cause edema, elevated blood pressure, weakness, dizziness, and headache.

Lily Root

(Bai He)

Lilium brownii

Taste: Sweet

Temperature: Cool

Zangfu organs: Lung, Heart

How it works: Tonifies Yin; cools heat; stops cough; calms the spirit and mind; harmonizes the middle jiao (abdomen).

Dose: 10 to 30 g

Notes: Not used in cases of cough due to wind-cold.

Longan Fruit

(Long Yan Rou)

Euphoria longan

Taste: Sweet

Temperature: Warm

Zangfu organs: Heart, Spleen

How it works: Tonifies Qi and Blood; increases energy and vitality; benefits sleep; tonifies Qi.

Dose: 10 to 15 g

Notes: Contraindicated if there is excess dampness or stagnation.

Loquat Leaf

(Pi Pa Ye)

Eriobotrya japonica

Taste: Bitter

Temperature: Cool

Zangfu organs: Lung, Stomach

How it works: Resolves phlegm; stops cough; clears heat; harmonizes the Stomach.

Dose: 10 to 15 g

Notes: Small hairs on the loquat leaf may irritate the mouth and throat, so strain tea well.

Lotus Seed

(Lian Zi)

Nelumbo nucifera

Taste: Sweet

Temperature: Neutral

Zangfu organs: Heart, Kidney, Spleen

How it works: Calms the spirit; nourishes the Heart, Kidney, and Jing (essence); astringent; stops leakage of diarrhea, premature ejaculation, and vaginal discharge.

Dose: 6 to 15 g

Notes: Do not take it when constipated with dry stools.

Mai Men Dong

(Ophiopogon Root)

Radix Ophiopogonis

Taste: Sweet, slightly bitter

Temperature: Cool

Zangfu organs: Spleen, Stomach, Heart

How it works: Tonifies Blood and Yin; cools heat; generates fluids; eases irritability and insomnia.

Dose: 10 to 15 g

Notes: It is listed in this book under its Chinese pinyin name to distinguish it from its use as an ornamental grass. Not used for cases of Yang-deficiency cold.

Marshmallow

Althaea officinalis

Taste: Sweet, slightly bitter

Temperature: Cold

Zangfu organs: Lung, Stomach, Kidney, Urinary Bladder

How it works: Tonifies Yin; clears heat; nourishes Yin; eases pain; benefits urination and digestion; emollient; expectorant.

Dose: 2 to 6 g

Notes: Use in moderation with Spleen Qi deficiency with dampness.

Mimosa Tree Bark and Flower

(He Huan Pi, He Huan Hua)

Albizia julibrissin

Taste: Sweet

Temperature: Neutral

Zangfu organs: Heart, Liver

How it works: Calms the spirit; benefits the Heart; resolves Qi stagnation; harmonizes the Liver; relieves pain; reduces swelling.

Dose: 10 to 15 g

Notes: Contraindicated in pregnancy because it stimulates the uterus.

Mint, Field Mint

(Bo He)

Mentha (mint); *Mentha haplocalyx* (Chinese field mint)

Taste: Pungent/spicy

Temperature: Cool

Zangfu organs: Lung, Liver

How it works: Regulates Qi; releases the exterior (wind-heat); cools heat; moves Liver Qi stagnation; benefits the head and eyes; aromatic.

Dose: 3 to 6 g

Notes: There are countless varieties of mint (*mentha*). The variety used most often in Chinese medicine, field mint (bo he), is very efficient for moving Liver Qi stagnation. However, all mints are interchangable in the recipes in this book.

Motherwort

(Yi Mu Cao)

Leonurus heterophyllus (Chinese motherwort); *Leonurus cardiaca* (Western motherwort)

Taste: Bitter, pungent/spicy

Temperature: Cool

Zangfu organs: Heart, Liver, Urinary Bladder, Small Intestine

How it works: Invigorates and moves Blood; calms the spirit; nourishes Heart Blood; calms the spirit; reduces water retention; cools heat; clears toxins; diuretic.

Dose: 9 to 15 g

Notes: Contraindicated in pregnancy because of blood-moving and a stimulating effect on the uterus. Western Motherwort (*Leonurus cardiaca*) is primarily used for postpartum healing.

Mugwort

(Ai Ye)

Folium Artemisia argyi (Chinese mugwort); *Artemisia vulgari* (Western mugwort)

Taste: Bitter, pungent/spicy

Temperature: Warm

Zangfu organs: Spleen, Liver, Kidney

How it works: Invigorates and moves Blood; dries damp; calms the spirit; eases pain and tension; benefits digestion; regulates menstruation; stops bleeding; heals skin.

Dose: 3 to 10 g

Notes: Do not take during pregnancy or while breastfeeding. The side effects of overdose (20 to 30 g) include thirst, nausea, vomiting, weakness, dizziness, tinnitus, tremors, and jaundice.

Mulberry Fruit

(Sang Shen Zi)

Morus alba

Taste: Sweet

Temperature: Cold

Zangfu organs: Heart, Liver, Kidney

How it works: Tonifies Yin and Blood; generates body fluids; benefits digestion and constipation with dryness.

Dose: 10 to 15 g

Notes: Due to sweetness, use in moderation with Spleen deficiency with diarrhea.

Mulberry Leaf

(Sang Ye)

Morus alba

Taste: Sweet, bitter

Temperature: Cold

Zangfu organs: Lung, Liver

How it works: Releases exterior wind (wind-heat); cools the Liver; moistens the Lung.

Dose: 4.5 to 9 g

Mullein

Verbascum Thapsus

Taste: Bitter, slightly pungent/spicy

Temperature: Cool

Zangfu organs: Lung, San Jiao, Kidney

How it works: Resolves and transforms phlegm; clears heat; stops cough; increases circulation of body fluids; reduces swelling; antiseptic; diuretic.

Dose: 3 to 10 g

Notes: Small hairs on mullein leaf may irritate the mouth and throat, so strain tea well.

Myrrh

(Mo Yao)

Commiphora myrrha

Taste: Bitter

Temperature: Neutral

Zangfu organs: Heart, Liver, Spleen

How it works: Invigorates and moves Blood; relieves pain; reduces swelling; heals skin.

Dose: 3 to 10 g

Notes: Similar action to frankincense, but myrrh is stronger for moving Blood and Qi stagnation pain. It is essential to source ethically harvested myrrh.

Nettle, Stinging Nettle

Urtica dioica

Taste: Salty, slightly pungent/spicy, sweet

Temperature: Cool

Zangfu organs: Liver, Lung, Urinary Bladder

How it works: Drains damp; reduces water retention; cools heat; nourishes Blood; softens hardness; relieves pain; astringent; diuretic; tonic.

Dose: 9 to 30 g

Notes: Contraindicated for edema caused by cardiac or renal failure.

Oat, Oat Straw, Milky Oat Top

Avena sativa

Taste: Sweet

Temperature: Neutral

Zangfu organs: Heart, Kidney

How it works: Tonifies Qi; calms the spirit; nourishes Yin; eases stress, tension, and insomnia; energizes.

Dose: 9 to 30 g

Notes: Use caution with a grain sensitivity or celiac.

Oolong Black Tea

(Wu Long Cha)

Camellia sinensis

Taste: Bitter, sweet

Temperature: Cool

Zangfu organs: Heart, Lung, Stomach, Small Intestine

How it works: Cools heat; drains damp; clears the head; benefits digestion after a heavy meal; moves food stagnation; diuretic.

Dose: 3 to 12 g

Notes: Take in moderation and with food in cases of Spleen Qi deficiency.

Passionflower

Passiflora incarnata

Taste: Sweet, bitter, sour

Temperature: Cool

Zangfu organs: Heart, Lung

How it works: Calms the spirit; nourishes the Heart Yin; cools Yin deficiency heat; sedative.

Dose: 3 to 9 g

Pearl

(Zhen Zhu)

Pteria martensii

Taste: Sweet, salty

Temperature: Cold

Zangfu organs: Heart, Liver

How it works: Calms the spirit and the Heart; benefits the eyes; heals skin.

Dose: 0.3 to 1 gram

Pearl Barley

(Yi Yi Ren)

Coix lacryma-jobi

Taste: Sweet

Temperature: Cool

Zangfu organs: Lung, Spleen, Stomach, Kidney

How it works: Drains damp; cools heat; benefits digestion; heals skin; eases pain.

Dose: 9 to 30 g

Plantain

(Da Che Qian)

Plantago major

Taste: Sweet

Temperature: Cold

Zangfu organs: Urinary Bladder, Spleen, Stomach

How it works: Drains damp; cools heat; stops bleeding; nourishes Yin; heals skin; anti-inflammatory; diuretic.

Dose: 5 to 15 g

Notes: Use in moderation in cases of Spleen-Qi deficiency. The different species in Asia and the United States can be used interchangeably.

Poria

(Fu Ling)

Poria cocos

Taste: Sweet

Temperature: Neutral

Zangfu organs: Heart, Spleen, Kidney, Lung

How it works: Drains damp; tonifies Spleen Qi; benefits digestion; reduces water retention; diuretic; calms the spirit.

Dose: 9 to 15 g

Notes: Use with caution in cases of Yin deficiency.

Red Clover

Trifolium pratense

Taste: Bitter, slightly sweet

Temperature: Cold

Zangfu organs: Liver, Heart, Lung

How it works: Cools heat; clears toxins; resolves toxins; tonifies and invigorates Blood; reduces swelling.

Dose: 3 to 9 g

Notes: Use caution if taking blood thinners, including ibuprofen, aspirin, and fish oil supplements.

Red Sage Root

(Dan Shen)

Radix Salviae miltiorrhizae

Taste: Bitter

Temperature: Cool

Zangfu organs: Heart, Pericardium, Liver

How it works: Invigorates, moves, and cools Blood; calms the spirit; eases pain; reduces swelling.

Dose: 5 to 10 g

Notes: Contraindicated for internal use during pregnancy. Use caution with bleeding disorders, including heavy periods and recurrent nosebleeds.

Reishi Mushroom

(Ling Zhi)

Ganoderma lucidum

Taste: Sweet

Temperature: Neutral

Zangfu organs: Heart, Liver, Lung

How it works: Calms the spirit; nourishes the Heart; tonifies Qi and Blood; increases vitality; benefits the immune system; anticancer and antitumor properties; adaptogenic.

Dose: 3 to 15 g

Safflower

(Hong Hua)

Flos Carthami

Taste: Pungent/spicy

Temperature: Warm

Zangfu organs: Heart, Liver

How it works: Invigorates, nourishes, and moves Blood; eases pain; regulates menstruation.

Dose: 3 to 10 g

Notes: Contraindicated for internal use during pregnancy. Overdose may cause bleeding.

Sage

Salvia officinalis

Taste: Pungent/spicy, slightly bitter

Temperature: Cool

Zangfu organs: Lung, Liver, Large Intestine

How it works: Releases the exterior (wind-heat); dries dampness; cools heat; stops sweating and lactation; antiseptic, astringent; diaphoretic.

Dose: 3 to 6 g

Notes: Should not be taken when lactating/breastfeeding.

Schisandra

(Wu Wei Zi)

Schisandra chinensis

Taste: Sour

Temperature: Warm

Zangfu organs: Kidney, Lung, Heart

How it works: Calms the spirit; astringent; stops cough and thirst; stops leakage of diarrhea and spontaneous sweating; nourishes Qi, Blood, and Yin; generates body fluids; adaptogenic.

Dose: 2 to 6 g

Notes: Can increase the effect of pharmaceutical medications when taken simultaneously.

Shiso

(Zi Su Ye)

Perilla frutescens

Taste: Pungent/spicy

Temperature: Warm

Zangfu organs: Lung, Spleen

How it works: Invigorates and moves Qi; harmonizes the middle jiao (abdomen); releases exterior wind (wind-cold); aromatic.

Dose: 5 to 9 g

Notes: Also known as perilla in the United States and kkaennip in Korea. Green shiso is more commonly used for medicine and as a food. However, red shiso leaves can be used for the same purposes. Contraindicated if diabetic because of effect on blood sugar.

Skullcap, Western

Scutellaria lateriflora

Taste: Bitter, pungent/spicy

Temperature: Cool

Zangfu organs: Liver, Heart

How it works: Calms the spirit; cools heat; resolves Qi stagnation; benefits the Liver; stops pain; nervine; sedative.

Dose: 2 to 9 g

Tangerine Peel

(Chen Pi)

Citrus reticulata

Taste: Pungent/spicy, bitter

Temperature: Warm

Zangfu organs: Lung, Spleen

How it works: Regulates Qi; dries damp; resolves Qi stagnation; relieves nausea, bloating, and diarrhea.

Dose: 3 to 9 g

Notes: Aged tangerine peel (chen pi) is traditionally aged for 1 to 2 years

and becomes dark green-brown and hard. This preparation is stronger for clearing dampness. However, the fresh and freshly dried peel has the same medicinal benefits, albeit more subtle.

Thyme

Thymus vulgaris

Taste: Pungent/spicy, slightly bitter

Temperature: Cool

Zangfu organs: Lung, Stomach, Liver

How it works: Releases exterior wind (wind-heat); stops cough; clears congestion; antiseptic; expectorant.

Dose: 2 to 6 g

Tulsi

Ocimum sanctum

Taste: Sweet, Pungent/spicy, bitter

Temperature: Warm

Zangfu organs: Stomach, Liver, Kidney

How it works: Calms the spirit; invigorates Qi; benefits circulation and digestion; eases pain; boosts the immune system; antimicrobial; adaptogen.

Dose: 3 to 12 g

Notes: It is also commonly known as holy basil. Contraindicated in pregnancy and when trying to conceive. Contraindicated if diabetic because of effect on blood sugar.

Umeboshi

(Wu Mei)

Prunus mume

Taste: Sour

Temperature: Neutral

Zangfu organs: Liver, Spleen, Lung, Large Intestine
How it works: Benefits digestion; stops leakage of diarrhea and spontaneous sweating; astringent; generates body fluids.
Dose: 10 to 30 g
Notes: Do not take for diarrhea caused by food poisoning or infections.

Vitex, Western

Vitex agnus-castus
Taste: Pungent/spicy, bitter
Temperature: Neutral
Zangfu organs: Liver, Heart
How it works: Regulates Qi; resolves Liver Qi stagnation; clears heat; eases pain; regulates hormonal balance, especially due to hormonal contraception.
Dose: 3 to 9 g
Notes: Contraindicated for postmenopausal women. This vitex is distinct from Chinese vitex (man jing zi), a cooling release-the-exterior herb used to treat cold and flu.

White Peony Root

(Bai Shao)
Paeonia Lactiflora
Taste: Bitter, sour
Temperature: Cool
Zangfu organs: Liver, Spleen
How it works: Tonifies Blood; cools heat; eases Liver Qi stagnation; regulates the menstrual cycle and PMS; eases pain.
Dose: 5 to 10 g
Notes: Not used in cases of Spleen-Qi deficiency with diarrhea.

White Wood Ear Mushroom, Tremella

(Bai Mu Er)
Tremella fuciformis
Taste: Sweet
Temperature: Neutral
Zangfu organs: Lung, Stomach
How it works: Tonifies Yin; cools heat; generates body fluids; moistens dryness.
Dose: 3 to 9 g

Yarrow

Achillea millefolium
Taste: Bitter, pungent/spicy
Temperature: Cool
Zangfu organs: Lung, Urinary Bladder, Liver
How it works: Releases exterior wind (wind-heat); clears damp heat; moves Liver Qi; cools Blood; stops bleeding; anti-inflammatory, diaphoretic, diuretic.
Dose: 3 to 9 g
Notes: Contraindicated in pregnancy. Use caution with any cold symptoms, including wind-cold, Yang deficiency cold, and feeling cold to the core.

RESOURCES

Where to Buy Herbs and Seeds

—

Herb Folk

My Asian American herb shop in Petaluma, California, specializing in organic herbal and green tea blends, broth herbs, regionally grown single herbs, moxibustion and holistic medicine supplies, and educational workshops. *HerbFolkShop.com*

Clear Source Herbs

My favorite source for high-quality single herbs common in Traditional Chinese Medicine and East Asian traditions. Their herbs are either certified organic or rigorously lot-tested and are traceable back to their growing area. *ClearSourceHerbs.com*

Five Flavors Herbs

Oakland, California herb shop offering consultations and specializing in extracts (tinctures) that integrate East Asian and Western herbalism. *FiveFlavorsHerbs.com*

Galen's Way

An independently owned and operated company handcrafting high-quality herbal extracts (tinctures) and herbal skin care. *Galenswaystore.com*

Herb Pharm

A certified organic farm making broad-spectrum herbal extracts (tinctures) and herbal products from herbs grown on their Southern Oregon farm. *Herb-pharm.com*

Kitazawa Seed Co.

An Asian-owned business offering heirloom seeds for Asian vegetables, herbs, and flowers. *KitazawaSeed.com*

Mountain Rose Herbs

An environmentally minded mail-order source for organic herbs, spices, oils, extracts, and medicine-making supplies. *MountainRoseHerbs.com*

Oshala Farm

A certified organic farm using regenerative, sustainable cultivation practices and offering an array of dried single herbs and herbal products. *OshalaFarm.com*

Pacific Botanicals

A medicinal herb farm and supplier of domestically grown herbs, with both fresh and dried herb offerings. *PacificBotanicals.com*

Root and Bones

A practitioner curated line and my go-to source for powder extracts of Chinese tonic herbs, medicinal mushrooms, and adaptogens. *RootandBones.com*

The Scarlet Sage Herb Co.

A San Francisco herb shop offering a wide variety of single herbs, natural remedies, and their own line of herbal medicine products. *ScarletSage.com*

Strictly Medicinal Seed Co.

A family-owned source for medicinal herb seeds, live plant starts, dried herbs, and tincture presses. *StrictlyMedicinalSeeds.com*

Traditional Medicinals

Certified B Corp offering a wide selection of organic teas and herbal products. *TraditionalMedicinals.com.*

Where to Buy Specialty Supplies

—

Asian Mart

Asian-owned online source for Asian groceries, household items, and beauty supplies. *Asianmart.com*

Clear Spring

Organic Japanese specialty food shop and where our family gets our favorite umeboshi plum, which is organic and free of artificial food dye. *www.clearspring.co.uk*

From Nature with Love
Online source with a great selection of medicine-making supplies, including clays, powdered herbs, oils, salts, and waxes.
FromNatureWithLove.com

The Japanese Pantry
High quality Japanese foods, ingredients, and supplies.
Thejapanesepantry.com

Koda Farms
Organic and traditionally farmed Japanese rice. My favorite is their Kokuho Rose medium grain heirloom rice. *Kodafarms.com*

Lanshin
Asian-owned, Brooklyn-based brand offering traditional Chinese skin care, gua sha, and massage products.
Lanshin.com

Mason Tops
Maker of fermentation tools that work with mason jars.
MasonTops.com

Strong Arm Farm
Source for sustainably, hand-harvested seaweed.
StrongArmFarm.com

Yang Face
Asian-owned business offering Traditional Chinese facial tools, including rollers and gua sha. Asian owned. *YangFace.com*

Education and Books
—

American Herbalists Guild
A non-profit organization that recognizes well-trained herbalists with a national registration and a directory of members.
AmericanHerbalistsGuild.com

Ancestral Apothecary Herbalism School
An herbal medicine school founded by educator Atava Garcia Swiecicki that centers the diverse cultural healing traditions of indigenous and BIPOC folk.
AncestralApothecarySchool.com

California Acupuncture Board
The California licensing board for acupuncturists and East Asian herbalists with a directory of schools and practitioners. *Acupuncture.ca.gov*

California School of Herbal Studies
One of North America's oldest and most respected herb schools, offering both online and in-person education.
CSHS.com

The Chinese Medicinal Herb Farm: A Cultivator's Guide to Small-Scale Organic Herb Production
A book by Peg Schafer on growing and harvesting Asian herbs in the various bioregions of the United States.

The Healing Garden: Cultivating and Handcrafting Herbal Remedies
A book by Juliet Blankespoor on growing and harvesting Western herbs.

The Land of Verse School of Herbal Medicine
An online herbal medicine certification program with a focus on ancestral and energetic medicine for beginning to advanced herbalists.
LandofVerse.com

National Certification Commission for Acupuncture
The United States licensing commission for acupuncturists and East Asian herbalists with a directory of schools and practitioners. *Nccaom.org*

Root Work Herbals–The People's Medicine School
An herbal certificate program based on the foundations of herbalism from a decolonial framework that centers BIPOC and QT experiences.
Rootworkherbals.com

The Science and Art of Herbalism Certification
A home study course to become a certified herbalist, by the godmother of Western herbalism, Rosemary Gladstar.
Scienceandartofherbalism.com

United Plant Savers
A non-profit organization dedicated to the preservation of native North American medicinal plants.
unitedplantsavers.org

Bibliography

Asian Pacific Institute on Gender-Based Violence. "Census Data & API Identities." 2004. https://www.api-gbv.org/resources/census-data-api-identies/.

Benjamin, Sarah Kate, and Summer Ashley Singletary. *The Kosmic Kitchen Cookbook: Everyday Herbalism and Recipes for Radical Wellness*. Boulder, CO: Roost Books, 2020.

Bennett, Robin Rose. *The Gift of Healing Herbs: Plant Medicines and Home Remedies for a Vibrantly Healthy Life*. Berkeley, CA: North Atlantic Books, 2014.

Benskey, Dan, Steven Clavey, and Erich Stöger. *Chinese Herbal Medicine: Materia Medica*, 3rd ed. Seattle, WA: Eastland Press, 2004.

Bliss, Nishanga. *Eat Real Food: Traditional Nutrition through the Seasons*. San Francisco, CA: Immune Enhancement Project, 2008.

Brown, Adrienne Maree. *Emergent Strategy*. Chico, CA: AK Press, 2017.

California State University San Marcos. "Defining Diaspora: Asian, Pacific Islander, and Desi Identities." Accessed February 2022. https://www.csusm.edu/ccc/programs/diaspora.html.

Caruso, Catherine. "Exploring the Science of Acupuncture." Harvard Medical School. November 1, 2021. https://hms.harvard.edu/news/exploring-science-acupuncture

Chen, John K. and Tina Chen. *Chinese Medical Herbology and Pharmacology*. City of Industry, CA: Art of Medicine Press, 2004.

Cheung, Rose and Genevieve Wong. *Healing Herbal Soups: Boost Your Immunity and Weather the Seasons with Traditional Chinese Recipes*. New York, NY: Simon Element, 2021.

De la Forêt, Rosalee. *Alchemy of Herbs: Transform Everyday Ingredients into Foods and Remedies That Heal*. New York, NY: Hay House, Inc, 2017.

Du Bois, W. E. B. (William Edward Burghardt). *The Souls of Black Folk: Essays and Sketches*. Chicago, IL: A. G. McClurg, 1903. New York, NY: Johnson Reprint Corp., 1968.

Flaws, Bob. *The Book of Jook: Chinese Medicinal Porridges: A Healthy Alternative to the Typical Western Breakfast*. Boulder, CO: Blue Poppy Press, 1995.

Flaws, Bob, and Honora Wolfe. *Prince Wen Hui's Cook: Chinese Dietary Therapy*. Brookline, MA: Paradigm Publications, 1983.

Friedman, Suzanne B., Lac, DMQ. *The Yijing Medical Qigong System*. Bloomington, IL: Xlibris Corporation, 2006.

Garran, Thomas Avery. *Western Herbs According to Traditional Chinese Medicine: A Practitioner's Guide*. Rochester, VT: Healing Arts Press, 2008.

Garran, Thomas Avery. *Western Herbs in Traditional Chinese Medicine: Methodology & Materia Medica*. U.S.A.: Passiflora Press, 2014.

Gladstar, Rosemary. *Family Herbal: A Guide to Living Life with Energy, Health, and Vitality*. North Adams, MA: Storey Publishing, 2001.

Haas, Elson M., MD. *Staying Healthy with the Seasons*. Berkeley, CA: Celestial Arts, 1981.

Hoffman, David. *Holistic Herbal: A Safe and Practical Guide to Making and Using Herbal Remedies*. London, England: Thorsons, 1983.

Jack, Alex and Gale Jack. *Amber Waves of Grain: American Macrobiotic Cooking*. New York, NY: Japan Publications, Inc., 1992.

Kaptchuk, Ted J., O.M.D. *The Web That Has No Weaver: Understanding Chinese Medicine*. New York, NY: McGraw Hill, 2000.

Keown, Daniel M.B., Ch.B., Lic. Ac. *The Spark in the Machine: How the Science of Acupuncture Explains the Mysteries of Western Medicine*. Philadelphia, PA: Singing Dragon, 2014.

Lee, Miriam. *Insights of a Senior Acupuncturist.* Boulder, CO: Blue Poppy Press, 1992.

Maciocia, Giovanni. *The Foundations of Chinese Medicine: A Comprehensive Text for Acupuncturists and Herbalists.* London, England: Churchill Livingstone, 1989.

Niedzwiecki, Max, and TC Duong. "Southeast Asian American Statistical Profile." *Southeast Asia Resource Action Center (SEARAC).* Washington, D.C., 2004. https://www.searac.org/wp-content/uploads/2018/04/Statistical-Profile-2010.pdf

Ono, Tadashi, and Harris Salat. *Japanese Soul Cooking: Ramen, Tonkatsu, Tempura, and More from the Streets and Kitchens of Tokyo and Beyond.* Berkeley, CA: Ten Speed Press, 2013.

Reichstein, Gail. *Wood Becomes Water: Chinese Medicine in Everyday Life.* New York, NY: Kodansha U.S.A., Inc., 1998.

Sacharoff, Shanta Nimbark. *Flavors of India: Vegetarian Indian Cuisine.* Summertown, TN: Book Publishing Company, 1996.

Sakai, Sonoko. *Japanese Home Cooking: Simple Meals, Authentic Flavors.* Boulder, CO: Roost Books, 2019.

Sato, Dwight, Namiko Ikeda, and Tomomi Kinoshita. "Home-Processing Black and Green Tea (Camellia sinensis)." The *University of Hawai'i at Mānoa, College of Tropical Agriculture and Human Resources, Food Safety and Technology* (March 2007): 1-2 https://www.ctahr.hawaii.edu/oc/freepubs/pdf/FST-26.pdf

Schafer, Peg. *The Chinese Medicinal Herb Farm: A Cultivator's Guide to Small-Scale Organic Herb Production.* White River Junction, Hartford, VT: Chelsea Green Publishing, 2011.

Scheid, Volder, Dan Bens?key, Andrew Ellis, and Randall Barolet. *Chinese Herbal Medicine: Formulas & Strategies.* 2nd ed. Seattle, WA: Eastland Press, 1990.

Tierra, Lesley. *Healing with the Herbs of Life.* Berkeley, CA: Crossing Press, 2003.

Wurchaih, Huar, Menggenqiqig, and Khasbagan. "Medicinal wild plants used by the Mongol herdsmen in Bairin Area of Inner Mongolia and its comparative study between TMM and TCM." *Journal of Ethnobiology and Ethnomedicine* 15, no. 32 (July 2019). https://doi.org/10.1186/s13002-019-0300-9.

Xiao-fan, Zong, and Gary Liscum. *Chinese Medicinal Teas: Simple, Proven, Folk Formulas for Common Diseases & Promoting Health.* Boulder, CO: Blue Poppy Press, 1996.

Zaurov, David E., James E. Simon, Chung-Heon Park, Wudeneh Letchamo, Qing-Li Wu, Mingfu Wang, Igor V. Belolipov, et al. "Medicinal Plants from Central and Western Asia." *Korean Journal of Medicinal Crop Science* 10, no. 4 (January 2022): 277–283. https://koreascience.kr/article/JAKO200203042347051.pdf

Index

Note: Page references in *italics* indicate photographs.

Acknowledgments

Making this book was a dream project, and I'm honored to have had the opportunity to bring this work to life. Although writing was a solitary process, I was supported by many folks along the way.

To my grandma and muse, Masako, whose unconditional love shaped me.

To my mom, Gail. You are the one who held my hand as I wrote this book. Thank you for meticulously editing every single word with your whole heart. Moreover, thank you for teaching me how to move through the world with integrity and confidence. Whether on behalf of your family, your community, or the earth, you aren't afraid to speak your mind and stand up for what is right.

To Derek, Thank you for seeing me and always encouraging me to go for it. Your love and steady presence hold our family together.

To my dad, John, for always listening to my stories and showing me that it's okay to dance to the beat of your own drum.

Thank you to everyone who contributed to the making of this book.

Kristen Murakoshi, your beautiful photographs captured not only the light but the nuance and shadows of this work.

Ayako Kiener, your illustrations brought a cultural vibe that reflects what it feels like to be Asian American.

To Kirstin Bickle, for showing up every step of the way and for helping to bring this book to life with style and laughter.

To Abby Rappoport, for sharing your extensive knowledge and meaningful edits, and for riffing with me on all things herbal.

To Mandy O'Doul, for letting us play in your flower fields, always.

To Melissa Nop, Sapho Flor, Sarah Koniak, and Kristi Quint, for helping me research each herb and different cultural foodways.

To Kristen Hewitt, Lauren Salkeld, Paul Wagner, Natalie Snodgrass, and the teams at Princeton Architectural Press and Chronicle Books.

And to my editor, Holly La Due. Thank you for believing in me. Your wisdom and enthusiasm for this project were a guiding light.

My sincere thanks to the community who lent me their support and cheered me on: Alysia Andriola, Kinyatta Reynolds, Summer Singletary, Tara Seymour, Dr. Areo Saffarzadeh, Tim Wilkins, Nora Wilkins, Sachiko Knappman, Sarah Deragon, Michelle Westling, Melissa Elysian, Sarah Kate Benjamin, Nina Jung, Mimi Cooper Lang Villa, Ann Gardner, Camille Esposito, Heather Baldini, Alyssa Melody, Dennis von Elgg, Aurora Richard, Paula Vielman-Reeves, Andrea Bouch Dimondstein, Rachael Bouch Dimondstein, Ella Lauser, Sarah Chung, Carrie Kane, and Timothy A. Gruneisen.

I am forever grateful to my teachers, including Dr. Xin Zhu (Hualing) Xu, Dr. Hideko Pelzer, Zhi-Bin (Benny) Zhang, Dr. Emmie Zhu, Daju Suzanne Friedman, Bettina Aptheker, and Angela Davis. To the authors whose work inspires me daily: Sonoko Sakai, Thomas Avery Garren, Andrew Ellis, Peg Schafer, Robin Rose Bennett, Lesley Tierra, Shanta Nimbark Sacharoff, Bob Flaws, and Rosemary Gladstar. And to all the acupuncture patients and herb students who have worked with me over the years—you are some of my greatest teachers.

Dear Weston and Zoë,

As I wrote this book, it was not lost on me that you were doing the work alongside me. I will never forget your sweet voices encouraging me and asking when it would finally be done. I am grateful to you both, because I know that it was not easy to share me with this book for a whole year. Now that we are on the other side of it, there are some things that I hope you know.

I hope that holding this book in your hands is a reminder that you can do anything. That your stories are meaningful. That your art has inherent value. And that when you raise your voice, it will speak to your community in ways that uplift and fulfill your own heart.

I hope this work helps cultivate a sense of pride in who you are and your Asian American heritage.

I hope that witnessing the arc of writing a book encourages you to go after your big dreams. Because when you do, your mom will always have your back.

Love,
Mama